NOURISHING
DIETS

Other Books by Sally Fallon Morell

Nourishing Fats: Why We Need Animal Fats for Health and Happiness

Nourishing Broth: An Old-Fashioned Remedy for the Modern World

Nourishing Traditions: The Cookbook that Challenges
Politically Correct Nutrition and the Diet Dictocrats (with Mary G. Enig, PhD)

The Nourishing Traditions Book of Baby & Child Care (with Thomas S. Cowan, MD)

The Nourishing Traditions Cookbook for Children (with Suzanne Gross)

Eat Fat Lose Fat (with Mary G. Enig, PhD)

NOURISHING DIETS

How *PALEO,* ANCESTRAL *and* TRADITIONAL PEOPLES *Really Ate*

SALLY FALLON MORELL

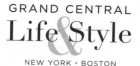

GRAND CENTRAL
Life & Style
NEW YORK · BOSTON

Grand Central Life & Style
Hachette Book Group
1290 Avenue of the Americas
New York, NY 10104
grandcentrallifeandstyle.com
twitter.com/grandcentralpub

First Trade Paperback Edition: June 2018

Grand Central Life & Style is an imprint of Grand Central Publishing.

The Grand Central Life & Style name and logo are trademarks of Hachette Book Group, Inc.

The Hachette Speakers Bureau provides a wide range of authors for speaking events. To find out more, go to www.hachettespeakersbureau.com or call (866) 376-6591.

The publisher is not responsible for websites (or their content) that are not owned by the publisher.

Library of Congress Control Number: 2018931666

ISBNs: 978-1-5387-1168-2 (trade paperback), 978-1-5491-6791-1 (audiobook, downloadable) 978-1-5387-1169-9 (ebook)

Printed in the United States of America

LSC-H

10 9 8 7 6 5 4 3 2 1

To Geoffrey

Contents

Preface

I first met Sally about twenty years ago through an article I read in a small magazine called *Spectrum*. By that time, I had been a practicing holistic and anthroposophical doctor for about fifteen years and had studied food and medicine for over two decades. I thought I knew a lot about food and the relationship between food and health. That small article quickly convinced me that no matter how much I thought I knew, this woman knew far more than I did. I resisted my first urge to go off and pout and decided to call her to talk about food, medicine and how she had learned about these subjects. That call led to Sally doing her first public Nourishing Traditions workshop in my small town in New Hampshire; it led me to become one of the founding board members of the Weston A. Price Foundation; it led to two books that we cowrote; and most importantly it led to a lifelong friendship.

After two decades of collaboration, I was honored to be asked to write this small preface to Sally's new book *Nourishing Diets*. I was surprised that I had two distinct reactions to reading her new book. The first was expected; the second surprised me.

The first reaction was that, in contrast to the inaccurate nonsense that is out there among bestselling books purporting to describe the dietary habits of healthy traditional people, Sally gives an in-depth and accurate depiction of what healthy diets *actually* were like. We have been led to believe that healthy Okinawans or Native Americans lived on low-fat animal foods, tree nuts and wild greens. The reality, as Sally describes in intimate detail, is that the healthy diets of the most successful humans on the planet were loaded with high-fat animal foods including insects and offal, as well as lots of fermented foods and drinks of all sorts. Traditional people eat many foods and parts of animals that most of us have never heard of, let alone eaten. Sally's depth of knowledge about what constitutes a real traditional diet surpasses by miles anything found in the popular books on this subject, including the usual "paleo" diet prescriptions.

Contrary to what we have been told, healthy traditional cultures, far from excluding this or that category of foods (like grains, dairy, beans, fats and organ meats), relished these foods, perhaps above all others. But they were meticulous about their preparation techniques to make foods healthy and palatable, many of which are now validated by modern science.

I often tell my patients the single most important health decision they have to make is to decide whether they think modern Americans are the healthiest people who have ever lived. This is what we are told, over and over again—we should all be grateful for the modern agricultural system, the wonders of the green revolution, the blessings of modern medicine, and the convenience of food fortification. If it were not for "progress" we would all live the nasty, brutish and short lives of our ancestors. The reality as Sally describes it is far different—the traditional diet conferred a level of health and vitality on these people that is unheard of for modern man. The key is to have an accurate description of the details of what this healthy nourishing diet entailed. For that, there is simply no resource even close to what Sally provides in *Nourishing Diets.*

My second reaction to Sally's book was a surprise. Reading the descriptions of the varied and unusual foods that comprise a healthy traditional diet I felt a profound sense of sadness for what we have lost. Even the most "foodie" of us living in the "foodie" capital of the United States (I live in San Francisco) live in a food desert compared to the incredible diversity afforded to traditional people. They ate hundreds of different foods, different textures, different and more robust flavors almost every day or week of their lives. Today we pay one hundred dollars a person to go to a top restaurant that has "discovered" bone broth, organ meats and wild vegetables. I felt this strong longing to live in a world where the traditional foods of my ancestors are freely available, to exercise my birthright to consume healthy, nutrient-dense food.

With Sally's able guidance it is possible that in time we can regain some of this lost diversity and flavor. Engaging in food diversity, as for example eating the organs and bones of an animal not just the "prized" muscle meat, is the key to regaining robust health. *Nourishing Diets* points the way to this rejuvenation and will serve as an invaluable guide for anyone interested in the reestablishment of the true human diet.

Thomas Cowan, MD
June, 2018

NOURISHING
DIETS

Modern Technology or Ancestral Wisdom?

THE MOST UNIVERSAL disease in the world is the decay of the teeth, and unfortunately we have not known the cause, until we have gone to the primitive* people to find how they prevent tooth decay," said Dr. Weston A. Price in the late 1930s, in the only video recording we have of him.[1] "Our difficulty is that we are adding too much white flour and sugar and do not get enough of the foods that carry the minerals and vitamins. When the primitive people adopt the foods of modern civilization, their teeth decay just as ours do."

Dr. Price continued: "I've spent several years studying the primitive people in various parts of the world, and I have come as a missionary from them to the people of modern civilization. And I beg of you to learn of their accumulated wisdom, and if you do, you, too, can have strong healthy bodies, without so much disease as we suffer from these days."

What an amazing thought—that the so-called "primitive" people of the world could come as missionaries to modern civilization, missionaries with the gift of their "accumulated wisdom," so that people today might live without disease—including the disease of tooth decay. Even today, explorers, anthropologists, government officials and medical practitioners believe that the transfer of knowledge can go only one way: from modern people with advanced technology to "primitive" people living a preindustrial lifestyle. The idea that the primitive people of the world can provide us with knowledge that could help us have strong, healthy bodies, freedom from tooth decay and resistance to disease…this idea is not one that finds acceptance in today's world.

---

* Dr. Price used the word "primitive" in a complimentary sense; he had great admiration for the nonindustrialized peoples he studied and their wisdom in food choices. Most anthropologists and explorers of his day referred to the people they encountered as "savages." Price studiously avoided the use of this derogatory term.

Yet the so-called civilized world is grappling with an epidemic of disease—not the infectious diseases that modern technology holds at bay, but chronic degenerative disease that is sapping the health and strength of industrialized nations, especially diseases that are now epidemic in the young: learning disorders, behavior problems, growth problems, asthma, allergies, digestive problems, obesity, addiction—even problems normally associated with adults such as arthritis, diabetes and cancer. A large portion of children born in the West today need braces, and treatment for pediatric tooth decay is the fastest growing medical profession. Few today realize that these problems will not be solved by modern medicine, but rather by embracing ancient wisdom on what to eat and how to prepare our food.

WHO WAS DR. WESTON PRICE? He was a Cleveland dentist who wanted to answer the question: what causes tooth decay? He also wanted the answer to its corollary: what causes poor physical development and poor health? In his lifelong search for the cause of the dental decay and physical degeneration that he observed in his dental practice, he turned from test tubes and microscopes to evidence among human beings. During the 1930s, Dr. Price sought the factors responsible for fine teeth among the people who had them—the isolated "primitive" people.

The world became his laboratory. As he traveled, his findings led him to the belief that dental caries and deformed dental arches resulting in crowded, crooked teeth and unattractive appearance were merely a sign of physical degeneration resulting from what he had suspected all along—nutritional deficiencies.

Price traveled the world over in order to study isolated human groups, including sequestered villages in Switzerland, Gaelic communities in the Outer Hebrides, Eskimos and Native Americans of North America, Melanesian and Polynesian South Sea Islanders, African tribes, Australian Aborigines, New Zealand Maori, and the Indians of South America. Wherever he went, Dr. Price found that beautiful straight teeth, freedom from decay, stalwart bodies, resistance to disease, keen eyesight and hearing and optimistic outlooks were typical of native peoples who ate traditional foods rich in essential food factors. As soon as these people began eating "the displacing foods of modern commerce," they began to suffer from tooth decay; and the children born to parents consuming modern foods had narrower facial structure, crowded and crooked teeth and increased susceptibility to disease.

The discoveries and conclusion of Dr. Price are presented in his classic volume *Nutrition and Physical Degeneration*, published in 1945. The book contains striking photographs of handsome, healthy native people and illustrates in an unforgettable way the physical degeneration that occurs when human groups abandon nourishing traditional diets in favor of modern convenience foods like sugar, white flour, pasteurized milk, and "shelf-stable" foods filled with extenders and additives.*

In Dr. Price's day, the medical profession considered good dental health a sign of good overall health, rejecting Army recruits based on the state of their teeth. Dr. Price's photographs and findings indeed indicate that strong bodies and freedom from degenerative disease go hand in hand with healthy teeth. In conversations with medical personnel in the communities he visited, he learned that those eating traditional foods did not suffer from the diseases that afflicted white people living on processed food nor native people who had adopted the white people's diet—they were free of tuberculosis, arthritis, heart disease and cancer. Childbirth was easy for those living on their native diets—a fact that many early explorers noted with amazement.[†]

WHEREAS NATIVE CULTURES with their accumulated wisdom clearly knew how to eat, modern man is drowning in confusion about what constitutes a healthy diet. Conflicting advice comes from every side. Should we be vegetarians? Avoid fat? Choke down skinless chicken breasts? Eat according to our blood type? Make juice out of kale?

And what about the so-called "paleo" or ancestral diets, which advise us to avoid grains and dairy foods? The paleo diet originated with Dr. Loren Cordain, a professor of exercise physiology at Colorado State University. His 2002 book *The Paleo Diet*[2] (the diet is now trademarked) launched the current dietary fad with claims of a diet tailored to the "foods we were designed to eat." The book and paleo diet website recommend lean grass-produced meat, fish and seafood, eggs, fruits and vegetables, nuts and seeds, and "healthful" oils (olive, walnut, flaxseed, macadamia, avocado and coconut). The diet is very high in protein and low in animal fats and proscribes all grains, legumes, potatoes, dairy foods (including butter), refined sugar, processed food, refined vegetable oils and all salt. In 2010, Robb Wolf, a student of Cordain, published a slightly different version of the paleo diet, *The Paleo Solution: The Original Human Diet*,[3] which eliminates *all* starches but allows small amounts of

---

* Unfortunately, even today governments everywhere are turning primitive tribes into "conservation refugees" by evicting them from their land in the name of environmental preservation. Globalist government policy follows John Muir, the grandfather of the American conservation movement, who argued that "wilderness" should be cleared of all inhabitants and set aside to satisfy the modern human's "need for recreation and spiritual renewal." This sentiment became national policy with the passage of the 1964 Wilderness Act, which defined wilderness as a place "where man himself is a visitor and does not remain." Expulsions from "nature preserves" continue to this day, especially in India and Africa.

† In his book, Dr. Price quotes the 1937 work *Safe Childbirth*, by Kathleen Olga Vaughan. Vaughan, a midwife, noted that wide pelvic structure was a requirement for easy birth; Dr. Price theorized that the same nutritious diet that resulted in wide facial structure also gave women wide pelvic structure.

salt. A typical meal includes a salad, 200 grams of lean beef, 300 grams of broccoli and fruit for dessert—a meal that would be very difficult to choke down without added carbohydrates, fat or salt, and one bound to result in cravings for sugar, fat and salt.*

The paleo diet is subject to a wide range of interpretation in hundreds of books, some of which do allow salt, carbohydrates and fats, but the common ground is avoidance of all grains, legumes and milk products on the premise that mankind has not adapted to these foods, which are new to his evolution.

As we shall see, the tenets of the paleo diet have little in common with the way our ancestors actually ate, and can lead to a number of nutrient deficiencies. We'll talk in detail about the principles of healthy traditional diets in chapter 9, but first, let's take a careful look at the diets of healthy people from around the world—the kind of people Dr. Price encountered during his research. What becomes clear is the welcome news that we don't need to deprive ourselves of grains, legumes, milk products, fats or salt in order to eat according to ancestral principles; the emphasis should not be on depriving ourselves of the foods we like to eat, but rather on choosing and preparing foods to maximize our intake of nutrients. As Dr. Price consistently emphasized, whatever specific foods native peoples ate, their diets were very high in

minerals and vitamins, particularly the "fat-soluble vitamins"—A, D and K_2— found uniquely in animal fats. In chapter 10, we'll provide guidance for implementing the principles of traditional diets in modern life—without having to eat foods that Westerners find unacceptable, like insects or weird fermented animal parts.

WE CAN'T GO BACK—we can't go back to a primitive lifestyle, nor would we want to. We must be careful not to romanticize tribal or village life with its constant specter of food shortages or even famine, the pressure to conform, the dread of ghosts, the ritual attached to all aspects of existence, the lack of comfort, the constant exposure to smoke. Dirt was a daily companion—even the fastidious South Sea Islanders suffered from lice. There was no room for individuality in the traditional tribe or village—it was a matter of survival for every member to conform to cultural norms and traditions. Many Western observers noted that the women, in particular, lived a life of drudgery. Some tribes engaged in cannibalism or even ritual torture.[4]

Modern man is an individualist and would have great difficulty returning to the narrow confines of tribal and village life; our consciousness has changed... but our bodies have not. We still have the same nutritional requirements as our

---

* Cordain and Wolf have a "20-percent rule," which allows paleo dieters to eat anything they want as 20 percent of their diet—presumably foods that would supply them with the salt, fat, and carbohydrates their bodies need.

ancestors, and these needs are only met with real, traditional food, chosen and prepared according to the patterns of pre-industrialized people, according to their accumulated wisdom.

Technology has freed us from constant manual labor and given us a life that is more comfortable and more free; but technology applied to our food hacks away at nutritional content in favor of long shelf life. The challenge for modern man is to use technology wisely, opting for wisdom over cleverness when it comes to how we farm, what we choose to eat, and how we prepare our food. Only traditional cultures can show us how.

Wrote Dr. Price,

In my studies I find that it is not accident but accumulated wisdom regarding foods that lies behind their physical excellence and freedom from our modern degenerative processes, and, further, that on various sides of our world the primitive people know many of the things that are essential for life—things that our modern civilizations apparently do not know. These are the fundamental truths of life that have put them in harmony with Nature through obeying her nutritional laws. Whence this wisdom? Was there in the distant past a world civilization that was better attuned to Nature's laws and have these remnants retained this knowledge? If this is not the explanation, it must be that these various primitive [peoples] have been able through a superior skill in interpreting cause and effect, to determine for themselves what foods in their environment are best for producing human bodies with a maximum of physical fitness and resistance to degeneration.[5]

CHAPTER 1

Australian Aborigines

The Most Paleo of Them All

ANY EXPLORATION OF ancestral foodways should begin with the native Australians. They provide us with a unique example of an isolated Paleolithic population, one that existed on the hunter-gatherer's lean-meat, grainless diet, without the practice of agriculture or animal domestication. They occupied temporary shelters and prepared their foods in the most primitive way; in short, they lived the life of the primitive nomad, wandering across the face of the earth. It was a life that was necessarily nasty, brutish and short.

An Australian government website asserts that the Aboriginal people in Australia lived by "roaming their vast continent in search of animals and eating seeds and roots of plants for survival...Foraging parties gathered enough food for their immediate needs and food was not often stored."[1]

According to this point of view, the Australian native survived because he lived on a continent blessed with abundance. Early colonists from Europe, who began arriving in Australia in 1788, described a land teeming with life, with soil of unusual loamy lightness and kangaroo grass so high as to conceal the sheep and cattle of the first settlers. Orchids, lilies and mosses flourished in the fertile ground. The settlers were astonished at the beauty of the country, which they considered completely natural and accidental. According to the early settler and diarist Sir Thomas Livingston Mitchell, writing in 1839, "We crossed a beautiful plain; covered with shining verdure, and ornamented with trees, which, although 'dropt in nature's careless haste,' gave the country the appearance of an extensive park."[2] Many other settlers noted that the land had the appearance of landscaped park, where tracts of pasture alternated with belts of timber in an artistic fashion, very pleasing to the eye.[3]

This beautiful continent abounded with fish and wildlife of every sort. "Newcomers commented endlessly on plains rich with life, skies dark with birds, seas black with fish…Kangaroos very numerous and easily caught…Newcomers heard possums grunting and saw glider possums flying."[4]

In the early 1840s, colonist Angus McMillan saw a lake "alive with swans, ducks and pelicans…The country was absolutely swarming with kangaroos and emus…In all ordinary seasons…they can obtain in two or three hours, a sufficient supply of food for the day. Even in the desert, people got food in four to five hours per day."*[5]

The problem with these descriptions of the native Australians is that they are misleading, if not completely wrong. The Aboriginal peoples did not live haplessly in a land fortuitously blessed by abundance; rather, through wise and ingenious land management, they *created* the landscape and the abundance that so amazed the European interlopers. And far from existing on a meager, dry diet of nuts, vegetables and lean meat, the Aborigines enjoyed a wide and varied diet that included everything from fatty animal food to grain flour made into cakes!

AGRICULTURE, PARTICULARLY THE cultivation of grain, is defined as the cultivation and breeding of plants and animals by largely sedentary human beings, thereby producing food surpluses that can be stored between harvests and for times of famine. Agriculture encompasses the domestication of animals, selection of seed, preparation of the soil, harvesting of crops, storage of surplus and water management. It requires large populations living in permanent housing. Contrary to the claims of paleo-diet enthusiasts, the Aboriginal Australians did all these things, a fact that emerges from a careful review of early colonial diaries, but one only reluctantly accepted by mainstream anthropologists.

"The whole country looks as if it had been carefully ploughed, harrowed, and finally rolled," wrote the colonist John McKinlay in 1861.[6] In crossing the Australian frontier, Thomas Mitchell marveled, "The grass is pulled…and piled in hayricks, so that the aspect of the desert was softened into the agreeable semblance of a hay-field…we found the ricks or haycocks extending for miles…the seed is made by the natives into a kind of paste or bread. Dry heaps of this grass, that has been pulled expressly for this purpose of gathering the seed, lay along our path for many miles. I counted nine miles along the river, in which we rode through this grass only, reaching to our saddle-girths, and the same grass seemed to grow back from the river, at least as far as the eye could reach through a very open forest."[7] In 1845, the colonist Charles Sturt saw harvested grain spread out in a "boundless field of stubble."[8]

On Cooper Creek in east central

_____

* This is a man describing the activities of men; the women spent much more time engaged in food gathering and processing.

Australia, the natives reaped millet from fields of one thousand acres. According to settler Augustus Greghory, "The natives cut it down by means of stone knives, cutting down the stalk half way, beat out the seed, leaving the straw which is often met with in large heaps; they winnow by tossing seed and husk in the air, the wind carrying away the husks. The grinding into meal is done by means of two stones."[9]

At times the Aborigines harvested through the use of fire. According to one settler, "Fire was set to the grass which was full in the ear yet green. While the fire was burning, the natives kept turning the grass with sticks all the time to knock the seeds out. When this was done, the fire burnt out, they gathered up the seed into a big opossum rug."[10]

IN ADDITION TO MILLET, the Aborigines cultivated a native wheat, oats, rye and bull Mitchell grass, which produced, according to botanist Fred Turner, "ears nearly six inches in length, well filled with a clean-looking, firm grain, which separates easily from the chaff."[11] Moreover, they also cultivated and harvested rice. One explorer-driver found two granaries, "one with about a ton of rice seed stored there in large dishes."[12]

So the Aboriginal peoples grew grain—lots of grain—which they harvested, winnowed, stored, soaked, ground into flour and baked into cakes. The Aboriginal grain belt stretched from east to west across the continent, with a wide band through the desert interior, whereas today modern agriculture only succeeds in growing grain in the wetter areas of southeast and southwest Australia.[13] The evidence indicates that the peoples of arid central Australia engaged in seed propagation, irrigation, harvest, storage and trade of seed across the region.[14] Several explorers and commentators witnessed grain traded to distant relatives in small sealed parcels.[15] In an 1860 expedition to the unexplored interior of eastern Australia, the Irish soldier John King found a store of grain estimated at four tons.[16]

Grindstones have turned up in Cuddie Springs, New South Wales and at Kakadu in the Northern Territory. In the 1940s, the explorer Hamilton Hume observed that "on the Darling [River] the Natives gather grain from the wild oats…and grind it between two stones and make a paste and eat it, the same is done by the Natives to the northward."[17]

The practice of agriculture includes the manipulation of grains through selection for desirable traits. When plants become "domesticated" as the result of a human-induced selection regime, they undergo changes in form and structure to such an extent that the plants become dependent on humans for the continuance of their life cycle. These changes include a tendency to ripen simultaneously and the development of a tough rachis,* which allows man to harvest the seed. Harvesting and winnowing techniques also contribute to changes in seed characteristics.

Aboriginal grains exhibited these qualities, and native seed-selection techniques were similar to those that led to the domestication of wild wheat and barley in Europe. According to some researchers, the tough rachis developed within just twenty to thirty years of this cropping style, to the extent that the grains required watering for germination to occur.[18] Aboriginal grains became dependent on the interventions of the Aborigines.

Grains grown in arid regions require water, and evidence of extensive irrigation systems and man-made wells is scattered throughout the desert areas of Australia. The Airaduri people in New South Wales built large dams to store water. Stories of ancestors teaching their people about selecting seed, sowing it and building dams are common in the grain areas.[19]

Many colonists saw dams and irrigation trenches, and even saw such structures in the process of construction: "The people would get in a line, using their digging scoops and larger *coolamons*.† The clay and earth was scooped into the larger *coolamons*, which were passed along the line.... with a line of people working the deepening of the favoured catchment area and the building of the bank could be done at the same time. When it was satisfactorily excavated, the people would trample the clay base. If ant nest material was nearby this was carried and trampled in to give a very firm base."[20]

A dam wall in the Bulloo River floodplain in southwest Queensland was over three hundred feet long, six feet high, and almost twenty feet at its base. The earthen embankment across the catchment of several streams was capable of holding almost two hundred thousand gallons.[21] A site in the Great Western Desert was estimated to hold over forty thousand gallons. In fact, today's empty and forbidding desert regions once hosted a considerable population of Aboriginal tribes, engaged in grain production without any

---

* The key difference between wild and domesticated grains is that domesticated varieties are "shatterproof." The grains are attached to a central axis known as the rachis. As wild grains ripen, the rachis becomes brittle, so that when touched or blown by the wind it shatters, scattering the grains as seeds, ensuring that the grains are only dispersed once they have ripened. In a small number of plants, however, a single genetic mutation ensures the rachis does not become brittle, even when the seeds ripen. This "tough rachis" mutation is helpful for humans gathering wild grains, who are likely to gather a disproportionate number of tough-rachis mutants as a result. If some of the grains are then planted to produce a crop the following year, the tough-rachis mutation will be propagated, and every year the proportion of tough-rachis mutants will increase.

† A wooden carrier called a *pitji* or *coolamon* is a valuable piece of equipment, especially for Aboriginal women. In addition to its use in construction, it served as a food carrier, water container and receptacle for carrying infants.

degrading impact on the environment. As one commentator observed: "Desert is a term Europeans use to describe areas where they can't grow wheat and sheep."[22]

The great advantage of Aboriginal crops was their development for harsh conditions through seed selection, direct planting and weeding. Many of the grains grew on sand and required a minimum of irrigation. They also had a very high nutritional value.[23]

Evidence of widespread and large-scale grain production by the "primitive" people in Australia makes it clear that the Aboriginal people were not reacting to the whims of nature, but directly affecting its production.[24] In Australia, the lines between the passive adaptation of the hunter-gatherer and exertive activities of the agriculturalist were blurred or even nonexistent.

While not all Aboriginal peoples cultivated and stored grain, the testimony of explorers indicates that most native Australians were, at the very least, in the early stages of an agricultural society and even ahead of many other parts of the world[25]—all without the advantages of metals, the wheel or domesticated beasts of burden.

THE ABORIGINES CULTIVATED many other species of plant foods besides grains, especially in areas of abundant rainfall. The east coast of Australia alone provides 250 species of edible plants, including tubers such as yams and grass potatoes, fern roots, palm hearts, legumes, nuts, seeds, shoots, leaves and a wide variety of fruits such as figs and berries.[26]

Chief among these was the *murnong*, or yam daisy, a native dandelion, which flourished with the help of human cultivation in areas blessed with moisture. In 1836, one settler saw "a vast extent of downs…quite yellow with *murnong*" and "natives spread over the field, digging for roots."[27]

The *murnong* seed does not last in the soil, so crops need continuous mature plants, yet "millions" grew in southeast Australia. Where women dug them, for mile on mile the ground looked plowed. The native women burned the grass to better see the roots. One settler met "open grassy country, extending as far as we could see, hills round and smooth as a carpet, meadows broad, and either as green as an emerald, or of a rich golden colour, from the abundance, as we soon afterwards found, of a little ranunculus-like flower…We went on our way rejoicing."[28]

Soon after the arrival of the Europeans in 1788, the yam daisy disappeared. According to colonist Isaac Batey, writing in 1846, "Where once abundant they have become quite extinct for the district where the writer was raised… [Today] they might be searched without discovering a solitary example…Elsewhere it has been intimated that our domestic animals had eaten them out, yet there was another factor of destruction in the soil becoming hardened with the continuous tramping of sheep, cattle or horses."[29] The flat feet of kangaroos were much gentler on the fragile soils of Australia!

Settler Edward Page observed, "When I first came here I started a vegetable garden, the soil dug like ashes." He described the soil as "a spot free of timber or scrub of any description, the soil reddish loam of great depth."[30]

Another important food plant was the nardoo or swamp fern, which grew in beds of shallow lakes. John Davis, an early settler, reported on the vast quantities of nardoo seed* waiting to be harvested on the dry floor of Lake Coogiecoogina in the Strzeleck Desert.[31] The Aborigines stored the nardoo seed and flour in ingenious vermin-proof vessels.[32] The nardoo is poisonous without careful preparation, a task that generally fell to the women.

The desert raisin or bush tomato comes from a small desert plant that grows naturally in many Australian dry areas. A species of tomato, the bushes grow quickly after summer rains, particularly after bushfires. The fruit provided food for the indigenous desert dwellers of central Australia for many thousands of years. The traditional harvesting method involves collecting the sun-dried fruit in the autumn and winter months. In dried form, the desert raisins can be stored for several years.

Another staple from desert regions was the *quandong*, a fruit of the semiparasitic *quandong* tree. Ripe red *quandong* fruits provided tasty treats whether eaten raw or dried for later use. Women collected the *quandong* fruit in *coolamons*, separated the edible fruit from the pitted stone, and then rolled the edible fruit into a ball.

Also in arid regions, spinifex grass produced large quantities of edible seed at certain times of the year. Edible fungus (*morabudi*), which the natives enjoyed both raw and cooked, was another desert bounty.

Onion grass provided flavoring for meat and grains. It was deftly harvested by the women, who would dig a trench at the edge of the patch, then work in a line, turning over the ground as they moved forward. Many early explorers witnessed this cultivation process and recognized its efficacy.[33]

The *cumbungi*, or bulrush, is a troublesome weed found in farm dams, creeks, ponds and slow-moving rivers, but for the natives it provided an abundant source of carbohydrates. Meal made from the *cumbungi* rush was similar to flour or potato meal. According to Thomas Mitchell, cakes made from the *cumbungi* flour "were lighter and sweeter than those made from common flour."[34] He observed huge mounds dotting the reed marshes near Swan Hill, which housed villages within the swamp

---

* Technically ferns do not produce seeds. The nardoo "seeds" are hard, nut-like objects up to [one-third] inch long called sporocarps, which grow from the plant's rhizome (underground stem or root). The sporocarp is a hard capsule full of spores in starchy packing.

to manage and harvest this valuable plant. Settlers were intrigued by these massive mounds and the fact that they were emitting steam. Upon examination, the mounds proved to be gigantic ovens for cooking *cumbungi*.[35] Thomas Mitchell described "the lofty ash hills of the natives, used chiefly for roasting the *balyan* (or bulrush)" and was astonished at the volume of starch produced.

One of the most remarkable sources of food for the Aborigines in eastern Australia was the mountain bunya pine. Once every three years, these huge trees bore enormous quantities of cones, the largest of which contain seeds over one inch long. Every third year, many tribes would travel to the Bunya Bunya festival—one of the few times when they were permitted to cross the boundaries of other tribes. The harvest was so plentiful that thousands could live for several weeks off the seeds. The nuts are described as having a delicious taste, something like roasted chestnuts.[36] The kernels were also pounded into a meal and baked in the ashes as a cake. The Aborigines stored bunya nuts by placing them in large cane baskets and burying them in a particular kind of mud. When exhumed—after many months of lying in the ground—the nuts had an offensive smell but nevertheless served as a popular food.[37]

Other trees that played an important role in Aboriginal culture included the many varieties of acacia, which provided flowers used in making sweet drinks, grubs collected from their trunks and roots, and bark used as a fish poison. Mangrove trees, which grew in freshwater swamps, or billabongs,* provided fruit and also harbored many creatures in their complex root systems: mangrove worms, freshwater oysters, mussels and crabs. Salt was collected from their leaves.[38] Gum trees or eucalyptus harbored grubs, beehives, koalas and possum, as well as a tasty insect exudate called *lerp*. Even galls that formed on their trunks were eaten. Some flowers provided nectar to make a sweet drink called *bool* by one tribe of Aborigines. The ribbon gum tree was a rich source of manna, a crumbly white substance with a pleasant taste, which exudes from the bark. As much as forty pounds could be collected from trees in one day.[39] Eucalyptus leaves were used to make herbal medicines, while the trees' gum could be used to fill the occasional dental cavity.[40] Melaleuca, or paperbark, tree flowers provided an ingredient for sweet drinks. More important, their bark was used in everything from cooking to canoe production. In short, far from wandering haplessly across the landscape, the Aboriginals nourished themselves from a complex web of cultivated food sources.

---

* A billabong is an oxbow lake, an isolated pond left behind after a river changes course. Billabongs are usually formed when the path of a creek or river changes, leaving the former branch with a dead end. Billabongs, reflecting the arid Australian climate in which these "dead rivers" are found, fill with water seasonally and are dry for a greater part of the year.

THE NUMEROUS AND varied aboriginal food preparation and storage techniques turned plants and seeds that were inherently inedible into foods that sustained life. Aboriginal women spent many hours washing, grinding, pounding, straining, grating, boiling and cooking plant foods. Bark troughs or large sea shells served as vessels for boiling water.[41] Tubers were stored in holes in the ground; bunya nuts were soaked in water or buried in bags; cycads were sliced, dried, wrapped in paperbark and buried in grass-lined trenches; water-lily corms were dried and stored; and portulaca were wrapped in mud, baked and stored—these methods made foods that were poisonous, bitter, or difficult to digest into nutritious bush tucker.

Most Australians today know about the poisonous nardoo seeds, which contain thiaminase, an enzyme that depletes the body of vitamin B_1 (thiamin). The nardoo seeds require careful sluicing, pounding, winnowing and baking in order to neutralize their thiaminase content and make them edible. The explorers Burke and Wills, who set about crossing the interior of Australia in 1860, died after consuming a diet of nardoo seed, a staple of the Aboriginal people.* Their symptoms indicated that they died of thiamin deficiency, known as beriberi, because they did not prepare the seeds in accordance with aboriginal food preparation methods. Despite eating plenty of food, the men got weaker and weaker. Wills wrote in his diary: "My pulse is at forty-eight and very weak and my legs and arms are nearly skin and bone. I can only look out like Mr. Micawber for something to turn up, but starvation on nardoo is by no means unpleasant, but for the weakness one feels, and the utter inability to move oneself, for as the appetite is concerned, it gives me the greatest satisfaction."[42]

Very often, the first step in the time-consuming process of plant preparation was the "yandying" process, used by women to separate seeds from stalks and other impurities with which they had been gathered. The process looks deceptively simple but is, in fact, extremely difficult, requiring deft movements and a great deal of skill. The gathered seeds are placed in a *coolamon*, and the various objects of differing density or characteristics are separated from each other by intricate and skillful rotating and jiggling movements.[43]

Fern roots formed a meal staple in many regions. Before enjoying them as food, the women dug them up, washed them, roasted them on hot ashes, cut them into lengths and pounded them between a pair of round stones. Other types of fern roots were dried in the sun, lightly roasted to remove the hair rootlets, peeled with the fingernails, chopped

---

* The explorers foolishly shot at the one native they saw, chasing away the only person who could have advised them on how to prepare the poisonous seeds.

on a log to break the fibers, mixed with water and other ingredients, and finally rounded into a lump for cooking. These fern root cakes accompanied fish, meat, crabs or oysters.[44]

The grass potato is a palatable fibrous root that was roasted and then pounded between two stones before eating. Some foods, such as orchid pseudobulbs, were dried first, then ground, mixed with water, and cooked. Yams were dug out with a stick—sometimes from a depth of three feet or more—and prepared by crushing and washing them in water and cooking them in ashes.[45]

Grain and legume preparation began with placing the seeds in "dilly bags" or leaching baskets and putting them in running water for anywhere from a number of hours to many days—a process that serves to remove the antinutrients and toxins found in many grains and legumes. The matchbox bean, for example, got a twelve-hour soaking,[46] while the jack bean was soaked for several days, then pounded, made into cakes and roasted.[47] Seeds of the zamia, a spiky, palmlike plant, were dried in the sun, then put in a dilly bag and suspended in running water for four to five days. Further processing involved crushing and pounding between two flat stones, grinding into a fine paste, wrapping the paste in paperbark, and baking under ashes.[48] Seeds of the pineapple palm were crushed into a flour, then washed in running water for a week and cooked in hot ashes.[49] Black beans were soaked in water for eight to ten days and dried in the sun. Then came roasting on hot stones, pounding into a coarse meal, mixing with water to make a thin cake, and then baking again on hot stones.[50]

Nuts from spiky pandanus (screw pine), which cling to the rocky headlands in eastern Australia, required six weeks of treatment to render them safe for eating. They were converted into a tasty and nutritious nut bread that was popular with the earliest European settlers.[51] Pandanus (screw pine) and *burrawang* (cycad) nuts went through stringent sluicing and immersion treatments to remove poisonous alkaloids. The roasted and pounded *burrawang* flesh needed two to three weeks of soaking to remove toxins.

As for fruit, the Australian flora provided many delicious and nutritious delicacies throughout the year, particularly in the humid coastal regions. Some of these were eaten raw just after picking, while others were processed. The wild orange was picked just before it was ripe, then buried for one day, during which it would become very sweet. The wallaby apple was likewise ripened by placing it in the sand for a day.[52] The taste of a type of wild plum improved after being stored or buried for a couple of days.[53] The fruit of the *quandong*, or native peach, was buried for four days. Dried figs were pounded into cakes and eaten with honey. Mangrove fruit was pulped, soaked and mashed through a basket.[54]

The Aborigines also used fruits like tamarinds and native lime to make refreshing beverages.[55] Acid drinks were made from the fruit of lawyer cane by squashing the fruit in water, and from breadfruit by soaking it in water.[56] Certain flowers rich in nectar were gathered in the early morning and steeped in water, which was drunk fresh or set aside to ferment.[57] Leaves of the red flowering *ti* tree were added to hot water to produce a tea-like beverage.[58]

An agricultural nation requires storage of food surpluses. Numerous early diarists describe the preservation of everything from grains, *quandong*, figs, plums, tubers, seeds and nuts to caterpillars, moths, meat, liver, eggs, fish, fish oil and even mussels! Drying and pounding transformed caterpillars into a kind of flour. Figs and *quandong* were pulped and mixed to form a product like quince paste.[59]

Storage vessels made of clay, straw, leaves and even gypsum kept grain and other foods dry and vermin-free. Early explorers found stone chambers with tight-fitting stone plugs. In the Great Sandy Desert, the tribes harvested acacia and eucalyptus seed and covered them with spinifex grass for consumption later in the year. Foods required stockpiling before ceremonies attended by hundreds or even thousands of people. Bunya trees fruited so heavily that large stores were set aside. Grain stores of more than fifty kilograms sewn up in animal skins lasted for months in perfect condition. Hollow trees and rock wells also served for food storage.[60]

Strict protocols and religious observation governed cooking, storage and food handling methods. For example, if a woman damaged the yam leaves or bruised the tuber during harvest, penalties would apply. These rules ensured the propagation and proliferation of edible and otherwise useful plants, while the ancestral preparation traditions ensured that they were edible. Modern science validates these traditions and demonstrates the need for more careful preparation of many of the foods—especially grains and legumes—we eat today.

NEITHER SALTY NOR SWEET tastes were lacking in the Aboriginal diet. Salt was collected from leaves of the river mangrove and was available from the salt flats in desert regions. Roasted leaves of a sodium-rich desert succulent called pigface also added salt to the diet.[61] Certain rushes and sedges, as well as seeds of the golden grevillea, some kinds of figs, the nonda plum and the bush tomato, contained reasonable amounts of sodium. Wild parsnip root and water chestnuts contain more than 4,500 milligrams of sodium per 100 grams.[62] Animal foods also supplied sodium, especially blood and certain organ meats, as did the goanna lizard, shellfish, snails and worms.[63] Ground seeds of the pepper vine added a peppery taste,[64] and aromatic leaves provided variety in cooking.

For sweetness, the Aborigines loved honey. They distinguished between two kinds. One was white and very sweet, and always found in small dead hollow trees. The other was dark, more plentiful and of a somewhat sour taste. Lerp, the sweet insect exudate found on certain trees, was collected and chewed or melted with warm water to form a jelly.[65] In the desert, the sweet taste came from eating the swollen abdomens of sugar ants. Children enjoyed tree gums dissolved in water and mixed with honey.[66]

Some tribes pounded flowers in a wooden dish, then drained the liquid into another dish and mixed this with the sugary parts of honey ants. The mixture was fermented for eight to ten days[67]—we have no descriptions of how it tasted or what effects it had!

THE CONTINENT OF AUSTRALIA teemed with animal life, and the Aboriginals ate it all—starting with marsupials such as kangaroo, wallaby, the smaller pademelon, duck-billed platypus and bandicoot. As the Aboriginals put it, "There's nothing like kangaroo to put strength into you."[68] Kangaroo rats, spiny anteaters, possums, koalas, bats, iguanas, lizards, frogs and snakes also provided nourishment. Bird life on the menu included emus, turkeys, swans, ducks, parrots, cockatoos, cassowaries and jabiru. Seafood including fish, shellfish, eels, turtles and shark. Sea mammals such as dugong and whale held an important place in the diets of seacoast tribes.

The traditional role for Aboriginal women was that of gatherer; they bore the responsibility for harvesting almost all plant foods, but also insects and shellfish. To the men went the duties of hunting large game, birds and fish.

Early colonists described stores of fish meal and fish flour; many commodities, including caterpillars, witchetty grubs, grasshoppers, meat and liver, called for individual preparation prior to storage. Dried animal foods were often coated in the ashes of particular woods and later mixed with seed flour before cooking.

Aboriginal people generally hunted kangaroo in groups. A number of hunters would spread out to herd the animals toward a net stretched across a pocket in the forest or brush near the animals' feeding area. Another group concealed itself near the net to catch the game with spears or clubs. In open country, they tracked and speared kangaroos while the animals were resting in the shade of a tree during the hot part of the day.[69]

An early settler has given us this description of a kangaroo hunt: "By the time the dew was dry on the grass and herbage—and they never hunt before—their spears were in readiness. Led by the chief, who took good care to keep me near him, they filed off into the scrub. A couple of miles brought us to a sudden halt. To my eye there was nothing visible, absolutely nothing. The native eye, and ear, and smell, have a keenness of perception of which civilized man knows nothing.* After a breathless pause of about two minutes, the chief raised his hand, making certain motions with his fingers, when the party flew off in different directions, while I was an admiring spectator of the strange maneuver. Presently they had formed a wide circle. Now they advanced a step or two. Then they were motionless as statues. Then they all moved a few steps again; and again were still; and all this while every eye seemed fixed on some central object which, to my unpracticed sight remained invisible. At length, however, I saw the game—two hundred kangaroo or more. The beautiful things were grazing among the scrub. They fed; the hunters advanced; they erected themselves to reconnoiter, and they of the chase were still."[70]

A key weapon in the kangaroo hunt was the iconic boomerang, which Europeans first encountered at Farm Cove (Port Jackson), Australia, in December 1804, where they witnessed its use as a weapon during a tribal skirmish: "The white spectators were justly astonished at the dexterity and incredible force with which a bent, edged waddy resembling slightly a Turkish scimitar, was thrown by Bungary, a native distinguished by his remarkable courtesy. The weapon, thrown at twenty or thirty yards distance, twirled round in the air with astonishing velocity, and alighting on the right arm of one of his opponents, actually rebounded to a distance not less than seventy or eighty yards, leaving a horrible contusion behind, and exciting universal admiration."[71]†

The Aborigines had ingenious ways of extracting nocturnal animals such as possum and koala—both prized foods—from their daytime resting places. They first detected the animal by its smell, claw marks or droppings, and then confirmed its presence by inserting a stick or frond tipped with honey into the hollow tree or log. If hairs stuck to the honey, they knew the animal was there. Then they either climbed the tree to drag out the animal or smoked it out of its resting place.

Bats such as the flying fox and grey glider were so numerous in certain places that they blocked out the stars and moon when they flew. Hunters caught them during the day as they slept in the scrub. Two or three people carrying about a dozen

---

* So skilled were the Aboriginal people in detecting movement in the brush that the Australian police frequently used them as trackers.

† The earliest known Australian Aboriginal boomerangs are ten thousand years old, but older hunting sticks have been discovered in Europe, where they seem to have formed part of the Stone Age weapon arsenal. One boomerang, discovered in Jaskinia Obłazowa in the Carpathian Mountains in Poland, made of mammoth's tusk, has been dated at about thirty thousand years old. King Tutankhamun of Egypt owned a collection of boomerangs of both the straight-flying (hunting) and returning variety.

small clubs would climb trees where the bats were sleeping. Standing on branches, they would frighten the bats and throw the clubs at them as they flew away.[72]

Reptiles including goannas (iguanas), lizards, frogs and snakes also found a place in the Aboriginal diet, as did birds of all sizes—emus, turkeys, swans, ducks, parrots and cockatoos. To catch flying birds such as parrots, the Aborigines set nets across trees and then threw boomerangs above a passing flock. Thinking these were hawks, the birds would dive down and find themselves caught in the nets. In the summer, hunters captured ducks by submerging themselves up to their necks in water holes and holding small branches to hide their heads. When a duck came close, the hunter would grasp its legs and drown it.[73]

Thomas Mitchell greatly admired the Aboriginal nets: "The meshes were about two inches wide, and the net hung down to within five feet of the surface of the stream…Among the few specimens of art manufactured by the primitive inhabitants of these wilds, none come so near our own as the net, which, even in quality, as well as the mode of knotting, can scarcely be distinguished from those made in Europe."[74]

One Queensland settler found a "kangaroo net fifty feet long and five and a half in width, made of as good twine as any European net."[75] Huge nets were used in combination with miles of brush fences or even stone walls. In central Victoria, a massive system of stone walls dates well before the period of European contact.[76]

During game drives, the hunters drove the animals across a twenty-mile front, an effort requiring the cooperation of several tribes and involving two thousand participants. The kangaroos were shunted into a series of holding pens where narrow apertures could direct animals designated for slaughter one way and those to be released in another. The hunters killed only the male animals, which kept overall population numbers high. Studies in South Australia found that the harvesting of ten thousand males a year over eight years led to an increase of animals from twenty to fifty per square kilometer. Emu harvests were conducted in the same way.[77]

Animal foods were generally cooked, either over an open fire or steamed in pits. Kangaroo, for example, was laid on a fire and seared for a short period so that the interior flesh remained practically raw; at other times, a kangaroo was placed in a large hole, surrounded by hot coals, and sealed from the air. Sometimes meat was wrapped in melaleuca bark. Flying fox bats were wrapped in the leaf of the Alexandra palm for cooking. When the bats were cooked, the leaves were unwrapped, pulling off the skin and fur at the same time.[78] Raw meat was sometimes tenderized by pounding.

No studies of the Aboriginal peoples make mention of any special preparation of bones into pastes or broths, as is commonly found among other traditional peoples throughout the world. Weston Price reported that the Aborigines made lime by burning seashells in a large fire for three to four days; Price speculates that the lime was probably used in food preparation. Insects eaten whole and ground-up moths provided calcium, as did the many plant foods properly prepared to neutralize calcium-blocking phytic acid. And perhaps they got calcium from milk, too. One traditional Aboriginal woman reported that if hunters could capture a female kangaroo carrying a joey, tickling the inside of the pouch produced a prodigious amount of milk, which they consumed with relish![79]

Aboriginal agriculture fits the description of "farming without fences." Various tribes cooperated in hunting methods that ensured an abundance of large animal foods, but smaller animals easily conformed to domestication. Village dwellers reared dingos (wild dogs), possums, emus and cassowaries; penned pelican chicks and let parent birds fatten them; moved rats and caterpillars to new breeding areas; and carried fish and crayfish stock across the country.[80]

Another area of land management involved the creation of havens for insect populations. The resourceful Aboriginals cultivated witchetty grubs by piling logs many feet high. Oak trunks pushed into the creeks and rivers attracted teredo grubs and harbored them until ready to harvest in a year's time. The task of harvesting this nutrient-dense food went to the women and old men.[81] Aborigines also ringbarked or girdled candlenut trees, removing a strip of bark around the trunk to make the trunks rot. White grubs would feed on the decaying wood and were then served as food.[82]

ANTHROPOLOGISTS TODAY grudgingly admit that the Aboriginal diet abounded in animal foods; but they continue to insist that their bush tucker was lean. Today's reigning medical paradigm holds that saturated animal fats—which are solid at room temperature—cause heart disease and many other ailments, while liquid polyunsaturated oils protect against these diseases. The discovery that traditional peoples consumed high levels of saturated animal fat—as much as they could get—while enjoying excellent health and freedom from heart disease poses a challenge to researchers at pains to impose political correctness on ancestral diets.

An example is a 1986 study published in the journal *Lipids*, titled "Animal foods in traditional Australian aboriginal diets: polyunsaturated and low in fat." From the abstract we read:

> Australian Aborigines develop high frequencies of diabetes and cardiovascular diseases when they make the transition to an urban lifestyle. The composition of the traditional diet, particularly its lipid components, is a most important aspect of the

hunter-gatherer lifestyle that would bear on the risk of these diseases. We have examined the fat content and fatty acid composition of a variety of animal foods eaten traditionally by Aborigines from different regions of Australia. The muscle samples of the wild animals from all over Australia were uniformly low in fat...with a high proportion of polyunsaturated fatty acids...The results of these analyses suggest that even when the traditional Aboriginal diet contained a high proportion of animal foods it would have been low in fat with a high proportion of polyunsaturated fatty acids (PUFA) and thereby could have protected Aborigines against cardiovascular diseases and related conditions through a combination of factors: low energy density, low saturated fat and relatively high PUFA content.[*83]

What these commentators miss are patterns of selective eating; game was so plentiful in Australia that the Aboriginals could pick and choose the choicest parts of the animal. They also observed nature and knew when animals were fattest. Except in times of drought or famine, the Aborigines rejected kangaroos that were too lean—they were not worth carrying back to camp.[84]

Kangaroos were fat when the fern leaf wattle was in flower; possums were fat when the apple tree was in bloom. Aborigines prized the highly saturated kidney fat from the possum and often ate it raw.[85] Other signs indicated when the carpet snake, kangaroo rat, mussels, oysters, turtles and eels were fat and at their best.[86] Fat from the intestines of marsupials and emus were favorites, and the yellow fat of the goanna lizard was considered a delicacy.[87] Aborigines prized the fatty organ meats. Dugongs and whales provided plentiful fat to natives on the coasts. They also ate eggs from reptiles and birds. Researchers have concluded that fatty smoked eel likely formed a basis of trade with other parts of Australia.[†]

One overlooked source of fat in the aboriginal diet is insects. Fifty to 60 percent of the weight of the dugong moth is fat. During the moth season, the natives collected these insects in vast numbers from rock crevices, swept into nets or whisked onto kangaroo skins. They were cooked in hot ashes for a short time until the wings and legs were singed away. They placed the moth carcasses on a bark platter until cool, then collected and sifted them in a net until the heads fell off. The body was eaten whole or ground into a paste and made into doughy cakes that were smoked to preserve them; or they were placed in an oven made

---

[*] Even Bruce Pascoe, author of the wonderful book *Dark Emu*, praises kangaroo flesh because it has a "low fat content." Elsewhere in this fascinating work, he describes feasts on fat-laden moths and other insects.

[†] Hollow trees served as smokehouses for eel. Analysis of the soil at their bases revealed eel fat, which may have been eight thousand years old.

of burning sand, covered up and cooked for a few minutes. Observers report that the cooked insects look like beautiful white kernels and have the flavor of marrow.[88] Settlers witnessed the Aboriginals returning from the moth harvest in great health, their bodies glistening with moth fat.

Crows assembled to take part in the moth feast, and they too became fat and so intent on their hunt, the festival participants could knock them on the head and eat them—a great delicacy, as the meat was plump and aromatic after the birds' diet of moth fat.

The witchetty grub, or moth larva, inhabits the rotting trunks of trees. These succulent treats—often over six inches long—were eaten both raw and cooked. Fat content of the dried grub is as high as 67 percent. The green tree ant was another source of valuable fat, with a fat-to-protein ratio of about twelve to one. Termites provided an additional source of fat.*

In contrast to the premise that the Aboriginal diet was low in fat, a most remarkable article appearing in the journal *Lipids* describes the "Fat, Fishing Patterns, and Health Among the Bardi People of North Western Australia."[89]

According to the authors, the Aborigines considered foods lacking fat as "rubbish." They fished for different species of fish when they had the most fat lining the intestines.† This fat was painstakingly removed, melted in a shell or tin can set on the coals, and then drunk or used as a dip for the flesh of the fish. The Bardi harvested rock oysters during spring tides; oysters taken at other times were "rubbish." An analysis found that the oysters harvested during spring tides were four times richer in fat. Analysis of fat from fish guts and livers, from oysters, and from turtle meat, fat and organ meats found that the predominant fat was saturated fat.

The Bardi peoples were fond of turtle, but only if the meat was fat. They could tell when a turtle was fat by the configuration of the crease in the front leg. But what if they were hunting at night? No problem. They waited for the turtles to come up for air at the water's edge and knew when the turtles were fat by the smell of their breath!

"THE ABORIGINALS WORKED the waterways of Australia with endless ingenuity," wrote Bill Gammage in his fascinating book *The Biggest Estate on Earth*. "They made nets of European quality, the mesh and knot varied to suit the prey. Duck nets with floats of reed and sinkers

---

* Insects also had medicinal uses. The bush cockroach provided a local anesthetic, and the green tree ant could be used to treat headaches and colds. The silk bag of the pine processionary caterpillar made a protective dressing for wounds and the honey from sugarbag bees helped "clear the guts out." Termites provided compounds that served as antibacterial agents.

† Unlike fish from cold regions, tropical fish have very little fat in their flesh.

of clay spanned the rivers; fish nets half a mile long circled tidal flats. On the coast and inland, thousands of weirs, dams and traps of stone, mud, brush or reeds made fishing easy. Permanent fences of stone, brush and stakes made zigzag patterns in the streams. Wicker gates or woven funnels let fish or crayfish upstream on in-tides and trapped them on the ebbs. Grass fronds laid over shallow edges gave fish shade and made them vulnerable to capture."[90]

Specialized nets for particular fish and crayfish required skill and patience to construct. Some took three years to make and were almost nine hundred feet long. Sturt saw a 300-foot net "of the very finest craftsmanship" strung across the Darling River.[91]

John McDouall Stuart came across people fishing at brush weirs in the harshest parts of the country.[92] Another method of capture involved adding certain poisonous plants to the water. When the fish rose to the surface, they could be speared or even captured by hand. Not that they needed poison to catch fish; according to Weston Price, "Their skill at fishing probably exceeds that of any other race. They are so highly trained in the knowledge of the habits of the fish and the type of movement that the fish transmits to the water and to the reeds in the water, that

one of their important contests between tribes is to see how many fish can be struck in succession with a spear, the fish never being seen, their only information as to its whereabouts being the change in the surface of the water and movement of grasses that are growing in the water as the fish moves...The experts bring up a fish six times out of eight."[93]

Settler James Kirby saw an automatic fishing machine near Swan Hill: "A [native] would sit near the opening and just behind him a tough stick about ten feet long was stuck in the ground with the thick end down. To the thin end of this rod was attached a line with a noose at the other end; a wooden peg was fixed under the water at the opening in the fence to which this noose was caught, and when the fish made a dart to go through the opening he was caught by the gills, his force undid the loop from the peg, and the spring of the stick threw the fish over the head" of the fisherman.*[94]

Thomas Mitchell witnessed massive fish traps on the Darling River at Brewarrina in New South Wales, which some claim are the oldest man-made structures on earth: one archeological team calculated their age at forty thousand years, and considered that to be a minimum.[95] Witnesses who saw the system in operation in the early 1800s were astounded

---

* Such were Kirby's preconceptions of the Aboriginal people that he described those who set up this ingenious machine, and the relaxed way in which they removed each fish from the loop, as "lazy."

by the efficiency of the traps, the efforts employed to maintain breeding stock and the enormous harvest. And the Brewarrina trap was only one of hundreds of such systems. Large numbers of people depended on fishing traps along most inland rivers. The structures incorporated ingenious engineering features that withstood regular floods. A stone locking system fixed the trap to the bed of the stream; the arch and keystone were two elements contributing to their strength.[96]

These large-scale fishing operations required considerable economic and social organization. The traps allowed breeding stock to pass through so that upstream fisheries could gain a share. Particular families managed and used particular ponds in the system, but those families had responsibilities to ensure fish to the families and systems upstream and downstream from their location. The system was integrated and sustainable.[97]

In arid regions, the resourceful Aborigines relied on wells capable of collecting water. Settlers described well covers made from large slabs of stone ground down to fit neatly over the wells to prevent animals from polluting the water.[98] In a remote area of South Australia, the colonist Charles Sturt found a well that was "twenty-two feet deep and eight feet broad at the top. There was a landing place...and a recess had been made to hold the water...Paths led from this spot to almost every point of the compass, and on walking along one

came to a village consisting of nineteen huts...Troughs and stones for grinding seed were lying about...The fact of there being so large a well at this point (a work that must have required the united labour of a powerful tribe to complete) assured us that this distant part of the interior was not without inhabitants."[99]

Of course, fresh, pure water was vital to the survival of the Aborigines, both in the subtropical coastal regions as well as in the arid interior. Except in times of extreme drought, the natives drank copious quantities of water. Researchers have found that "In one of the driest habitats on earth, these people use about twice as much water per unit of mass as Europeans in the same environment." An adult Aboriginal male could drink almost three quarts of water in thirty-five seconds.[100] During times of drought, they obtained water from water-holding frogs and from certain plants.[101]

Kangaroo-skin water bags served for carrying quite large volumes of water. Paradoxically, these were not used in the driest areas, perhaps because kangaroos are relatively rare in the desert, and the animal's vital nutrients—particularly fat-soluble nutrients—are lost if it is not cooked in its skin.[102] Up to a gallon of water could be carried in certain large leaves folded up in ingenious ways.

As for seafood on the coasts, many Europeans observed large organized fishing expeditions in canoes, rafts, outriggers and boats with small sails. The women dove to capture mutton fish or abalone* which they cooked in their shells on hot coals or removed and pounded until tender. Dried, pounded abalone could be stored in large quantities for festivals; it also served as an important article of trade for these tribes. And it was the women and their children who constructed and farmed extensive clam gardens.

Crayfish catching was men's work; the men would swim to a reef and hang on to the kelp while feeling for crayfish feelers with their feet. Once they detected the feelers, they would dive down and grab them, pulling the crayfish from its cave.[103]

Most amazing are reports of Aboriginals fishing in partnership with dolphins— observed by Foster Evans, a police magistrate in Geelong, as well as others at many Australian beaches, including Moreton Bay. The dolphins drove the fish ashore to make catching them easy for the men.[104]

Similar practices characterized the long tradition of whale hunting off the coast of New South Wales. Several observers documented ritualized interaction with killer whales, which encouraged the mammals to herd larger whales into the harbor, where they would be driven into shallow water and harvested. The local tribe set up this interaction with the killer whales with a ceremony where a man would light two fires on the beach and pretend to limp between them as if he were old and frail. They believed that this encouraged the whales to take pity on the man and bring the bigger whales to the bay for his use.[†105]

SETTLERS WERE ASTOUNDED by the order and beauty of the Australian countryside. "The face of the country is such as to promise success whenever it shall be cultivated," wrote one admirer. "The trees being at a considerable distance from each other and the intermediate space filled, not with underwood, but a thick rich grass growing in the utmost luxuriency."[106] Most attributed such artistry to "careless nature," little suspecting—or rather, reluctant to acknowledge—the part the Aborigines played in creating the pleasing landscape.[107] There were exceptions: Edward Curr, pioneer squatter on the Murray River wrote, "It may perhaps be doubted whether any section of the human race has exercised a greater influence on the physical condition of any large portion of the globe than the wandering

---

* Aboriginal women would often develop abnormal bone growth or "surfer's ear," in which irritation from cold wind and water exposure causes the bone surrounding the ear canal to develop lumps of new bony growth, which constrict the ear canal.

† This relationship between the lead killer whale and the humans on the shore continued for many years after the Europeans arrived, until a disgruntled whaler shot the lead killer whale. That was the last time the cetaceans cooperated with men.

savages of Australia." He knew that linking "wandering savages" to widespread land management contradicted everything Europeans thought about "primitive" people. He deliberately defied the European belief that the Aborigines were wanderers barely touched the land and were playthings of nature.[108]

Along with the digging stick, the main Aboriginal land management tool was fire. Ethnobotanists are only beginning to appreciate the vital role that fire played in increasing the food supply of the Aborigines. Early explorers often reported Aboriginal land fires. Many of the important Aboriginal food plants require regular burning if they are to attain their maximum production. Some desert plants require more frequent burning than others, resulting in what many have described as a "mosaic" of plant communities, all in different stages of fire recovery.[109]

According to Bill Gammage, "Fire was used to shape the land...It was a major totem, a friend. People knew when to use it and when not to. They knew if they released it according to universal law and local practice it would do what they wanted. If it did not then they, not it, had offended...Like songlines,* fire unified Australia. It locked the landscape into long-term widespread patterns, because neighbours obeyed the same law, and coordinated their burning or non-burning."†[110]

Fire management—where and when to burn, and how hot the fires should be—came under strict control of the elders. They avoided the growing season of particular plants at all costs and advised neighboring tribes of any fire activity. These skillful burn techniques were responsible for the look of the landscape—from open plains to small copses with clear forest floors to belts of trees gracefully alternating with pastureland, even cul-de-sacs

---

* Within the animist belief system of the indigenous Australians, a songline is one of the paths across the land that mark the route followed by localized "creator-beings" during the "Dreamtime" of long ago. The paths of the songlines are recorded in traditional songs, stories, dances and paintings. A knowledgeable person is able to navigate across the land, often for hundreds of miles, by repeating the words of the song, which describe the locations of landmarks, water holes and other natural phenomena.

† Surprisingly—or not surprisingly—Gammage's book delineating his findings about Aboriginal land management has not met with acceptance in the scientific community: critics claim there is no evidence for Aboriginal fires. According to one professor, "In this racial fantasy it is white men, not black, who are barbarous and ignorant...While this romantic cant highlighted Aboriginal moral superiority, it bore no resemblance to the manner in which human beings actually live on the planet." According to Gammage, "I have not found a single scientist who takes into consideration the fundamental Aboriginal conviction that people risk their souls if they do not manage every inch of ground they are responsible for." Others have insisted that it is impossible that people widely dispersed over a huge continent could all have the same idea about land management; and they dismiss the Aboriginal beliefs about the Dreaming as ignorant superstition. They take offense at the notion that our main purpose in life is to care for the earth and not to pillage and poison the planet and its inhabitants. To the modern scientist, the idea that the "primitive" Aboriginal people could collectively receive such wisdom from the supersensible world is nonsense. In fact, everything about the Aborigines presents a challenge to the mind-set of the materialistic scientist.

into the untouched brush where small animals found shelter to breed and large animals like kangaroos could be corralled and killed.

The natives burned great tracts to make sure the grass would come up "green and sweet" with the first rains, and to drive out game for hunting purposes.[111] Frequent fires explained the absence of underbrush that gave Australia its parklike appearance.

No species could threaten or overrun another. Too many animals or plants prompted open season; too few led to temporary bans. Settlers described massive slaughter of kangaroos* or huge piles of dead eels—the Aboriginal method of keeping various species in check when they became too numerous. By contrast, widespread law insisted that no plant that was bearing seed could be dug up after it had flowered.

Burning also helped maintain the desert, increasing dry-adapted vegetation. In areas that have been abandoned, where burning of the country is no longer carried out and where the water holes are not kept open by digging and clearing, animal and bird life have largely disappeared.[112]

Even the practice of abstaining from hunting and gathering in the area of sacred sites contributed to the overall ecology of the Aboriginal environment. Such sites served as sanctuaries for animal life. According to anthropologist P. K. Latz,

"These areas would be vitally important for the long-term viability of an area as immediately after droughts they would be a source of plants and animals to restock depleted areas, thereby ensuring a more rapid recovery of the home range's biota."[113]

Another area of land management involved the creation of havens for insect populations. Oak trunks were pushed into the creeks and rivers to attract teredo grubs.[114] Sometimes wood was piled many feet high, allowing the creation of a harvest in a year's time.

The land required constant maintenance or it reverted back to wilderness, something the indigenous Australian detested. Land not burned was not "looked after." Land not cared for was "dirty country."[115]

According to Thomas Mitchell: "Where a man might gallop whole miles without impediment and see whole miles before him ... the omission of the annual periodic burn by natives of the grass and young saplings has already produced in the open forest lands nearest to Sydney thick forests of young trees ... Kangaroos are no longer to be seen there, the grass is choked by underwood; neither are there natives to burn the grass, nor is fire longer desirable among the fences of the settlers."[116]

Without fire and with the introduction of sheep, the vast yellow fields of yam daisy disappeared. Without clearing the

---

* After the Europeans dispossessed the Aboriginals from their land, many parts of the country became overrun with kangaroos. Caterpillars, locusts and mosquitos increased to plague conditions after the Aborigines were no longer allowed to burn.

brush through fire, the country became threatened by large, disastrous fires, as the Australians in Victoria suffered in 2009.*

To the Aboriginal, land care was the main purpose in life. He felt an overwhelming affection for his ancestral territory. Mountains and creeks and springs and water holes were the handiwork of ancestors and required homage in the form of constant care. According to the Aboriginals, the white man defiled this land. As one Aboriginal woman put it, "No longer do men pluck up the grass and weeds and sweep the ground clean around it, no longer do they care for the resting place of Karora."[117]

According to Gammage, "The land is part of the Dreaming and must be cared for. This might require dramatic or spasmodic change (burning forests, culling eels, banning or restricting a food) and it certainly demands active intervention in the landscape. Ancestors do this still, obeying the Law and seeking balance and continuity. Humans should do no less."[118]

SO THE NATIVE AUSTRALIANS had a highly organized social and economic structure, one that included construction of water complexes, ingenious land management, sustainable agriculture, trading and food storage—all of which allowed them to enjoy a plentiful, varied and nutrient-dense diet. What about the premise that the Aboriginals were largely nomads, wandering from place to place and living in the most rudimentary shelter?

THE TRADITIONAL VIEW holds that the Aborigines lived in simple lean-to shelters made of bark and sticks, but Thomas Mitchell described the houses as large and circular, "made of straight rods meeting at an upright pole in the centre; the outside had first been covered with bark and grass, and then entirely coated over with clay. The fire was made in the center and a hole left in top for the chimney."[119]

In 1829, the explorer George Grey came upon a village on the Gascoyne River where the houses were "built of large-sized logs, much higher, and altogether of a very superior description to those made by the natives of the south-westerly coast."[120]

Charles Sturt came upon a village of seventy domed huts, each capable of housing up to fifteen people. The houses had a coating of clay over grass and leaves. Smoky internal fires kept mosquitos away and small doorways served as a fly deterrent. Sturt described a peaceful evening scene where he heard the whirring

* The fire resulted in 173 fatalities and the destruction of more than two thousand houses. Laws forbidding homeowners from cutting away brush around their homes had gone into place several years earlier. Authorities blamed the fires on "record-high temperatures and strong winds after a season of intense drought" and warned that "drier, warmer conditions and more people living in high-risk areas suggest a future with more disastrous fire events." The Aboriginals understood that disastrous fires only occurred when they did not take care of the landscape through fire management; any destructive fire was a fault of their own, not of the weather.

of hundreds of mills grinding grain into flour: "The natives...sat up to a late hour at their own camp, the women being employed beating the seed for cakes, between two stones, and the noise they made was exactly like the working of a loom factory. The whole encampment, with the long line of fires, looked exceedingly pretty, and the dusky figures of the natives standing by them, moving from one hut to the other, had the effect of a fine scene in a play. At eleven all was still, and you would not have known that you were in such close contiguity to so large an assemblage of people."[121]

Often the Aboriginals had two seasonal camps and two different styles of housing: large thatched, waterproofed and domed houses served for the wet season, and lighter, airier buildings for the dry. Houses on stilts made living comfortable in wet areas. While clay over grass and leaves was the most common building style, one settler sketched a village where the houses had stone foundations.[122] On the southeast of the continent, whale bones served to support the domes. One account mentions a dome seven meters in diameter.[123]

Occasionally domed dwellings had a small veranda attached over the entrance with a single wall to provide protection for a fire lit in the doorway; small walls created yards for dogs or domestic animals and even sheltered areas for outdoor seating. Many had internal raised sleeping platforms, and some houses had partitions to create several rooms. Typically, each round house had a smaller round structure for food storage. Dedicated spaces outside the building were reserved for sleeping and resting during fine weather.

All large buildings and villages had cooking ovens and food preparation facilities, some as large as ten feet per side. Ovens and grain storage huts had walls that combined stones with clay mortar.[124]

When colonist Charles Sturt and his parched, hungry companions came upon an Aboriginal village in the 1840s, the natives offered water to the men and their horses and fed them with roasted ducks and some cakes; they gave them a large new hut to sleep in and sticks for making a fire. Compared to the suffering Europeans, the Aboriginals were living off the fat of the land and even eating cake![125]

OF ALL THE PEOPLES visited by Dr. Weston A. Price during his historic research expeditions of the 1930s, none elicited more awe than the Australian Aborigines, whom Price described as "a living museum preserved from the dawn of animal life on the earth." For Price, the Aborigines represented the paradigm of moral and physical perfection. Their skills in hunting, tracking and food gathering were unsurpassed. He marveled at their social organization, which allowed for the schooling of children from a young age, and respect and care for a sizable number of old people, for whom special foods that were easy to gather and hunt were reserved.*

Price's photographs of Aborigines on their native diets illustrate dental structures so perfect as to make the reader wonder whether these natives were wearing false teeth.[126] Early explorers reported the Aborigines to be "well formed; their limbs are straight and muscular, their bodies erect; their heads well shaped; the features are generally good; teeth regular, white and sound. They are capable of undergoing considerable fatigue and privations in their wanderings, marching together considerable distances."[127] Many observers reported their great dexterity and acute eyesight, which enabled them to see stars that others might see only with a telescope and animals moving at a distance of a mile away, which most people cannot see at all.

An early Australian settler named Philip Chauncy reported several examples of the extraordinary "quickness of sight and suppleness and agility of limb and muscle" in the Aborigines, including an Aborigine who stood as a target for cricket balls thrown with force by professional bowlers from only ten to fifteen yards away and who successfully dodged them or parried them off with a small shield for at least half an hour. Other natives threw cricket balls at great distances, and outdid "the best circus performers by bounding from a spring board in a somersault over eleven horses standing side by side."[128]

Weston Price consistently found that healthy nonindustrialized peoples consumed a diet very high in vitamins and minerals and containing at least ten times the fat-soluble activators—vitamins found only in animal fat—of the typical American diet of his day. The Aboriginals obtained these from animal fat, organ meats of game animals (they ate the entire animal, even the entrails), as well as insects, fish and especially shellfish, including lobster, crab, crayfish, prawns, snails, oysters, mussels, mud whelk, abalone, scallops, sea urchins and periwinkles.[129]

Nevertheless, the vast materia medica of the Aborigines indicates they were not entirely free from aches and pains. Australian plants provided Aborigines with remedies for diarrhea, coughs, colds, rheumatism, ear infections, toothache, upset stomach, headache, sore eyes, fevers, sores, rashes, hemorrhaging of childbirth, warts and ulcers—as well as for treatment of wounds, burns, insect bites and snake poison.

The Aborigines also used herbs for contraception and sterilization, thus allowing them to space their children and prevent overpopulation. Men often had more than one wife, sometimes five or six. According to the escaped convict William Buckley, "If a family increases too

---

* In South Australia, tradition forbade young men from eating twenty types of easy-to-obtain foods and boys from eating thirteen types, in order to reserve these for the elders.

rapidly, for instance, if a woman has a child within twelve months of a previous one, they hold a consultation amongst the tribe she belongs to, as to whether it shall live or not; but if the father insists upon the life of the child being spared, they do not persist in its destruction, and especially if it is a female."*[130]

W. V. MacFarlane studied desert Aboriginal people in transition but still living mostly—but not completely—on native foods, and found that every member of the tribe suffered from chronic conjunctivitis, a sign of vitamin A deficiency.[131] Even the smallest changes in diet and lifestyle made them vulnerable to disease. Like all the other indigenous groups Weston Price studied, the Aborigines succumbed to rampant tooth decay and disease of every type soon after they adopted the "displacing foods of modern commerce"—white flour and sugar, jams, canned foods and tea—that began to arrive after 1788. Children born to the next generation had irregularities of the dental arches with conspicuous facial deformities—patterns that mimicked those seen in white civilizations.[132]

The Aboriginal artist Yukultji Napangati, perhaps the youngest living person to have lived the nomadic desert life, made her first contact with modern Australia in 1984, when she and a group of young people were "discovered" and driven to a community of native people in Kiwirrkurra. She and her sister, Yalti, were interviewed for *The Weekend Australian Magazine* in 2014. Yalti recalls "the shock of sugar on the tongue, the sweetest thing she had ever tasted. 'I ate it like this,' Yalti says, picking up a 1 kg supermarket container of sugar…and tipping it to her mouth."[133] Sugar is the serpent's apple, the expulsion from paradise.

Like many indigenous peoples around the globe, the modern Aborigine suffers greatly from the modern diet. He is prone to weight gain, diabetes, tuberculosis, alcoholism and gasoline sniffing, a major source of illness and death in modern indigenous communities. Many Aborigines recognize the need to return to native foods. Listen to this story from the Aboriginal storyteller Daisy Kanari:

> Long time ago when Aboriginal people lived on the good and healthy bush foods in the bush, they lived without any sickness: they lived a strong and healthy life. But now it is different. This is what we think: when we were children our parents looked after us and fed us on *quandongs*, witchetty grubs, honey ants, rabbits and many more. These foods are good and it is what we grew up eating.

---

* The Aboriginal initiation rites for boys appear to have been mild, involving neither circumcision or subincision. Some tribes celebrated manhood by knocking out one front tooth, and indicated marriage in women by cutting off the two lower [end] sections of the little finger on the left hand. Dr. Price noted that a series of initiations for the boys helped instill both fearlessness and respect for the welfare of the entire tribe.

Then the Europeans came with their loads of food: of sugar, flour, milk, tea leaves and tins of meat. From then to now, people still live on European food. Today things are bad with petrol and alcohol. When our sons drink alcohol, they keep going and wander aimlessly. They do not come back to their mothers. Also with petrol: when children smell petrol over a long period of time, they die forever. Petrol and alcohol are bad things that have recently come into our country and lives.[134]

Some groups of Aborigines have returned to the bush—both in the desert regions and in reserves in coastal and mountainous areas. They may hunt with twenty-twos and carry water in buckets, but they have relearned the foodways of their ancestors. Some of their products have potential commercial value—from bean cakes and fermented drinks as snack foods, to insect powders as a nutritious food additive for both people and livestock, to medicinal preparations. Enlightened government policy would educate the Australian population as to the value of these items and create a market for them, thus allowing the Aborigines to support themselves with dignity of purpose in their traditional lifestyle.

And when it comes to land management, what an inspiring proposition than the idea that our main purpose in life is to make every inch of our earth, from deserts to arctic regions, teem with abundance, and superbly beautiful? We may need to use front-end loaders, movable electric fencing, and pigs rotated through the woods rather than fire to accomplish this goal, and we do this with a fully developed sense of our own individuality rather than as a tribal group with access to the Dreamtime, but the goal of both Aboriginal and modern people should be the same: to create beauty and abundance on the earth by honoring and supporting the natural world.

CHAPTER 2

Native Americans

Guts and Grease

THE NATIVE AMERICAN hunter-gatherer's dinner became front-page news in the late 1990s. Drawing from the writings of Dr. Boyd Eaton and Loren Cordain, experts in the so-called Paleolithic diet, columnists and reporters began spreading the word about the health benefits of a diet rich in protein and high in fiber from a variety of plant foods.[1] It's actually amusing to see what the modern food pundits came up with as examples of the "Paleolithic Prescription," the diet that Native Americans from both continents supposedly ate during their long prehistory. Columnist Jean Carper offered a "Stone Age Salad" of mixed greens, garbanzo beans, skinless chicken breast, walnuts and fresh herbs, mixed with a dressing made of orange juice, balsamic vinegar and canola oil.[2] Elizabeth Somer, MA, RD, "a leading nutrition expert," suggested whole wheat waffles with fat-free cream cheese, coleslaw with nonfat dressing, grilled halibut with spinach, grilled tofu and vegetables over rice, nonfat milk, canned apricots and mineral water, along with shrimp and clams. Her Stone Age food pyramid included plenty of plant foods, extra-lean meat and fish, nonfat milk products, and honey and eggs in small amounts.[3]

Above all, the food writers told us—and still tell us—avoid fats, especially saturated fats. The hunter-gatherer's diet was highly politically correct, they insisted, rich in polyunsaturated and monounsaturated fatty acids, but relatively low in overall fat and very low in that dietary villain—saturated fat. Cordain (who, as noted earlier, owns the trademark for The Paleo Diet) provides the following monkish regimen for a correct paleo diet: eat grass-produced beef (which is typically lean), fish and seafood, eggs, fresh fruits and veggies, nuts and seeds, and "healthful oils" (olive, walnut, flaxseed, macadamia, avocado, and coconut), while avoiding cereal grains, legumes, dairy (including butter), refined sugar, potatoes, processed foods, refined vegetable oils and salt. He makes no mention of organ meats or fermented foods and frowns on fatty meats like bacon.*[4]

Robb Wolf, author of *The Paleo Solution*, aims the paleo message at millennials with a similar prescription, recommending a strict plan of lean meat, fruits, vegetables, seafood, nuts and seeds (including chocolate), and the same "healthy fats," while denouncing dairy, grains, processed food and sugars, legumes, "starches" and alcohol.[5]

Fortunately for modern mankind, the diet that supported robust health among "Paleolithic" and indigenous people of the Americas, although regional and seasonal, was a lot more varied, satisfying and interesting than what passes for the hunter-gatherer diet in the pages of modern magazines and diet books.

THE HUNTER-GATHERER WAS healthier than modern man—of that there is no doubt. Focusing on Native American tribes from several regions, Dr. Weston A. Price noted an almost complete absence of tooth decay and dental deformities among those who lived as their ancestors did.[6] They had broad faces, straight teeth and fine physiques. This was true of the nomadic tribes living in the far northern territories of British Columbia and the Yukon, as well as inhabitants of the Florida Everglades. Skeletal remains

of the Vancouver Indians that Price studied were similar, showing a virtual absence of tooth decay, arthritis and any other kind of bone deformity. Tuberculosis was nonexistent among tribes who ate as their ancestors had done, and the women gave birth with ease.

In 1933, Price interviewed Dr. Joseph Romig, a physician who had spent three decades in Alaska, and noted, "In his thirty-six years of contact with these people he had never seen a case of malignant disease among the truly primitive Eskimos and Indians, although it frequently occurs when they became modernized." He found, similarly, that the acute surgical problems requiring an operation on internal organs, such as the gallbladder, kidney, stomach and appendix, did not tend to occur among the primitive people but were very common problems among the modernized Eskimos and Indians. "Growing out of his experience in which he had seen large numbers of the modernized Eskimos and Indians attacked with tuberculosis, which tended to be progressive and ultimately fatal as long as the patients stayed under modernized living conditions, he sends them back when possible to primitive conditions and to a primitive diet, under which the death rate is very much lower than under modernized conditions. Indeed, he reported that a great majority of the afflicted recovered

* Dark chocolate gets Cordain's blessing, even though a typical dark chocolate bar can contain almost one tablespoon of sugar per ounce. Cordain recommended diet sodas in his first book, but now reckons they are not good for you.

under the primitive type of living and nutrition."[7]

The early explorers across the continent consistently described Native Americans as tall and well formed. Of the tribes in Florida, the explorer Álvar Núñez Cabeza de Vaca* wrote, "[They] are of large build and go about naked, from a distance they appear to be giants. They are a people wonderfully built, very lean and of great strength and agility."[8]

"They are so skilled in running," he marveled, "that without resting or tiring they run from morning until night following a deer."[9]

"They boast and brag of being strong and valiant," wrote a later observer of the Gulf of Mexico's Karankawa people, "because of this they go naked in the most burning sun, they suffer and go around without covering themselves or taking refuge in the shade. In the winter when it snows and freezes so that the water in the rivers is solid and the pools, lakes, marshes and creeks are covered with ice, they go out from the ranch at early dawn to take a bath, breaking the ice with their body."[10]

Far to the north, the First Nations peoples of Canada often surpassed six feet. According to a diarist writing in the early 1770s, "I have seen two northern Indians who measured six foot three inches and six feet four inches."[11]

In South America, European descriptions of their encounters with native peoples swelled with admiration. According to the explorer Francisco Dominguez, the Native Americans were "nimble and vigorous, swift of foot, and so long-winded that they tire out the deer, and catch them with their hands, besides slaying many more with their arrows."[12]

Another early observer noted their dexterity, "not only in running, but also in swimming, which they all can do... As for the Brazilians, they are so natural in this trade, that they would swim eight days in the sea, if hunger did not prevent them, and they fear more that some fish should devour them, than to perish through weariness."[13]

Others noted that the men were "tall and muscular, but never corpulent, with finely formed facial features and limbs of perfect proportion." The women were "truly handsome as to features and proportion." Writing in 1768, one observer noted that the Yuracaré of the mountain regions were "the tallest of the mountain peoples, and their women are finely proportioned. Everything about the Yuracares indicated force and suppleness... Their proud and arrogant gait accords

---

* Cabeza de Vaca spent eight years traveling across the American Southwest as part of the Narváez expedition. He was one of only four of the original company to return after the journey, during which he occasionally submitted to slavery by the local tribes in order to survive. Later he became a trader and a reluctant faith healer to the more welcoming tribes along the Rio Grande. After returning to Spain in 1537, he wrote an account of his travels and the peoples he encountered. Cabeza de Vaca qualifies as a notable "protoanthropologist" for his detailed accounts of American Indian customs.

perfectly with the character and the lofty idea they have of themselves. Their features are very fine and their faces full of vivacity and pride and not wanting a certain expression of gaiety."[14]

Of another mountain tribe, the Guaraní, the missionary fathers noted their thick black hair, "which retained its color until extreme old age, and only rarely was any baldness to be seen among them."[15]

One explorer reported that the Patagonian men of the Argentine Pampas averaged over six feet tall and measured four feet around the chest. Their strength was prodigious—it took nine or ten Europeans to hold down one Patagonian man.[16] "They appear to be subject to no diseases," wrote another explorer, "and enjoy remarkable uniformity of health, and many of them are very athletic and capable of great endurance."

The stoic Native American men and women could endure great hardship. "The strength and boldness of the women comes from the little tenderness they are bred with," wrote Alonso de Ovalle, a procurator for Rome in Santiago, Chile, "for they avoid neither heat nor cold; and in the coldest winters, when birds are killed with cold, they wash their heads in cold water, and never dry their hair, but let it remain wet, and dry itself in the air; and as for their children, they wash them in the rivers, when they are yet very young."

In Tierra del Fuego, Charles Darwin found the indigenous people to be "quite naked, and even one full-grown woman was absolutely so. It was raining heavily, and the fresh water, together with the spray, trickled down her body...At night five or six human beings, naked and scarcely protected from the wind and rain of their tempestuous climate, slept on the ground."[17] Weston Price reported, "They can sleep comfortably through the freezing nights with the ponchos wrapped about their heads and their legs and feet bare."[18]

Dr. Price and many others also noted the ease of childbirth among native women. "The indigenous Brazilian women are very fruitful, and have easy labors, on which occasions they retire to the woods, and bring forth alone, and return after bathing themselves and their child."[19] "When a woman is delivered of her first child," wrote one observer, "she presently goes about her duties as before."[20]

However, not every indigenous group enjoyed good health. In Cabeza de Vaca's travels along the Gulf Coast, he found several tribes suffering from hunger "because they do not have maize or acorns or nuts...[and were] confined to gathering small fruit from trees while waiting for the prickly pears to ripen. We found these Indians to be very sick, emaciated and bloated."[21] He reported on one village where, although the people were "very well proportioned and of very good features.... the majority of them are blind in one eye from a clouded spot that they have on it,"[22] a sign of vitamin A deficiency. The people living along the Gulf of Mexico consumed mostly grubs, worms and seafood, having little access to game, except for the occasional deer. Once Cabeza de Vaca entered into the Rio Grande area of Texas where buffalo were plentiful, he found people who were much more robust and of "a better disposition."[23] These were the first Native Americans he came upon who lived in permanent settlements, wore "robes of cotton," and practiced an established agriculture that supplied them with beans, squash and maize.[24] He noted, "They are the people with the most well-formed bodies we saw and of the greatest vitality and capacity and who best understood us and responded to what we asked them. And we called them the people of the cows because the greatest number of those cows [buffalo] are killed."[25]

WHAT KIND OF foods produced such fine physical specimens? The diets of the American Indians varied with the locality and climate but all were based on animal foods of every type and description. They pursued large game like buffalo, deer, wild sheep and goat, antelope, moose, elk, caribou, bear, peccary, llama and alpaca (in the Altiplano of Peru), monkeys and tapirs (in the Amazon rain forest), as well as smaller animals such as beaver, rabbit, squirrel, skunk, muskrat and raccoon. They ate reptiles including snakes, lizards, turtles and alligators; fish and shellfish; wild birds including ducks and geese; and wild dogs (but not wolves

and coyotes, which were taboo).[26] Those tribes living in coastal areas also ate sea mammals. They enjoyed insects including locust, crickets, worms, spiders and lice. Although the Native Americans did not domesticate large animals for milk, they did eat "the curdled milk taken from the stomachs of suckling fawns and buffalo calves," and milk (along with blood) sucked from the slashed udders of lactating animals.[27]

According to Boyd Eaton and Loren Cordain, these foods supplied plenty of protein but only small amounts of total fat, and this fat was high in polyunsaturated fatty acids and low in saturated fats. The fat of wild game, according to Eaton, is roughly 38 percent saturated, 32 percent monounsaturated, and 30 percent polyunsaturated.[28] This breakdown may help promote polyunsaturated vegetable oils as healthy and natural, but it does not jibe with the fat content of wild animals in the real world.

The table on page 40 lists fat content in various tissues of a number of wild animals found in the diets of American Indians. Note that only squirrel fat contains the level of polyunsaturated fatty acids that Eaton claims is typical for wild game. On a continent noted for the richness and variety of its animal life, it is unlikely that squirrels would have supplied more than a tiny fraction of total calories in any group's diet. Seal fat, consumed by coastal tribes, ranges from 14 to 24 percent polyunsaturated. The fat of all the other animals hunted and eaten by Native Americans contains less than 10 percent polyunsaturated fatty acids, some less than 2 percent.

Most prized was the internal kidney fat of ruminant animals, which can be as high as 65 percent saturated.

Sources of Fat for the American Indian[29]

	% Saturated	% Monounsaturated	% Polyunsaturated
Antelope, kidney fat	65.04	21.25	3.91
Bison, kidney fat	34.48	52.36	4.83
Caribou, bone marrow	22.27	56.87	3.99
Deer, kidney fat	48.24	38.52	6.21
Dog, kidney	25.54	41.85	7.69
Dog, meat (muscle)	28.36	47.76	8.95
Elk, kidney	61.58	30.10	1.62
Goat, kidney	65.57	28.14	0.00
Moose, kidney	47.26	44.75	2.11
Peccary, fatty tissues	38.47	46.52	9.7
Reindeer, caribou, fatty tissues	50.75	38.94	1.25
Seal, harbor, blubber	11.91	61.41	13.85
Seal, harbor, adipose tissue (fat)	14.51	54.23	16.84
Seal, harp, blubber	19.16	42.22	15.04
Seal, harp, meat (muscle)	10.69	54.21	23.51
Sheep, mountain, kidney fat	47.96	41.37	2.87
Sheep, white-faced, kidney fat	51.58	39.90	1.16
Sheep, intestine, roasted	47.01	40.30	7.46
Snake, meat (muscle)	26.36	44.54	0.09
Squirrel, brown, adipose tissue (fat)	17.44	47.55	28.6
Squirrel, white, adipose tissue (fat)	12.27	51.48	32.3
Game fat, according to Eaton	38	32	30

USDA data, prepared by John L. Weihrauch with technical assistance of Julianne Borton and Theresa Sampagna.

Politically correct paleo dieters also ignore the fact that Native Americans hunted animals selectively—just like their counterparts in Australia. The explorer Vilhjalmur Stefansson, who spent many years with the indigenous peoples of Canada, noted that they preferred "the flesh of older animals to that of calves, yearlings and two-year olds…It is approximately so with those northern forest Indians with whom I have hunted, and probably with all caribou-eaters." They preferred the older animals because they had built up a thick slab of fat along the back. In a thousand-pound animal, this slab could weigh forty to fifty pounds. Another twenty to thirty pounds of highly saturated fat filled out the cavity, especially around the kidneys. This fat was saved, sometimes by rendering, stored in the animal's cleaned bladder or large intestine, and consumed with dried or smoked lean meat. Used in this way, Stefansson estimates that fat contributed up to 80 percent of total calories in the diets of the northern tribes.[30]

Beaver was a treat, especially the fat-rich tail, but smaller animals like rabbit and squirrel provided sustenance only when nothing else was available because, according to Stefansson, they were so low in fat. In fact, small animals called for special preparation. The meat was removed from the bones, roasted, and pounded. The bones were dried and ground into a powder. Then the bones were mixed with the meat and any available grease from other animals, a procedure that would greatly lower the percentage of polyunsaturated fatty acids while raising the total content of saturated fat.[31]

When a scarcity of game forced the Native Americans to consume only small animals like rabbits, they suffered from "rabbit starvation." "The groups that depend on the blubber animals are the most fortunate, in the hunting way of life, for they never suffer from fat-hunger," wrote Stefansson. "This trouble is worst, so far as North America is concerned, among those forest Indians who depend at times on rabbits, the leanest animal in the North, and who develop the extreme fat-hunger known as rabbit-starvation. Rabbit eaters, if they have no fat from another source—beaver, moose, fish—will develop diarrhoea in about a week, with headache, lassitude and vague discomfort. If there are enough rabbits, the people eat till their stomachs are distended; but no matter how much they eat they feel unsatisfied. Some think a man will die sooner if he eats continually of fat-free meat than if he eats nothing, but this is a belief on which sufficient evidence for a decision has not been gathered in the North. Deaths from rabbit-starvation, or from the eating of other skinny meat, are rare; for everyone understands the principle, and any possible preventive steps are naturally taken."[32]

In some locations, scarcity of game led to extreme eating. Cabeza de Vaca encountered tribes along the Gulf of Mexico who existed on the edge of starvation: "Their sustenance is chiefly roots of two or three kinds, and they hunt for them throughout the land. They are very bad and the men who eat them bloat. They take two days to roast, and many of them are very bitter. The hunger that those people have is so great that they are forced to eat them, they roam up to two or three leagues looking for them. Sometimes they kill some deer, and sometimes they take some fish, but this is so little and their hunger so great that they eat spiders and ant eggs and worms and lizards and salamanders and snakes and vipers, and they eat earth and wood and everything that they can find, and deer excrement and other things that I refrain from mentioning. They keep the bones of the fish they eat and of snakes and other things in order to grind up everything afterward and eat the powder it produces... The women are very hard working and endure a great deal, because of the twenty-four hours there are between day and night, they have only six of rest, and the rest of the night they spend in firing their ovens in order to dry those roots they eat." Although these people struggled to survive, they did not succumb to rabbit starvation thanks to the fat contained in reptiles, insects and worms.

IN HIS EARLY TWENTIES, Samuel Hearne of the Hudson's Bay Company traveled with indigenous northern Canadians for several years between 1769 and 1772, seeking a fabled copper mine north of the Arctic circle.* His diaries contain the first reports of the foodways and customs of the northern indigenous peoples, who inhabit one of nature's harshest environments.

Like so many others, he was impressed by the hardiness and fortitude of the native people. Food came in waves—feast or famine. When the hunting was good, "Nothing is more common with those Indians, after they have eaten as much at a sitting as would serve six moderate men," often to the point of making themselves sick.[33] "Notwithstanding the Northern Indians are at times so voracious, yet they bear hunger with a degree of fortitude which...is much easier to admire than to imitate. I have more than once seen the Northern Indians, at the end of three or four days fasting, as merry and jocose on the subject, as if they had voluntarily imposed it on themselves."[34] Sometimes a piece of an old half-rotten deerskin or a pair of old shoes "were sacrificed to alleviate extreme hunger."[35] Hearne reported that they appeared to eat human flesh "when driven by necessity."[36]

The practice of pounding and drying meat when game was plentiful helped forestall hunger during lean times—a tedious job that usually fell to the women—and this dried meat was always eaten with fat. Hearne was the first European to describe pemmican, a mixture of dried meat and rendered fat: "To prepare meat in this manner, it requires no farther operation than cutting the lean parts of the animal into thin slices and drying it in the sun, or by a slow fire, till, after beating it between two stones, it is reduced to a coarse powder...

---

* It took Hearne three years to find the mine, after which he reported that it was too remote and inaccessible to be of use to the colonists.

When fat is plentiful this shredded dry meat is often packed into a sack made of hide, and boiling fat is poured over and into it."[*][37] The native tribes of Texas preserved pemmican as a sausagelike product, often mixed with pecan meal and stuffed into animal intestines.

The Dakota made pemmican by breaking up and boiling long animal bones to extract the fatty marrow, and mixing it with dried meat, cornmeal, or pounded chokecherries.[38] However, a tribe on the move did not usually go to the trouble of making pemmican, but instead carried fat and pounded meat. Hearne described it as "portable, palatable, all the blood and juices are still remaining in the meat, it is a very nourishing and Wholesome food; with care may be kept a whole year without the least danger of spoiling. It is necessary, however, to air it frequently during the warm weather, otherwise it is liable to grow mouldy; but as soon as the chill air of fall begins, it requires no farther trouble till next Summer." Said Hearne, "I could travel longer without victuals, than after any other kind of food."[39]

According to Hearne, the dried meat of the northern indigenous peoples was superior to that of the southern. "All the dried meat prepared by the Southern Indians is performed by exposing it to the heat of a large fire, which soon exhausts all the fine juices from it, and when sufficiently dry to prevent putrefaction, is not more to be compared with that cured by the Northern Indians in the Sun, or by the heat of a very slow fire, than meat that has been boiled down for the sake of the soup is to that which is only sufficiently boiled for eating; the latter has all the juices remaining, which, being easily dissolved by the heat and moisture of the stomach, proves a strong and nourishing food."[40]

Hearne and his companions seemed fixated on getting plenty of fat from a variety of sources. He notes the practice of selective eating: when game was plentiful, they "frequently killed several merely for the tongues, marrow and fat." At one point, they found plentiful musk ox and bison, "many of which the Indians killed, but finding them lean, only took some of the bulls' hides for shoe soals [soles]."[41] Unborn calves, pulled from their mothers' bellies, provided flesh "being so equally intermixed with fat and lean, is reckoned among the nicest bits...The tongue is also very delicate...the young calves, fawns, beaver, etc. taken out of the bellies of their mothers are reckoned most delicate food....and in the same may be said of young geese, ducks, etc. in the shell."[42]

---

[*] According to Lawrence J. Barkwell, in an article entitled "Pemmican," a bag of buffalo pemmican weighing about ninety pounds was called a *taureau* (French for "bull") by the Métis people of Canada. Bags of *taureau* mixed with fat from the udder were known as *taureaux fins*; when mixed with bone marrow, they were known as *taureaux grands*; and when mixed with berries, *taureaux à grains*. It generally took the meat of one buffalo to fill a *taureau*.

Regarding moose, Hearne said, "the fat of the intestines is hard, like suit [suet], but all the external fat is soft, like that of a breast of mutton, and when put into a bladder, is as fine as marrow. In this they differ from all the other species of deer, of which the external fat is as hard as that of the kidneys."[43]

He observed that "the flesh of the musk ox noways resembles that of the western buffalo, but is more like that of the moose or elk; and the fat is of a clear white, slightly tinged with a light azure. The calves and young heifers are good eating."[44]

According the Hearne, "the flesh of the porcupine is very delicious, and so much esteemed by the Indians, that they think it the greatest luxury."[45] Mallards, he noted, are good in the fall when they are fat; swan flesh is "excellent eating, when roasted equal in flavor to young heifer-beef."[46] He praised "a large kettle of broth, made with the blood, and some fat and scraps of meat shred small, boiled in it. This might be reckoned a dainty dish at any time, but was more particularly so in our present almost famished condition."[47]

When foul weather prevented making a fire, they ate their meat and fish raw.[48] Said Hearne, "I have frequently made one of a party who has sat round a fresh-killed deer and assisted in picking the bones quite clean...I thought that the raw brains

and many other parts were exceedingly good."[49] Organ meats of the kill were always the first choice; the kidneys of both moose and buffalo were usually eaten raw, but tripe* was cooked. "The tripe of the buffalo is exceedingly good, cooked by removing the honey comb and boiling three quarters of an hour. The lesser stomach or as some call it, the many-folds, either of buffalo, moose or deer, are usually eaten raw, and are very good. But that of the moose, unless great care be taken in washing it, is rather bitter, owing to the nature of their food."[50] No part of any beast was wasted: "They are also remarkably fond of the womb of the buffalo, elk, deer, etc., which they eagerly devour without washing or any other process, but barely taking out the contents[51]...The parts of generation belonging to any beast they kill, both male and female, are always eaten by the men and boys; and though those parts, particularly in the males, are generally very tough, they are not, on any account, to be cut with an edge-tool, but torn to pieces with the teeth."[52]

One uncooked delicacy "is made of the raw liver of a deer, cut in small pieces of about an inch square and mixed up with the contents of the stomach of the same animal; and the farther digestion has taken place, the better it is suited to their taste; It is impossible to describe or conceive the pleasure they seem to enjoy

---

* Tripe is the muscle wall (the interior mucosal lining is removed) of the first three chambers of a cow's stomach.

with eating such an unaccountable food." Hearne apparently enjoyed the dish with relish, but could not bring himself to join in a feast of maggots: "I have even seen them eat whole handfuls of maggots that were produced in meat by fly-blows."[53]

Deerskin thongs, according to Hearne, served mainly as a food, along with tiny inhabitants living in the hide: "When the hair is taken off and all the warbles are squeezed out, if they are well boiled, they are far from being disagreeable. The Indians, however never could persuade me to eat the warbles, of which some of them are remarkably fond, particularly the children. They are always eaten raw and alive, out of the skin, and are said, by those who like them, to be as fine as gooseberries." The Indians also relished lice. Hearne admired "the wisdom and kindness of Providence in forming the palates and powers of all creatures in such a manner as is best adapted to the food, climate and every other circumstance which may be incident to their respective situation."[54]

Hearne especially enjoyed a special preparation of caribou: "Of all the dishes cooked by the Indians, a *beeatee*, as it is called in their language, is certainly the most delicious that can be prepared from caribou only, without any other ingredient. It is a kind of haggis, made with the blood, a good quantity of fat shred small, some of the tenderest of the flesh, together with the heart and lungs cut, or more commonly torn into small shivers; all of which is put into the stomach and toasted by being suspended before the fire on a string...it is certainly a most delicious morsel, even without pepper, salt or any other seasoning."[55]

Like all other indigenous peoples, the northern tribes consumed dried fish and fish roe, and valued train oil (oil from whales or other sea mammals) "as a cordial and as sauce to their meat."[56]

Samuel Hearne provides us with the best information we have about how Native Americans really ate, and although the modern individual could not be expected to consume such high-yuck-factor foods, it's clear that he doesn't have to eat lean meat and skinless chicken breasts, either.

BORN ON THE BLOOD INDIAN reserve in Alberta, Canada, Beverly Hungry Wolf interviewed her female relatives and tribal elders to collect information about food preparation, child rearing and myths and legends, which she published in *The Ways of My Grandmothers* (1980).[57] Beverly's grandmother prepared the cow "as she had learned to prepare buffalo when she was young." Again, the emphasis is on removing and preserving the fat. Her first step: removal and rendering of the large pieces of fat from the back and cavity. The lean meat was cut into strips and dried or roasted, pounded up with berries, and mixed with fat to make pemmican. Most of the ribs were smoked and stored for later use. All the excess fat inside the body was hung up so the moisture would dry out of it. It was later served with dried meat.

Some fats in the animal were rendered into lard instead of dried.

Beverly Hungry Wolf's kinfolk consumed all the organs of the animal, including heart, kidneys and liver, prepared by roasting or baking, or laid out in the sun to dry. They did not cook the lungs, just sliced them and hung them up to dry. Intestines were also dried. *Sapotsis* or "crow gut" is a Blackfoot delicacy made from the main intestine, which is stuffed with meat and roasted over coals. Tripe was prepared and eaten raw or boiled or roasted. Brains made a delicious raw delicacy. If the animal was a female, the teats or udders would be boiled or barbecued. If the animal carried unborn young, this was fed to the older people because it was so tender. The guts of the unborn were removed and braided, then boiled, too. The tongue was always boiled if it wasn't dried. "Even old animals have tender tongues," Beverly Hungry Wolf recalls.

Hooves and blood got special attention. The hooves were boiled down until all their gristle softened. Beverly Hungry Wolf saved the blood, often mixing it with flour or meat to make sausages in the guts.

The second stomach was washed well and eaten raw, but certain parts were usually boiled or roasted and the rest dried. "Another delicacy is at the very end of the intestines—the last part of the colon. You wash this real good and tie one end shut. Then you stuff the piece with dried berries and a little water and you tie the other end

shut. You boil this all day, until it is really tender and you have a Blackfoot Pudding."

Lakota holy man John (Fire) Lame Deer, author of the 1972 book *Lame Deer Seeker of Visions*, describes the eating of guts as a contest: "In the old days we used to eat the guts of the buffalo, making a contest of it, two fellows getting hold of a long piece of intestines from opposite ends, starting chewing toward the middle, seeing who can get there first; that's eating! Those buffalo guts, full of half-fermented, half-digested grass and herbs, you didn't need any pills and vitamins when you swallowed those."[58]

The marrow was full of fat and was usually eaten raw. Native Americans knew how to strike the femur bone so that it would split open and reveal the delicate interior flesh. Boyd Eaton and other paleoapologists report that the marrow is rich in polyunsaturated fatty acids, but Vilhjalmur Stefansson describes two types of marrow, one from the lower leg that is soft and "more like a particularly delicious cream in flavor," and another from the humerus and femur that is "hard and tallowy at room temperatures."[59] According to Beverly Hungry Wolf, the grease inside the bones "was scooped out and saved or the bones boiled and the fat skimmed off and saved. It turned into something like hard lard." More saturated fat the professors have overlooked!

Beverly Hungry Wolf's people considered certain parts of the animal as appropriate for men or women. The male organs were for the men, as well as the ribs toward the front, which were called "the shoulder ribs, or the boss ribs. They are considered a man's special meal." For women, a part of the "intestine that is quite large and full of manure...the thicker part has a kind of hard lining on the inside. My grandmother said that this part is good for a pregnant mother to eat; she said it will make the baby have a nice round head. Pregnant mothers were not allowed to eat any other parts of the intestine because their faces would become discolored."[60]

IN NATIVE AMERICAN tradition, all foods considered sacred or important for reproduction were animal foods, rich in fat. Beverly Hungry Wolf tells us that pemmican made with berries "was used by the Horns Society for their sacred meal of communion." Boiled tongue was an ancient delicacy, served as the food of communion at the Sun Dance. A blood soup, made from a mixture of blood and corn flour cooked in broth, provided as a sacred meal during the nighttime Holy Smoke ceremonies.*[61]

Bear was another sacred food—altars of bear bones adorn many Paleolithic sites. According to American colonist William Byrd II, writing in 1728, "The flesh of bear hath a good relish, very savory and inclining nearest to that of Pork. The Fat of this Creature is least apt to rise in the Stomach of any other. The Men for the most part chose it rather than Venison."[62] According to the Chippewa, bear grease gave resistance by making them physically strong.† According to a report on the Chippewa by Inez Hilger "We eat it sometimes now and everybody feels better."‡[63]

Bear was an important food for reproduction. When William Byrd asked why the Chesapeake squaws were always able to bear children, he learned that "if any Indian woman did not prove with child at a decent time after Marriage, the Husband, to save his Reputation with the women, forthwith entered into a Bear-dyet for Six Weeks, which in that time makes him so vigorous that he grows exceedingly impertinent to his poor wife

---

* In the context of a healthy traditional diet, some Native Americans, usually men, practiced ritual fasting to obtain spiritual or mysterious powers. Young warriors, especially, would separate themselves from the tribe and fast until their totem animal appeared to them; shamans also fasted or used consciousness-altering plants like peyote to gain access to the spirit world. But the daily diet contained animal foods of all types.

† Preliminary analysis indicates that bear fat is extremely high in vitamin K_2.

‡ Bear grease was a popular treatment for men with hair loss from at least as early as the seventeenth century until the First World War. Nicholas Culpeper, the English botanist and herbalist, wrote in 1652, in his book *The English Physician*, "Bears Grease staies [stops] the falling off of the hair."

and 'tis great odds but he makes her a Mother in Nine Months."[64]

Fish roe was another important fertility food. Native Americans living in coastal areas consumed large amounts of fish, including the heads and roe, and dried roe provided high levels of nutrients throughout the year. Weston Price found that indigenous Peruvians living high in the mountains, twelve thousand feet above sea level, carried dried fish roe in their backpacks. When asked why, they told Dr. Price they ate it "for high perfection of offspring."[65]

Another important food, presented as a gift during gatherings and ceremonies, was the oil from the ooligan* or candlefish. Price reported that in the area of Vancouver, the candlefish was collected in large quantities and its oil removed and used as a dressing for many seafoods. Shellfish were eaten in large amounts when available.

Animal fats, organ meats and fatty fish all supply fat-soluble vitamins A, D and K_2, which Dr. Price recognized as the basis of healthy primitive diets.[†] These nutrients are catalysts to the assimilation of protein and minerals. Without them, minerals go to waste and the body cannot grow tall and strong. When tribes have access to an abundance of fat-soluble vitamins, their offspring will grow up with "nice round heads," broad faces, and straight teeth.

In addition, certain fatty glands of game animals provided vitamin C during the long winter season in the north. The indigenous tribes of Canada revealed to Dr. Price that the adrenal glands in the moose prevented scurvy. When a moose was killed, the adrenal gland and its fat were cut up and shared with all members of the tribe. The walls of the second stomach also supplied vitamin C, to prevent "the white man's disease."[66]

NATIVE AMERICAN PEOPLES were omnivores, eating a variety of plant foods to accompany a diet of meat and fat.

---

* The state of Oregon gets its name from the ooligan fish.

† An exception to the Native American diet high in animal foods seems to be the diet of the Tarahumara, known as the "running" Indians of the Southwest, described as the "finest natural distance runners in the world." A 1971 article by Dale Groom, MD, published at the height of the low-fat diet craze in the *American Heart Journal*, described the diet as based on corn, with "relatively little meat...seldom is livestock slaughtered for food except on occasions of fiestas." It turns out that these fiestas occur very frequently. In the next paragraph, Groom notes that the Tarahumara run after game such as deer and wild turkey. A 1989 book, *The Running Indians*, claims without reference that the Tarahumara diet is 10 percent protein, 10 percent fat, and 80 percent complex carbohydrates; yet the author acknowledges that the people live by keeping sheep and goats, and consume fish and also insects; a dish of ground corn with a slimy, yellow appearance contained caterpillars. They refrain from certain foods, including fat, before races—with the implication that they eat fat at other times. The Tarahumara use several narcotic plants before racing, have a short life span, and often suffer from malnutrition and disease.

Moreover, the plant foods they ate, most notably hundreds of varieties of corn, a staple crop throughout North and South America, were cultivated, not just gathered.* Indeed, many American Indian groups practiced sophisticated farming methods, similar to modern permaculture. With corn, the civilized world first confronted the need for proper preparation of plant foods to ensure nutrient availability and palatability. When nonnative American people began to cultivate corn and consume it as a staple crop, the problem of malnutrition soon appeared. For example, in the late nineteenth century, the niacin-deficiency disease pellagra reached epidemic proportions in parts of the southern United States, where corn served as a major source of calories.† Scientists found this a mystery, since these types of malnutrition did not occur among the indigenous Americans, for whom maize was the principal staple food.

The problem was that nonindigenous Americans adopted maize without the necessary cultural knowledge of its proper preparation. Native Americans knew they needed to soak maize in alkali water—made with ashes and lime (calcium oxide)—a process called nixtamalization, resul-ting in a product called *nixtamal* or masa. The soaking liberates the B-vitamin niacin; niacin deficiency leads to pellagra. Nixtamalization also removes virtually all the aflatoxins from mycotoxin-contaminated corn, renders it easier to grind, and improves its flavor and aroma. Interestingly, cornmeal made from untreated ground maize will not form a dough when water is added, but the chemical changes in masa allow a dough to form easily.

But nixtamalization was only the beginning of the complex process that turned corn into a nutritious, life-sustaining food. The indefatigable Native American women mixed nixtamalized corn with water to form a thick dough and then cooked it in a pot. The cooked dough was then wrapped in a corn husk and underwent an acid fermentation period of up to two weeks.[67] This was the original tamale (made with *nixtamal*)—a fermented food! A ball of fermented dough, flattened on a hot rock, made a nutritious tortilla. Often these preparations were then fried in bear grease or other fat. Added to water, the dough worked its magic to produce a refreshing fermented beverage.

As an adjunct to their meat-based diet, corn provided variety and important

---

* Indeed, corn cannot grow without the action of man planting it in the ground.

† Medical researchers debated two theories for the origin of pellagra: the deficiency theory said that pellagra was due to a deficiency of some nutrient, while the germ theorists argued that pellagra was caused by a germ transmitted by stable flies. (A third theory, promoted by the eugenicist Charles Davenport, held that people only contracted pellagra if they were susceptible to it due to certain "constitutional, inheritable" traits of the affected individual.)

calories. But when the proportion of corn in the diet became too high, as happened in the American Southwest, the health of the people suffered. Skeletal remains of groups subsisting largely on corn reveal widespread tooth decay and bone problems.[68]

In the jungles of Central America, the indigenous tribes followed a similar procedure, wrapping the nixtamalized dough in banana leaves for two weeks and then adding the dough balls to water to make a thick fermented drink called *pozol*.* Europeans described *pozol* as a beverage that allowed the indigenous people to resist the heat of the tropical zones.[69]

In South America, the Kaingang people of Brazil prepared a fermented corn product called *jamin-bang*. They put corn in wicker baskets and immersed the grain in a stream for several days. The soaked kernels were then ground into a pulp, placed in baskets lined with leaves, covered with leaves, and allowed to ferment for three to six days. The product was then rolled into flat cakes and baked to make a nutritious bread. A similar Brazilian fermented food is *polvilho azedo*, a fermented and sun-dried cassava starch product.[70]

Another important native grain was wild rice—a grain of the genus *Zizania* and more akin to oats than rice—which grows in running water and along lakeshores, not only in the Great Lakes region and New England but as far south as the Patuxent River in Maryland; another species grew in Texas and New Mexico. Typically, Native Americans paired wild rice with beaver tail fat, stewed it in deer broth or maple syrup, or prepared it into stuffing for wild birds.

Many Native American groups cultivated or collected legumes—in fact, legumes were a mainstay for a large number of tribes, "paleo" diet proscriptions notwithstanding. Typically, the women planted bean seed together with a corn seed in little mounds in their fields—the corn stalk and bean vine grew together and their fruits were consumed together—often as succotash (see page 206), a dish composed of beans, corn, dog meat and bear fat. *Shuco*, a sour bean and corn porridge, provided nourishment in Central America. The plentiful harvest of the leguminous mesquite tree, which grows throughout the Southwest, was ground into flour and added to many foods, providing a nutritious staple.

As for "starches"—another "not recommended" item in the paleo diet—Native Americans had lots to choose from, starting with tubers like the Jerusalem artichoke or sunchoke (the root of a type of sunflower). These were cooked slowly for a long time in underground pits until the hard, indigestible root was transformed into a highly digestible

---

* Not to be confused with *pozole*, a kind of Aztec stew made with fermented corn dough and meat—originally the meat of human sacrifices, and later of pork, said to taste very similar to human flesh.

gelatinous mass. Cultivated squash of myriad varieties, and cactus and yucca gathered through the Southwest, are high-starch foods. Indigenous tribes from the Amazon and Central America ate bananas and many other tropical fruits.

Various species of agave nourished the tribes of the southwestern United States, not only with the fermented drink pulque,* prepared from the agave juice, but also with starch from the bulbs of the cacti. The bulbs required special preparation in which they were roasted for several days in underground pits, pounded into thin sheets, ground into flour, and formed into cakes, "which made a very good substitute for bread."[71]

Wild potatoes in North America and cultivated potatoes in South America added carbohydrates to the indigenous diet. The domestic potato grows in the Andes Mountains, with some varieties cultivated above ten thousand feet. The indigenous varieties of potatoes contain glycoalkaloids, a toxin common to the nightshade family, especially those growing in the more hostile high-altitude environments. The glycoalkaloids concentrate in the skin of the potato, which the Native Americans removed and discarded. Drying, freezing and leaching techniques also helped reduce the glycoalkaloid content. The resultant potato powder was easy to transport and could be stored for many years.

And then there is the *wapato*, or duck potato—chestnut-size corms (the swollen stem base) produced by the aquatic plant genus *Sagittaria*. They grow in shallow waters and swamps in all the non-desert regions of North America, from Florida to the northwest. In the late fall or early spring, the women harvested these "swamp potatoes" by disturbing the mud with their feet, causing the corms to float to the surface. They could be eaten raw, but were less bitter when cooked.† Varieties that do not produce starchy corms have lots of starch in the stalk.

Throughout the North American continent, nuts like acorns were made into gruel or little cakes after careful preparation to remove tannins. In the southeast, pecans contributed important calories from fat and carbohydrates. The starchy chestnut flourished throughout the forests of the eastern part of North America. Ground and sifted chinkapin and hickory nuts served to thicken venison broth.[72]

---

* Pulque is the milk-colored, slightly viscous, slightly foamy fermented sap of the agave plant; its production dates at least from the Aztec period. The characterization of pulque as an alcoholic beverage ignores the complex character of the drink. The traditional brew has a sour, vomitlike smell, the definite mark of bacterial fermentation (which produces lactic acid) in addition to yeasted fermentation (which produces alcohol). The beverage is rich in B vitamins, vitamin C and many other nutrients.

† According to their diaries, Lewis and Clark consumed mainly elk and *wapato* while they explored the Columbia River region, now in present-day Oregon.

Staples like corn and beans were stored in underground pits, ingeniously covered with logs and leaves to prevent wild animals from finding or looting the stores. The women protected corn against vermin by hanging it in baskets in the smoky part of their dwellings.[73] Birch bark was used to make trays, buckets and containers, including kettles. Water was boiled by putting hot rocks into the vessels. Southern and Southwestern tribes used gourds or clay pots for the same purpose. Even animal skins were put to work as cooking vessels. The Dakotas would fasten an animal skin to four stakes in the ground, then add water and finely cut meat. Heated stones added to the water would cook the meat. In times of want, a woman could make a stew of a single squirrel or bird, boiled in water with old bones to flavor the "liquor," and no other condiment but salt.[74]

In general, fruits were dried and used to season fat, fish, and meat—dried blueberries flavored moose fat, for example. Beverly Hungry Wolf recalls that her grandmother made pemmican by mixing wild mint with fat and dried meat. The mint would keep the bugs out and also prevent the fat from spoiling. Wild onions served as a common flavoring for meat dishes and, in fact, were an important item of commerce.

In northern Canada, plant foods were limited to summer berries and moss; the moss was consumed in peculiar ways. According to Samuel Hearne, "The stomach of no other large animal beside the deer is eaten by any of the Indians that border on Hudson's Bay. In Winter, when the deer feed on fine white moss, the contents of the stomach is so much esteemed by them that I have often seen them sit round a deer where it was killed, and eat it warm out of the paunch. In summer the deer feed more coarsely and therefore this dish, if it deserves that appellation, is then not so much in favour."[75]

A "black, hard, crumply moss" was sometimes boiled "into a gummy consistency...It is so palatable that all who taste it generally grow fond of it. It is remarkably good and pleasing when used to thicken any kind of broth; but it is generally most esteemed when boiled in fish liquor."[76]

Native Americans also enjoyed sweet-tasting foods. Maple sugar or pine sugar served as sweetener for meats and fats. In the Southwest, they chewed the sweet heart of the agave plant. In fact, the Spanish noted that where agave grew, the indigenous population had bad teeth.[77]

On the James River in Virginia, an early colonist described a dinner menu served by the wife of a chief: hominy, boiled venison, roasted fish and dessert of melons and other vegetables[78]—a sophisticated meal with a balance of protein, fat and carbohydrates!

USE OF SOUR-TASTING fermented foods is a characteristic of all indigenous diets, including the diet of Native Americans across the continent. As noted, the Cherokee "bread" consisted of *nixtamal* wrapped in corn leaves and fermented for two weeks.[79] Beans, tubers, berries, and other plant foods underwent "special preparation," usually fermentation. Many observers commented on the habit of eating gamey, rotten meat or fish.

Samuel Hearne described a fermented dish consumed by the Chippewa and Cree:

> The most remarkable dish among them...is blood mixed with the half-digested food which is found in the caribou's stomach, and boiled up with a sufficient quantity of water to make it of the consistence of pease-pottage. Some fat and scraps of tender flesh are also shred small and boiled with it. To render this dish more palatable, they have a method of mixing the blood with the contents of the stomach in the paunch itself, and hanging it up in the heat and smoke of the fire for several days; which puts the whole mass into a state of fermentation, which gives it such an agreeable acid taste, that were it not for prejudice, it might be eaten by those who have the nicest palates...most of the fat which is boiled in it is first chewed by the men and boys, in order to break the globules that contain the fat; by which means it all boils out, mixes with the broth; whereas if it were permitted to remain as it came from the knife, it would still be in lumps, like suet. To do justice, however, to the cleanliness in this particular, I must observe, that they are very careful that neither old people with bad teeth, or young children, have any hand in preparing this dish.[80]

A number of reports indicate the Native Americans preferred broth and herbed beverages to water. The Chippewa boiled water and added leaves or twigs to make a flavored beverage.[81] In the eastern part of North America, sassafras was a favorite ingredient in teas and medicinal drinks.[82] Sassafras powder, corn silk and dried pumpkin blossom flavored and thickened broth into gourmet sauces. California Indians added lemonade berries to water to make a pleasantly sour drink.[83] Refreshing sour drinks were produced from fermented corn porridge.[84] In the Southwest and South America, a drink called *chicha* is made with little balls of corn dough that the women impregnate with saliva by chewing and then add to water to produce a delicious, sour, fizzy fermented beverage.

Indigenous people usually cooked their grains after fermenting them, but raw fermented beverages and even raw fermented meat foods provided beneficial bacteria for the digestive process on a regular basis—a practice that modern science has only recently validated as healthful.

THE EXPLORER HERNANDO DE SOTO led the first European expedition deep into the territory of the modern-day United States during the 1540s. They landed in Florida and traversed Georgia, Alabama and possibly Arkansas, and saw the Mississippi River. The records of the expedition are the only European description of the culture and habits of North American native tribes before these peoples encountered other Europeans—de Soto's men were both the first and nearly the last Europeans to witness the villages and civilization of the Mississippian culture.

Anthropologists have sometimes insisted that the American Indians did not consume salt,* but de Soto received "an abundance of good salt" as a gift from the Mississippian tribes, and observed the production and trade of salt in the southeastern part of the country. In the lower Mississippi Valley, he met traveling native merchants selling salt. According to the de Soto records, lack of salt could lead to a most unfortunate death: "Some of those whose constitutions must have demanded salt more than others died a most unusual death for lack of it. They were seized with a very slow fever, on the third or fourth day of which there was no one at fifty feet could endure the stench of their bodies, it being more offensive than that of the carcasses of dogs or cats. Thus they perished without remedy, for they were ignorant as to what their malady might be or what could be done for them since they had neither physicians nor medicines. And it

was believed that they could not have benefited from such had they possessed them because from the moment they first felt the fever, their bodies were already in a state of decomposition. Indeed, from the chest down, their bellies and intestines were as green as grass."[85]

The most important sources of salt were the salt springs that dotted northwestern Louisiana, western Arkansas and the Ohio River Valley. Archeological remains in these areas indicate that the indigenous people evaporated the brine water from salt springs in shallow clay salt pans, most likely by adding hot rocks to the brackish water. They also retrieved salt from the ashes of certain plants and from salt-impregnated sand, and sometimes gathered rock salt. Well-defined salt trails allowed the transport of salt to the east. Coastal tribes generally got their salt through trade rather than the evaporation of seawater, as wood for fire-making is sparse near the ocean beaches and the moist climate is not conducive to evaporation. Salt roads stretched hundreds of miles over South America, connecting the Amazon and the Andes with sources of salt, and a heavy salt trade crisscrossed the Yucatán, Belize and Honduras.[86]

Salt traders traveled New Mexico as well. The traders did not belong to any tribal group but traveled alone from group

---

* No added salt is allowed on Loren Cordain's version of the paleo diet, although adherents may consume modern foods for 20 percent of their meals and can presumably get the salt they need during binges on potato chips and salted nuts.

to group carrying baskets of salt gathered from salt lakes, along with other goods.[87] Nor did the inhabitants of California lack salt. Mysterious basins carved out of the granite in the Sierra Nevada allowed the evaporation of salty water from nearby saline streams. Similar basins were discovered in 1891 by geologist Henry W. Turner in what is now Sequoia National Park.[88]

American Indians used salt as a condiment for flavoring stews and corn dishes, and possibly in rituals, but not for salting meat as the Europeans did. Salt may have also served medicinal functions.*

IN THEIR PREFERENCE for fat, their choice of organ meats over muscle meats, their use of a large variety of plant foods, and the inclusion of salt in the diet, Native American foodways resembled those of the Australian Aborigines in many ways. But did the natives of the American continents engage in land management like the Aborigines? Or—as archeological authorities in America have insisted—were they "at best complex hunter-gatherers and at worst 'wealthy scavengers,' incapable of the sophisticated cultural development associated with agricultural societies"?[89]

Leaving aside the mysterious civilizations that planted pyramids in Mexico and Central America, and perched impossible stone fortresses high in the Andes Mountains, what about the iconic teepee-dwelling Native Americans? Were they treading lightly over the landscape, living in a wilderness "untrammeled by man," in the words of the Wilderness Act of 1964, never changing their environment from its original untamed state?

The Americas may have appeared as untamed wilderness after huge numbers—something like 90 percent—of the indigenous population succumbed to smallpox and other diseases,† leaving few to tend their fields and orchards, but the earliest Europeans to set foot in the new world described the woods as "park like." They also noted the coastline and riverbanks dotted with innumerable villages, the land agreeably sculpted into fields of corn and other crops, the air smoky with brush fires, the rivers chevronned with weirs to shepherd fish for easy capture, orchards tended for chestnuts and other useful

---

* Dr. William Todd, physician for the Hudson's Bay Company Swan River district in 1837, described two American Indians who were able to recover from smallpox by floating in a salty lake for almost twenty-four hours. Christened Little Manitou Lake, or Lake of the Healing Waters, the body of water was later found to contain high concentrations of minerals, in addition to salt, and became an important spa center during the 1920s and '30s.

† The rapid demise of the well-nourished, well-formed American Indian to smallpox and other diseases is a mystery still seeking solution. The effects of the white man's diseases were catastrophic—carrying off up to 95 percent of the population in some areas—whereas plagues of the same diseases among more poorly nourished Europeans killed no more than one-third of the population.

trees, and, above all, woods cleared of underbrush.

According to Charles C. Mann, author of *1491: New Revelations of the Americas Before Columbus*,

At the time of Columbus the Western Hemisphere had been thoroughly painted with the human brush. Agriculture occurred in as much as two-thirds of what is now the continental United States, with large swathes of the Southwest terraced and irrigated. Among the maize fields in the Midwest and Southeast, mounds by the thousand stippled the land. The forests of the eastern seaboard had been peeled back from the coasts, which were now lined with farms. Salmon nets stretched across almost every ocean-bound stream in the Northwest. And almost everywhere there was Indian fire.

Even in the Amazon, the local tribes had converted about a quarter of the rain forest into farms and agricultural forests.[90]

Samuel Hearne described controlled burning above the Arctic circle: "In the preceding Summer, when they were in those parts, they had set fire to the woods; the moss still burning in some places."[91] He marveled that "strawberries known to be more plentiful in such places as have formerly been set on fire...after moss and underwood have been set on fire, raspberry bushes and hips have shot up in numerous spots where nothing of the kind had ever been seen before.... This is a phenomenon that is not easily accounted for; but it is more than probable that Nature wanted some assistance, and the moss being all burnt away, not only admits the sun to act with more power, but the heat of the fire must, in some measure, loosen the texture of the soil, so as to admit the plants to shoot up, after having been deep rooted for many years without being able to force their way to the surface."[92]

And then we have the example of California. California schoolchildren are taught that the indigenous peoples, the so-called "digger Indians," were the "most primitive" of all the American Indian tribes, living in an ecosystem naturally blessed with abundance; for when the early European explorers and settlers came to California, they found a land of beauty and bounty. The descriptions compiled by M. Kat Anderson in her defiant book, *Tending the Wild*,[93] recount hills, valleys and plains filled with elk, deer, antelope, hare, rabbit and quail, with bear and mountain lion abounding, the sea shores crowded with seal and otter, and the skies congested with birds, sometimes so thick they blocked out the sun. One observer noted a flock of white geese that covered an area of four square miles when they landed. The lakes and rivers were swarming with salmon, trout and other fish, and their beds and banks were covered with mussels, clams and other shellfish. Shrimp thronged the San Francisco Bay!

Early observers were even more impressed with the profusion of California's varied flora. The forests yielded pine nuts and pine sugar; California's massive oaks produced prodigious amounts of acorns; the prairies and meadows were covered with wildflowers, often with just one species, creating a mass of color for hundreds of acres. Carefully tended mesquite trees yielded bushels of pods with just a few hours of gathering. Vast wetland regions yielded *yampahs*—an edible potato-like tuber. Even more amazing, the landscapes seemed magically clear of brush—oak trees grew in sprawling savannas and the Yosemite Valley was clear of undergrowth so you could see from one end of it to the other.

The Europeans assumed they had discovered an untouched wilderness that just happened to resemble a garden, populated by "primitive" native tribes who profited from nature's bounty simply by hunting and gathering. But in fact, California was not so much a wilderness as a true garden, full of beauty and abundance because wise guardians had tended it for thousands of years. For untold generations, the California tribes had shaped the landscape by pruning, coppicing, cultivating, transplanting, weeding, selecting cultivars— and above all by controlled burning.

Controlled burning served as the main tool for creating California's parklike landscape. Through periodic burning, they cleared brush under trees and enlarged meadows and prairies. Burning broke down dry vegetation, returning nutrients to the soil—everything grew better after a burn, the local tribes told the white man. Burning under the oak trees eliminated insects—without burning every year or two under the oaks, the acorns became infested with pests. Burning encouraged straight shoots to come up from bulrushes and from small trees, supplying material for basket making. Burning encouraged certain useful species above others. Burning could be used to corral wildlife— masses of grasshoppers moving ahead of controlled burns, for example, were nutritious and easily gathered morsels. Above all, frequent small fires prevented the buildup of brush that could fuel a catastrophic fire; while controlled burning helped to preserve trees and encouraged them to grow, uncontrolled fire could wipe out forests and, therefore, the food supply.*

Like the Aboriginal tribes of Australia, the California Indians cultivated vast tracts of edible grains. Corn seems not to have traversed the Rocky Mountains, but wild rye, wheat and oats grew in abundance in California's fire-managed prairies. This bounty was gathered with wicker seed-beaters into large baskets—so

---

* The demise of the American chestnut tree, which grew everywhere in profusion in the eastern United States, is blamed on an Asian bark fungus accidentally introduced into North America on imported Asiatic chestnut trees in the early 1900s. Perhaps the trees were more susceptible to the blight because they had not received periodic burning for many years.

abundant were wild grains in some places that many bushels could be gathered within hours. The grains were winnowed and sifted with special baskets, ground on flat rocks, roasted and made into gruels and cakes. The seeds of wildflowers, particularly the chia seed, were also gathered and consumed as staples. Gathering methods always dispersed some seeds, enlarging the area of cultivation and increasing yield over the years.

Like the Australian Aborigines, the California Indians saw their role as guardians of nature, agents for improving nature's appearance and increasing her abundance; the plants and animals were their relatives, needing support and care, just like human relatives. By contrast, the European colonists viewed nature as something outside—unpredictable and often dangerous; nature was there for exploitation or, in the case of naturalists like John Muir, to be left "pristine" and untouched. Interestingly, modern Native Americans often use the word "wilderness" as a negative label for land that humans have not taken care of for a long time, a land where dense understory shrubbery or thickets of young trees block visibility and movement. Indeed, this is exactly what happened in Yosemite Valley when the white man took over: the valley became filled with brush and the beautiful vistas through the oak trees disappeared.* The indigenous people believed that a hands-off approach to nature—above all the prohibition on controlled burning—promoted wild and rank landscapes that were inhospitable to life. "The white man sure ruined this country," said James Rust, a Southern Sierra Miwok elder. "It's turned back to wilderness."

The white man also ruined the traditional foodways. Today the American Indians still living on reservations—some three hundred thousand of them—get most of their food from the government store. The National Nutrition Monitoring and Related Research Act of 1990, also known as Public Law 101-445, states that all federal agencies shall promote the current U.S. Dietary Guidelines in carrying out any federal food, nutrition or health program. These low-fat, high-carb recommendations that have replaced the Native American diet of guts and grease are more than voluntary guidelines; for Native Americans, they are a federal prescription for diabetes, obesity and other diseases.

The foods that the long industrial supply lines deposit on the reservations are the cheapest foods that modern technology can produce, and the multinational giants that produce them are equipped with lawyers and lobbyists to ensure that their products are the ones our government buys.

American Indians on reservations are hit harder and faster than the general population by this onslaught of processed food

---

* The term conservationists use to describe this process is "rewilding."

because their choices are so limited. Uncle Sam will never admit that the native populations were tall, strong and healthy just three or four generations ago. Today a large proportion suffer from chronic disease. Addiction is common. Yet many American Indians remember stories or even have vivid memories of life before federal handouts, a time when diabetes and other diseases of civilization were unheard of. A few are indeed returning to native ways—hunting, fishing, and gardening—learning the hard way that the white man's food trinkets come at a terrible price.

CHAPTER 3

The Far North

Seal Oil and Whale Blubber

BEFORE WE LEAVE the Americas, it is important to take a close look at the foodways of the Eskimos or Inuit*—people who lived in excellent health in the extreme conditions of Alaska, northern Canada and Greenland as long as they followed the exacting parameters of their indigenous diet. The Eskimo territory stretches over half the Arctic, crossing four international boundaries—a vast territory united by genetics, a common language base, similar cultural practices, similar implements and preserving equipment, and a marine mammal diet.

Dr. Weston A. Price visited the hardy Native Alaskans in 1933 and wrote a glowing report of the robust good health enjoyed by this true hunter-gatherer population. Those living on their native diet in Alaska suffered none of the white man's diseases—not even scurvy, in spite of a lack of plant foods. Price and others marveled at the absence of tooth decay, resistance to illness, ease of childbirth and cheerful disposition of these Arctic-dwelling peoples.[1]

"By the common testimony of observers," wrote Arnold de Vries in his 1952 book *Primitive Man and His Food*, "they laugh as much in a month as civilized people do in a year."[2] He noted that the Eskimos are not as tall as the typical American Indian,† but "broad and well-formed...Deformity is very rare among

---

* Eskimos and Inuit are racially distinct from American Indians, and the Eskimo-Aleut languages are unrelated to any American Indian language groups. "Eskimo" is a blanket term used to refer to indigenous people living in the polar regions of the world. However, the generic word "Eskimos"—meaning "eaters of raw flesh"—is considered a negative term in Canada and Greenland. In fact, the Canadian government passed an act in 1982 giving recognition to the word "Inuit" over Eskimo to refer to the indigenous people of Canada. Thus, the term "Inuit" applies to the indigenous people of Canada and Greenland but not to all the indigenous people living in and around Siberia and Alaska.

† Vilhjalmur Stefansson, on the other hand, describes the Eskimos as tall, with many at six feet or taller, although he notes that the women are shorter than the average European woman.

them. They have great endurance and are very strong in the prime of life. Observers tell us that the adult Eskimo can carry a hundred pounds in each hand and a hundred pounds in his teeth and walk with ease for a considerable distance."[3]

Collections of Eskimo teeth housed at the Smithsonian National Museum of Natural History in Washington, D.C.; Dalhousie University in Canada; and the American Museum of Natural History in New York contain not one example of decay in hundreds of teeth.[4] Dr. Price noted that even in teeth worn down to the gums from chewing on leather and biting sandy grit lodged in dried fish, "the pulp chambers are never open, but always filled with secondary dentine," an indication of extreme immunity to decay.[5]

LIVING IN THE FAR NORTH, where the ground is frozen eight months of the year, the Eskimo peoples naturally rely on the surprising abundance of Arctic animal life: sea mammals such as seal, whale and walrus; land mammals such as bear, moose, musk ox and especially caribou; birds including duck, goose, loon, owl and ptarmigan; eggs from ducks and seagulls; small mammals like rabbits and squirrels; shellfish including crab, conch and clams; and fish including salmon, whitefish, tomcod, pike, char, flounder, herring and smelt.

In addition to the muscles (meat) of land animals, Eskimos enjoy their fat, organs (especially liver and kidney), marrow, stomach lining and stomach contents, and the liver, liver oil, head, tail, fins, bones and roe of fish.*

When Eskimo hunters kill a seal, they often eat the raw liver, mixed with small pieces of fat. Intestine, fresh or wind-dried, is a delicacy. Dried strips of meat are spread with rendered fat.[6] Cod liver is placed in a container to allow the oil to run off, or the oil may be extracted by heating the liver in a pot. The oil is eaten with dishes low in fat, such as dried capelin (a type of smelt), which is dipped in the cod liver oil.[7]

The Eskimos also like to chew bones and sinews, and eat fish and meat both raw and cooked. In the old days, boiling of meat and fish took place in carved-out soapstone pots. The feeble flame of an oil lamp would slowly heat the cooking water. "The woman in charge of the cooking chews a piece of blubber and spits it out into the pot so that the water becomes covered with a film of fat," observed Arne Høygaard, who studied the Greenland

---

* Very little of killed animals goes to waste. According to Hugh Brody in *The Living Arctic* (1978), typically only the lungs, genitals and small amounts of entrails are left on the ice. Brains rubbed into hides serve as a skin softener and preservative; spinal and leg tendons make sturdy thread; seal windpipes and intestines make igloo windows; fish skins can be fashioned into needle and fishhook cases; ptarmigan bladders make children's balloons; fish eyes and boiled duck feet make delicious snacks; the bones of a seal flipper provide all the pieces for an elaborate Inuit game; and a goose or ptarmigan wing serves as an excellent feather duster.

Eskimos during the 1930s, speculating that this custom prevents unnecessary evaporation and waste of heat.[8]

The Eskimo people have many ways of preserving food. In the warm months, large quantities of seal meat and organs are dried in the sun. "The dried muscles are quite black, of a very firm consistency, and cannot be chewed by a man with weak jaw muscles."[9] Fish can also be preserved by drying, or are eaten raw, usually with blubber or blubber oil.[10]

Another important food preservation method is storage in specially prepared "pokes" or blubber bags to produce *imigarmit*. The preparation of a good *imigarmit* is a great art. The skin of the seal, with the blubber attached, is sewn into a bag, which is dried in the sun for a number of days. Additional blubber, cut into strips, washed and dried several hours, goes into the bag along with additional foods such as dried seal meat and organs, berries and other plant foods, boiled seal flippers, boiled narwhal skin and dried marine algae. As described by Høygaard, "After some days the blubber will have changed into oil. The skin bag is sewn together very carefully to prevent the access of air. It must then be kept in the shade and in a place where the ground is dry."[11] Care taken to prevent exposing the contents to light, moisture and air prevents rancidity of the fragile omega-3 oils found in the fat of marine animals.

The Eskimo preserves his catch by drying, smoking, freezing, submerging in oil and above all by fermenting. Meat, skin, fat, whole birds, fish and fish eggs can all be fermented into "stink" foods. Typically, meat and fish are placed in baskets or sewn sealskin pokes and fermented in underground pits until the flesh and bones soften to the consistency of ice cream. The softened bones of fermented fish served as an important source of calcium for the Eskimos before they were introduced to dairy foods.

Fermented fish is not "rancid" but has a different texture, with rich and complex flavors—often compared to the flavors of ripe cheese. Any yellow scum of rancid oil on the surface of fermented fish, which does become rancid, is rinsed or scraped away.

Vilhjalmur Stefansson learned to like fermented fish while living with the Eskimos on the Mackenzie River in Alaska in the early 1930s. In a community of three or four families, fifteen or twenty individuals engaged in fishing, pulling in dozens to hundreds of pounds of salmon per day. In the warm months, they consumed the fresh fish after boiling. As the weather became colder, they transitioned to frozen fish.

In the morning, winter-caught fish, frozen so hard that they would break like glass, were brought in to lie on the floor till they began to soften a little. One of the women would pinch them every now and then until, when she found her finger indented them slightly, she would begin preparations for breakfast. First she cut off the heads and put them aside to be boiled for the children in the afternoon. Eskimos are fond of children, and heads are considered the best part of the fish. Next best are the tails, which are cut off and saved for the children also. The woman would then slit the skin along the back and also along the belly and getting hold with her teeth, would strip the fish somewhat as we peel a banana.

Thus prepared, the fish were put on dishes and passed around. Each of us took one and gnawed it about as an American does corn on the cob. An American leaves the cob; similarly we ate the flesh from the outside of the fish, not touching the entrails. When we had eaten as much as we chose, we put the rest on a tray for dog feed.

Stefansson became "as fond of raw fish as if I had been a Japanese. I liked fermented (therefore slightly acid) whale oil with my fish as well as ever I liked mixed vinegar and olive oil with a salad."

"There were several grades of decayed fish," explained Stefansson. "The August catch had been protected...from animals but not from heat and was outright rotten. The September catch was mildly decayed.

The October and later catches had been frozen immediately and were fresh. There was less of the August fish than of any other and, for that reason among the rest, it was a delicacy—eaten sometimes as a snack between meals, sometimes as a kind of dessert and always frozen, raw." When Stefansson got up his courage, "I tried the rotten fish one day, and if memory serves, liked it better than my first taste of Camembert. During the next weeks I became fond of rotten fish."[*][12]

Stinkhead or *tepa* is a common Inuit dish of fermented whitefish heads, traditionally prepared by placing them in a wooden barrel—or, in more modern iterations, in a plastic bag or bucket—which is then buried in the ground and left for a few weeks, allowing the heads to decompose. Flippers from the *oogruk*, or bearded seal, make a tasty treat when fermented in rendered fresh blubber. After a two-week fermentation, hungry eaters pull the fur off the flippers, cut them into small pieces, and then enjoy the repast. Beaver paws get a similar treatment.

With modernization, Alaska has witnessed a steady increase of botulism contamination, with more cases of botulism than any other state in the United States. Botulism has occurred in many traditional Eskimo fermented foods including

---

[*] Stefansson compared the enjoyment of rotten fish to the fondness "among nobility and gentry to like game and pheasant so high that the average Midwestern American or even Englishman of a lower class, would call them rotten." He reckoned that a taste for mild cheese was "somewhat plebian," whereas a liking for odiferous fermented foods was a characteristic of the upper classes.

fermented whole fish, fish heads, walrus, sea lion, whale flippers, beaver tails, seal oil and birds. The risk is greatest when a plastic container is used for fermenting instead of the old-fashioned, traditional vessels, such as a grass-lined hole, as the botulinum bacteria thrive in the anaerobic conditions created by the airtight enclosure in plastic. The Eskimos have reverted to fermenting fish heads and other foods directly in the ground or in sealskin pokes, after learning the hard way to respect the traditional food preparation methods of their ancestors. In fact, fermenting food, especially animal foods, is a delicate, complex process, and every step of the preparation process must be carefully executed to ensure a highly acidic environment that makes the food safe to eat.

Fish roe, livers and heads, important, nutrient-dense parts of most fish, are prepared in a variety of ways. For example, *tinaulik* combines lightly boiled and mashed fish livers with blackberries; *aanaalik* is dried salmon with the roe inside. Eating boiled fish heads is a skill that starts with eating the large cheek muscles and the fatty part behind the ball of the eyes, and then involves removing each bone, one at a time, chewing up the soft parts, and licking it clean. According to Anore Jones, who lived with the Eskimos during the 1990s, "Each bone has a slightly different and delicious taste, unusually rich with healthy oils, which tempts you to keep trying the next bone to get a new flavor."[13] For every type of fish, there is an optimum time to harvest for best flavor and fatness, a traditional process for drying, and a safe way to ferment to avoid oxidation and botulism.

Kiviak is a festival food for the Inuit of Greenland. Described as "the world's most disgusting meat dish," it is actually an ingenious way to store the bounty of warm months for winter. The ingredients: four to five hundred dead birds (preferably auks) and one dead seal. Preparation time: three to eighteen months. Instructions: skin the seal, removing all the meat until only a thick layer of fat remains lining the skin, stuff the birds into the sealskin and sew it shut; smear fat over the seams to keep the flies away; place under a rock to ferment for as long as a year and a half. The innards of the birds liquefy, taking on the consistency of soft cheese; the most authentic way to eat the dish is to cut the head off the birds and devour the insides. The bones will be soft and edible; the fermented bird hearts become deliciously sweet due to glycogen stores.[14]

Modern readers may not be up for these challenging foods, but the principles mirror those found in other cultures—a preference for organ meats and fats, and for fermented foods. Western man has his own versions of these delicacies: such as pâté, butter, cheese and caviar.

TWO STAPLES OF the Eskimo diet have bewildered spokespersons for dietary correctness: seal oil and whale blubber.

The basic process of making seal oil (or any marine oil) unifies all of Eskimo culture. Following the kill of seal, *oogruk*, walrus, narwhal, beluga or bowhead whale, the hunters remove the skin with the blubber from the carcass and separate the meat and organs. The meat and organs are variously dried, fermented, frozen or cooked; some of the dried meat is packed in oil. The blubber is separated from the skin during the drying process, cut into strips, and stored in a poke or barrel to render the oil slowly by autolysis—essentially fermenting the tissues so they release the oil without heat—which happens during the summer or when the poke is kept in a warm dwelling.* Seal oil serves for cooking and as a dip or dressing; typically, pieces of fish—either raw or cooked—are dipped in seal oil before consumption, and many foods are preserved in seal oil.

The other signature food is muktuk, whale skin with the thick layer of blubber attached, usually consumed raw or pickled. "*Mattaaq* (fat and skin) is the best thing you can have," says an elderly woman quoted in a January 2006 *National Geographic* article, "Living on Thin Ice." "White man food isn't good. If you want to live up here, you have to be a hunter." The article described a dinner of walrus heart soup, followed by slices of walrus fat "to keep us warm."[15] Described as tasting of hazelnuts,[16] muktuk is considered a great delicacy.

Another delicacy is *mamit*, fat scraped from the inside of the skin. The scraped blubber is boiled in fresh water for about an hour and becomes jellylike after cooling. The Eskimos consider this gelatin-rich food especially good for children.

PROFESSOR ERIC DEWAILLY of Deval University is one of many researchers to tackle the "Eskimo paradox," namely, the fact that Eskimos on their native diets consume anywhere from 55 to 80 percent of their calories from fat, but have low rates of heart disease. Even those Eskimos getting only half their calories from native foods have a rate of cardiac disease that is half that for the west. According to Dewailly, the key difference is that the fats in the Eskimo diet come from wild animals, which, he claims, are lower in saturated fat than domestic animals. According to Dewailly, whale blubber consists of 70 percent monounsaturated fat and close to 30 percent omega-3 fatty acids[17]—percentages that leave no room for the villainous saturated fat.

In fact, recent careful analyses by lipid scientists indicate that both whale blubber and seal oil composition are similar: about 18 percent saturated, 58 percent monounsaturated, 2 percent omega-6, and 20 percent omega-3.[18]

Danish researchers studied consumption of seal meat and blubber during the early 1900s. Between 1897 and 1910, the

---

* Vilhjalmur Stefansson reported that the Eskimo sod house was as warm as any house heated by modern methods. In fact, when meals were being cooked, the indoor temperature could reach 95° or even 100°F. Even in winter, the inhabitants slept naked under cotton blankets.

average consumption of seal blubber was 570 grams per day.[19] If seal blubber is actually 18 percent saturated fat, then consumption of saturated fat would be about 103 grams per day—almost 7 tablespoons, or close to a half cup of saturated fat per day. That is nearly twice the amount of saturated fat found in a whole stick of butter.

But Eskimos do not live on whale blubber and seal oil alone—in addition, they eat the meat of land animals whenever they can—lots of meat. The Russian ethnologist Waldemar Bogoras studied the Chukchee peoples of northeastern Siberia in 1904. He noted that "the staple food of the Reindeer Chukchee is reindeer meat, and that of the Maritime people 'sea meat'—the meat of sea mammals." He observed that the Reindeer Chukchee were capable of eating enormous quantities. "The principal meal of the Chukchee is in the evening... At this time the Chukchee eats much and ravenously. They swallow large quantities of meat, gnaw the bones, and try to outdo each other in quickness... There are some exceptionally great eaters among the Chukchee. I was told about one Reindeer Chukchee... who was able to consume at one eating a two-year-old reindeer buck... He could stay without food for two or three days. Then, after a sumptuous meal, his stomach would be enormously distended, so that the skin would look quite smooth, and he would spend a whole day motionless, digesting."[20] That dainty meal would include organ meats and fat, of course.

According to the American John Murdoch, writing in 1885, the Eskimos burned most of their blubber for light and cooking, preferring to consume the more saturated fat of reindeer, or the higher omega-6 fat of birds. "We found, indeed, at Point Barrow, that comparatively little actual blubber either of the seal or whale was eaten, though the fat of birds and the reindeer was freely partaken of. Seal or whale blubber was too valuable—for burning in the lamps, oiling leather, and many other purposes, especially for trade."[21]

If our heart-healthy Eskimo is eating caribou, then the fat he consumes will be much more saturated—often more saturated than that of domestic animals, with some prized pieces, like the kidney fat, as much as 65 percent saturated. In the Inuit language, the words for "fat"—*uksuk* and *tunnuk*—distinguish between the fat of sea and land animals, respectively,[22] indicating Eskimo awareness of the need for both types of fat—the softer fat of sea animals and the harder fat of land animals.

In 2002, Paal Røiri, a Norwegian, analyzed the diets of Eskimos living entirely on native foods and found that 33.6 percent of dietary fat was saturated with 56.6 percent as monounsaturated. The remaining 9.7 percent was polyunsaturated, with the balance of omega-6 and omega-3 fatty acids at 1 to 1, with most of the omega-3 fatty acids as the beneficial elongated versions (EPA and DHA).[23] So omega-3 consumption in the Eskimo diet is indeed high, and the ratio of omega-6 to omega-3 considered beneficial, but overall consumption of omega-3 fatty acids is hardly the 30 percent claimed by Eric Dewailly and others.

Is the Eskimo diet a very low-carb diet as paleo dieters or traditionalists contend? Paal Røiri estimates the carbohydrate intake at 2 percent of calories;[24] however, others put Eskimo carbohydrate intake at about 10 percent of calories, largely in the form of glycogen from raw meat, raw organ meats and raw fat.[25] For example, when blubber is analyzed by direct carbohydrate measurements, the results indicate that it contains as much as 8 to 30 percent carbohydrate.*

While the literature contains considerable debate on the levels of fat, saturated fat and carbohydrate in the Eskimo diet, of one observation there can be no doubt: the Eskimos on their native diets eat huge amounts of cholesterol, with intakes ranging from 420 milligrams to as high as 1,650 milligrams per day.[†] Yet a 1972 study showed that serum cholesterol levels within the population average 221 mg/ 100 ml, levels that are perfectly normal.[26] Are the Eskimos genetically adapted to tolerate more cholesterol than other human groups, or should the whole theory be discarded like seal entrails on the ice?

A signature Eskimo dish that combines *uksuk* and *tunnuk* is *akutuq* or "Eskimo ice cream." Traditionally prepared for funerals, potlatches or other celebrations—such as when a boy kills his first animal—*akutuq* requires great skill to prepare, with many subtle tricks to get good results. The five ingredients are fat (from caribou, sheep or moose, typically a combination of hard fat from the back or interior and softer fat from the animal belly), seal oil, sweetener (traditionally berries, although today honey or sugar is used), liquid (water or berry juice), and other ingredients, such as fish, fish eggs, meat, and cooked or fermented greens. The preparation begins with careful rendering of about 1 pound hard fat and ½ pound softer fat by chopping the fat, pounding it into thin sheets, and gently warming it until liquid. About 1 cup seal oil is added to the melted fat and the mixture is stirred for up to two hours. With the addition of water, the mixture begins to fluff; by alternating the addition of small amounts of water and seal oil, the skillful cook can achieve an *akutuq* that is fluffy and white. Berries or other ingredients flavor the final product.[27]

This final confection (before the addition of other ingredients) contains about

---

* The first food item that Eskimos adopted when they had contact with Europeans was flour to make "bannock bread," a habit so widespread that some observers have claimed that bannock bread is a traditional Eskimo food. This practice would of course raise the carbohydrate level of the diet considerably.

† For reference, until recently, the U.S. Dietary Guidelines recommended no more than 300 milligrams cholesterol per day, the amount found in two eggs. ·

40 percent of calories from saturated fat. If the Eskimo partygoer eats a small serving weighing about 100 grams, he will imbibe just under 3 tablespoons of saturated fat, the same amount of saturated fat found in about three-quarters of a stick of butter—and that's just in his dessert!

The diet of the traditional Eskimo was hardly politically correct; moreover, the high-protein high-fat diet of the Eskimo does not cause ketosis, nor even high levels of nitrogen in the blood. Early investigators attributed the Eskimo's healthy protein metabolism to exceptionally high levels of dietary fat.[28]

PLANT FOODS COMPRISE an estimated 1 to 2 percent of the Eskimo diet; nevertheless, Eskimo women and children spend many hours during the summer months gathering edible leaves, roots and berries. Nature makes up for the long winters with profuse growth between May and September.* After all, the long winter nights give way to long summer days, when there is sunlight even at midnight. In fact, Vilhjalmur Stefansson described productive gardens and potato plants growing profusely north of the Arctic Circle.

Willow leaves and buds, sea lovage, wild celery, pink plume, brook saxifrage, fireweed and wild chive are eaten raw, or preserved or fermented in seal oil; the leaves of wild rhubarb, sourdock and beach greens are cooked. Lamb's-quarters make a good salad or a hot vegetable dish. A kind of Eskimo sauerkraut is cooked sourdock leaves fermented with berries. Sourdock is acidic enough to pickle fatty fish or meat, including walrus skin. Cooked wild rhubarb mixed with *akutuq* makes a fine sauce for cooked fish. A recipe for *kinuluk* calls for whitefish stomachs and roe, blubber, cranberries, and wild rhubarb to be cooked together and then pickled for several days. Rosewood roots also get pickled and then eaten with blubber.

Plant foods can be fermented in large sealskin pokes, or smaller pokes made of the seal flipper. Wooly lousewood flowers can be fermented with water in a seal flipper poke. As an elder Eskimo woman explained, "Let them lie out in the sun and get old. They get real sweet. It is the sun that makes them good."[29]

Seaweed is another important plant food, eaten raw or dipped into boiling meat stock. The complex carbohydrates of seaweed require specific intestinal flora to digest. According to Høygaard, the Inuit of Greenland "state that they get stomach

---

* According to Stefansson, before road-building came to the frozen north, Eskimos, especially those living in the interior, had to endure the warm months from May to September almost as prisoners. Rushing rivers were difficult to cross and lakes required detours. The ground was marshy, making walking difficult; wet clay stuck to the feet. Clouds of mosquitos brought misery to everyone and the weather was often sweltering. When the fall frosts arrive, all changes. The insects die; the lakes and rivers freeze over and become passable. Snow covering the land allows sledding. And the Eskimos' clothes and houses ensure that they are always comfortable and warm.

pains from eating large quantities of sea-weed after a long period without it. But after a few days' training they can again eat it without stomach pains."[30]

Many northern plants, including ledum, sage, willow and spruce tips, make fine tea.

The pride of the Alaskan summer is berries, including salmonberries, blueberries, blackberries, cranberries, rose hips, bear berries, wild strawberries and red currants, all prepared in various ways and often mixed with fish, meat and fat.

Humans cannot eat moss, twigs or grass—but the caribou can, and the half-digested contents of some caribou stomachs can be fermented to provide nourishment for people and dogs—always dressed with oil or fats.[31]

HOW THE ESKIMOS avoided scurvy, especially during the winter months, was long a mystery. Writing in 1935 in reference to the Eskimo diet, Vilhjalmur Stefansson noted that "Specifically it was believed...that without vegetables in your diet you would develop scurvy. It was a 'known fact' that sailors, miners and explorers frequently died of scurvy 'because they did not have vegetables and fruits.' This was long before vitamin C was publicized." Yet the Eskimos on their native diets were immune to scurvy, and Stefansson and others lived many months in the Arctic consuming only fish and meat (including organ meats and fat) without adverse effects.

Stefansson points to the example of the Arctic explorer Robert Scott, who set out for his first expedition to the South Pole in 1901 carrying lime juice, fruits and vegetables. "He saw to it that the diet was 'wholesome,' that the men took exercise, that they bathed and had plenty of fresh air. Yet scurvy broke out...to the believers in the virtues of lime, the onset of scurvy was a baffling mystery."

One of the Shackleton expeditions, undertaken in 1907, was less well organized. "They were as careless as Scott had been careful; they did not have Scott's type of backing, scientific or financial. They arrived helter-skelter on the shores of the Antarctic Continent, pitched camp, and discovered that they did not have enough food for the winter, nor had they taken such painstaking care as Scott to provide themselves with fruits or other antiscorbutics...compared with Scott's, their routine was slipshod as to cleanliness, exercise and several of the ordinary hygienic prescriptions."

But Shackleton's lack of planning turned out to be a blessing. According to Stefansson, "What signified is that Scott's men, with unlimited quantities of jams and marmalades, cereals and fruits, grains, curries, and potted meats, had been little inclined to add seals and penguins to their dietary. With Shackleton it was neither wisdom or acceptance of good advice but dire necessity which drove to such use of penguin and seal.

"In spite of the lack of care...Shackleton had better average health than Scott. There was never a sign of scurvy; every man retained his full strength."

On Scott's last expedition, in 1910, he proved he had learned nothing from Shackleton's example, again placing reliance on medical advice—with tragic results:

> The men lived on the foods of the United Kingdom, supplemented by the fruit and garden produce of New Zealand. Because they had so much which they were used to, they ate little of what they had never learned to like, the penguins and seals.
>
> Once more they started their sledge travel after a winter of sanitation. The results had previously been disappointing; now they were tragic. While scurvy did not prevent them from reaching the South Pole, it began to weaken them on the return and progressed so rapidly that the growing weakness prevented them, if only by ten miles, from being able to get back to the final provision depot.[32]

The answer to the mystery of why the Eskimos don't develop scurvy came one year later, in 1911, when a Danish researcher named Bertelsen discovered the antiscorbutic properties of muktuk.[33] Later analysis found a respectable 38 mg of vitamin C in 100 grams of muktuk.*[34] Seal liver and arctic char also contain considerable amounts, and small amounts occur in other fish and raw meat, especially organ meats. Raw adrenal glands are especially high in vitamin C, as is fish roe—both of which the Eskimos make a point of eating.[35]

Researchers Geraci and Smith studied traditional Inuit families of the Northwest Territories in 1979 and described their eating patterns. In addition to three small meals of dried meat or dried arctic char, the fourth and largest meal of the day "was usually a stew, made with flesh, bones, marrow and selected viscera of terrestrial and marine mammals and birds... the broth was always consumed as part of the meal." They found that the average vitamin C intake ranged between 11 and 118 mg per day, including some vitamin C in the broth. Vitamin C intake was much higher when muktuk was available.[36]

Once the traditional diet of raw meat and fish, raw fat and organ meats was abandoned, or even just diminished, scurvy became a problem. Geraci and Smith found that 80 percent of town dwellers, who consumed a more modern diet, had poor ascorbic acid levels.

A RELATED MYSTERY concerns salt: unlike every other traditional diet, the traditional Eskimo diet contained no salt.

---

* For comparison, oranges contain about 53 mg per 100 grams.

According to Stefansson, the Eskimo word for "salty," *mamaitok*, is synonymous with "evil-tasting." Stefansson reports that the Eskimos disliked salt intensely. "I was somewhat reconciled to going without salt," wrote Vilhjalmur Stefansson after many months on his Eskimo diet, "but I was nevertheless overjoyed when one day Ovayuak, my new host in the eastern delta, came indoors to say that a dog team was approaching which he believed to be that of Ilavinirk, a man who had worked with whalers and who possessed a can of salt. Sure enough, it was Ilavinirk, and he was delighted to give me the salt, a half-pound baking-powder can about half full, which he said he had been carrying around for two or three years, hoping sometime to meet someone who would like it for a present. He seemed almost as pleased to find that I wanted the salt as I was to get it. I sprinkled some on my boiled fish, enjoyed it tremendously, and wrote in my diary that it was the best meal I had had all winter. Then I put the can under my pillow, in the Eskimo way of keeping small and treasured things. But at the next meal I had almost finished eating before I remembered the salt. Apparently then my longing for it had been what you might call imaginary. I finished without salt, tried it at one or two meals during the next few days and thereafter left it untouched. When we moved camp the salt remained behind."[37]

Salt provides sodium and chlorine, both necessary for digestion and many other processes. Lean beef contains about 50 milligrams sodium per 100 grams, and seafood can be a good source of chlorine, so the seafood and meat of the Eskimo diet can provide adequate amounts of these nutrients without the addition of salt. When carbohydrate foods, especially flour, entered into the diet of the modernized Eskimo, salt became a necessity—additional sodium is essential for the breakdown of carbohydrates.[*]

One overlooked source of salt in the Eskimo diet is blood. Inuits believes that seal blood fortifies human blood by replacing depleted nutrients and rejuvenating their own blood supply. According to anthropologist Kristen Borre, when hunters kill a seal, "one of the hunters slits the abdomen laterally, exposing the internal organs. Hunters first eat pieces of liver or they use a tea cup to gather some blood to drink."[38] Blood contains about 85 percent of the sodium in human and mammal bodies; indeed, the taste of blood is salty."[39]

The Arctic researcher Arne Høygaard reported that the Greenland Eskimos took great care to store and preserve *akaq*, or seal blood: "Blood is usually poured into empty stomachs or sections of mammalian gut, then dried and stored for the winter. Sometimes it is roasted by the side of the oil lamp to a crisp powder, or prepared as a soup."[40] He noted that sea mammals have a great deal of blood, and this blood

---

[*] The need for salt is greater in herbivores than in carnivorous animals.

does not coagulate for some time after the death of the animal. *Akaq* is black in color. Said Høygaard, "It has a disgusting taste and smell, and sticks to the teeth to such an extent, that it is impossible to get rid of the taste until several hours afterwards. *Akaq* was the only Eskimo food which I personally found repulsive. But the Eskimo takes another view of the matter: '*Akaq* is a good and wholesome food. When I have eaten much *akaq*, I feel delightfully warm and sleepy. Afterwards I sleep heavily and feel well when I wake up.'"[41]

Høygaard also noted the practice of adding seawater to the pot when boiling meat, especially during the summer months. Sometimes it is even added to *akaq*, making a dish that would be decidedly salty.

DIETITIANS HOLD UP the Eskimo diet as "The Inuit Paradox," described in a 2004 *Discover Magazine* article as "an example of how high levels of omega-3 fatty acids can counterbalance the bad health effects of a high-fat diet."[42] However, the high omega-3 content of this extreme diet can be a problem, especially when a diet of fish, seal oil and whale blubber is not balanced with more saturated fat from caribou and other land animals. Vilhjalmur Stefansson, for all his insistence on complete satisfaction from his all-fish diet while living with

the Eskimos, eagerly participated in a long trip to obtain caribou. The Eskimos are prone to nosebleeds, bleeding from the lungs and hemorrhagic stroke,[43] all of which can be side effects of too much omega-3. Even the tendency to age early—Høygaard stated that an Eskimo of forty years looked ten years older than inhabitants of Norway living in a similar climate[44]—can be attributed to a surfeit of omega-3 fatty acids in the diet. Premature skin wrinkling has been linked to overconsumption of polyunsaturated fatty acids,[45] and this would be especially true of the highly unsaturated omega-3 fatty acids in marine animals. Høygaard also found arteriosclerosis, another condition that has been associated with overconsumption of polyunsaturated fatty acids, in X-rays of Eskimos as young as thirty years of age.[46]

The Eskimo on his native diet consumes huge amounts of vitamin A, the vitamin that modern dietitians love to hate. One estimate puts vitamin A consumption among the Eskimos at 50,000 IU per day.[*][47] Seal oil contains almost 4,000 IU vitamin A per cup,[48] and the Eskimos consumed seal oil not by the teaspoonful but by the cupful. Liver from fish and land animals and fish heads are also very high in vitamin A.

Vitamin A gets the blame for the phenomenon called Arctic hysteria, or

---

[*] The Recommended Daily Allowance (RDA) for vitamin A in Americans is a mere 3,000 IU (just 6 percent of the average Eskimo intake), with an upper limit of 10,000 IU (only 20 percent of average Eskimo intake).

pibloktoq. Most commonly occurring in winter, especially in women, according to anthropologist Edward Foulks, "the condition begins with several days of irritability or withdrawal, a sudden excitation wherein the victim flees the camp and engages in irrational and dangerous behavior, followed by convulsive seizures, a twelve-hour period of coma or stuporous sleep, and finally a return to normal behavior. During the attack, the individual appears to be in a daze, out of conscious contact with those around him—similar to the behavior of the Eskimo shaman. The episodes can last from a few minutes to several hours, and often terminate in an epileptic seizure with uncontrolled muscle contractions. Typically, the victim has no memory of the attack."[49]

First documented in 1820, the disorder appears to be common to all Arctic regions. One observer, Admiral Robert Peary, described the symptoms during an expedition to Greenland.

The theory of vitamin A toxicity was introduced in a 1985 paper.[50] The author reported—probably relying on Vilhjalmur Stefansson's observation—that the Inuit consider polar bear liver, which is an extremely rich source of vitamin A, to be toxic; explorers who eat polar bear liver out of necessity may experience drowsiness, irritability, headaches and nausea within hours of consuming it; and case reports of vitamin A toxicity involve irritability, drowsiness, double vision and anorexia. However, the Inuit considers seal liver, which contains half as much vitamin A, safe to eat in unlimited quantities, and considers even the meat of polar bear—which is not especially high in vitamin A—to cause indisposition and headache when eaten in large quantities.[*][51] The fact that photophobia—intolerance to light—often precedes a *pibloktoq* attack argues against vitamin A toxicity as a cause of the condition, as photophobia is a sign of vitamin A *deficiency*.

Psychologists have offered many explanations for the baffling condition, starting with the premise that "the Eskimo disorder was basically no different than those seen in the clinics of Charcot and Freud."[52] However, *pibloktoq* also occurs in dogs, a fact that rules out a psychoanalytic explanation.[53] The most reasonable hypothesis ties *pibloktoq* to tetany—an observation made by the earliest explorers[54]—which occurs with severe deficiencies of calcium and vitamin D.[55] Tetany is often accompanied by sporatic episodes of "emotional and cognitive disorganization" and

---

* The Eskimo avoids several foods that are toxic, including the flesh of the Greenland shark and the liver of the bearded seal. Vilhjalmur Stefansson found that about one polar bear liver in five or six made people ill but noted that there is no record of a man nor a dog dying from eating polar bear liver. H. R. Thornton, a missionary in Wales, Alaska, in 1890–1893, reported that the Eskimos "say that if the lining membrane of the [polar bear] liver be taken off, it loses its poisonous properties and may be eaten with impunity." Yet university nutrition courses invariably tell students that vitamin A can be toxic because Arctic explorers got sick when they ate vitamin A-rich polar bear liver.

convulsive seizures, just like *pibloktoq*. Eskimo children are particularly prone to cramps and tetany.[56]

Getting enough calcium is a real challenge in Arctic regions; a key source is dried or fermented fish bones; fish skin also contains moderate amounts of calcium. Eskimos eating mostly land and sea mammals make a point of chewing on and making broth from the bones; still, average calcium intake among the Eskimos is estimated at 500 milligrams per person,[57] far less than the recommended 1,000 to 1,300 milligrams per day.

Furthermore, in winter months and in regions where the Eskimos have little access to fish, vitamin D intake can also be low. Populations in areas of the Arctic where fishing is limited or the weather is unsuitable for drying fish may lack not only calcium but also vitamin D, needed for calcium absorption. Vitamin D works synergistically with vitamin A, and because vitamin A consumption is very high in the Arctic, it is likely that vitamin D requirements are also high.

The Eskimo prefers meat to fish—in fact, the word for "eat" in the Eskimo and Inuit languages, *neqe*, is the same as the word for "meat." Fish serves as an appetizer or snack, but the preferred main meal is meat.[58] And when fish is scarce—which happens often in the winter months—vitamin D and calcium deficiencies present a real danger.

BALANCE IS KEY to the success of the native Eskimo diet—the balance of seafood rich in vitamin D with organ meats of land animals, rich in vitamin A, and the balance of sea mammal fat rich in omega-3 fatty acids with land mammal fat rich in saturated fat. Foods vital to Eskimo health include dried or fermented fish bones for calcium, raw meat and fat for vitamin C, and blood for sodium. When these foods are absent, due to scarcity or trends to modernization, health problems ensue.*

But the main danger for the Eskimo, as for most indigenous peoples, is modern, sugary, processed foods. Rates of cardiovascular disease are relatively low for Eskimos living on their native foods—in spite of high levels of fat, including saturated fat. In Ammassalik on the western coast of Greenland, these rates doubled during the years 1948 to 1960 with the influx of sugar and cereals. By 1978, the Inuit were consuming 128 pounds of grain food (mostly white flour) and 117 pounds of refined sugar per year, or ⅔ pound per day.[59] And these days, the Eskimos make *akutuq* with Crisco.

---

* Unfortunately, interfering public health organizations today are urging the Eskimos not to eat organ meats in order to avoid pollutants; but the vitamin A and other compounds in organ meats are exactly the nutrients needed to protect the body from toxins.

CHAPTER 4

The South Seas

Abundance and Beauty

DR. WESTON A. Price visited the South Seas during the mid-1930s, calling in at the Marquesas Islands, Tahiti, Rarotonga, Nuku'alofa, New Caledonia, Fiji, Samoa and Hawaii. In a separate trip, he visited New Zealand.

On every island he was able to confirm the impressions of early navigators, that the Polynesians and Melanesians were "exceedingly strong, vigorously built, beautiful in body and kindly disposed." They had broad shoulders, wide facial structure, straight white teeth and graceful, splendid bodies. The Tongans, in particular, were very tall; their queen at the time was six feet three inches. Those living on native foods suffered only about 0.14 percent tooth decay. Price reported that they were magnificent singers: "A large native chorus at Nukualofa, in the Tongan Group, sang without accompaniment 'The Hallelujah Chorus' from Handel's Messiah with all the parts and with phenomenal volume and modulation."[1]

Many early visitors commented on the cheerful, buoyant disposition of the islanders, their tendency to sing joyfully while working, and their frequent festivals; they were harmonious and hospitable, yet they could also be fierce warriors* and in some areas, as reported by Price and many others, engaged in ritual cannibalism. "They especially prized the livers" of their foes, as Price put it.

The South Sea Islanders lived from fishing and agriculture, using tools made from stone, bone, shell and wood. In general, the men engaged in planting, harvesting, fishing, cooking, house construction and canoe building; the women

---

* For example, during his second voyage to Tahiti, Captain James Cook and his men witnessed a war fleet of 160 double canoe vessels crowded with rowers and fighting men armed with clubs, pikes and stones, and wearing turbans, breastplates and helmets. Flags streamed in the wind. One hundred seventy smaller double canoes served for transport and supplies. Cook estimated that the fleet could have held almost eight thousand men.

tended the fields and animals (generally pigs and chickens), gathered food and fuel, prepared food before cooking, and made clothes and household items.

The indigenous islanders tended to live in scattered dwellings rather than villages. However, early explorers found complex social structures on some of the islands, with a rigid class system of nobility and workers. Some areas (New Zealand, the Cook Islands, and Mangareva) had slaves, and many of the cultures were dominated by land-owning aristocrats, headed by a king or queen.

Life in the balmy, breezy Pacific could be highly ritualistic, with specific ceremonies and taboos linked to the foods they ate. The kava* ceremony, for example, took place at important events, including the installation of new chiefs, with specific gestures and phrases used at specific times. At ceremonial kava rituals in Rotuma, Fiji, the kava was chewed by virgin girls (marked by caked limestone on their hair) before it was mixed with water to make the drink and then served to individuals according to rank.

The South Sea Islanders generally cooked most of their food in iconic underground pits or earth ovens called *imu* or *umu*, but consumed mangoes, custard apples and coconut meat raw; they chewed raw sugarcane for its juice. Breadfruit, tubers and roots joined the flesh of pigs, dogs, domestic poultry and wild birds in the ovens, often wrapped in leaves. Liquid foods were baked in the same ovens in coconut shell halves. The islanders consumed fish either marinated or cooked, and consumed some small fish and shellfish raw.

AS NOTED BY Dr. Price, seafood was the main source of protein throughout the Pacific—fish and shellfish of every type, including edible tortoise, crustaceans, sand langoustes, crabs, sea centipedes, sand beetles, sea urchins, sea slugs, octopus and eels. Many islands provided freshwater fish as well. Some seafood, such as octopus, sea crab and sea cucumber, were eaten raw; others were cooked in underground ovens.

Early visitors described ingenious fishing methods, including the use of nets, weirs in streams, poisoning, spearing, trapping and use of fishhooks. Some men could catch fish by hand. One colonist described eels kept in holes two or three feet deep and fed by hand as pets.

---

* Kava or kava-kava is a beverage produced from the roots of *Piper methysticum* (from Latin for "pepper" and Latinized Greek for "intoxicating") and consumed throughout the South Pacific. The tea, which tastes "like muddy water with a hint of bitterness," has sedative anesthetic, and euphoriant properties. Its active ingredients are called kavalactones. A Cochrane systematic review concluded that kava was likely to be more effective than a placebo at treating short-term anxiety. Early visitors to the islands took a dimmer view, noting that it led to "befuddlement" and immobilized the limbs; some islanders drank kava in excess and went into convulsions, or lost their appetites, stopped eating, and developed a skin condition resembling leprosy. The ability to pull oneself out of a kava-induced stupor was regarded as an attribute of heroes.

Early writers had great admiration for the South Sea fishing nets, some of which were 30 to 40 fathoms (180 to 240 feet) long and 12 fathoms (36 feet) deep, the bottom edges weighted with stones wrapped in coconut fibers and the top edges held afloat with short pieces of dry hibiscus wood.[2]

Dr. Price was the first colonist to describe the coconut crab,* which migrates in great numbers from the mountains to the sea. The islanders catch the crabs and feed them coconut. "In two weeks' time the crabs are so fat that they burst their shells," said Price, who called them "delicious eating."

In his chapter on the South Seas, Price noted that one French colony was massacred by the islanders in retaliation for cutting off access to the sea. "They believe they require sea foods to maintain life and physical efficiency," he noted. On the Fijian island of Viti Levu, Price witnessed piles of seashells in the hills.

My guide told me that it had always been essential, as it is today, for the people of the interior to obtain some food from the sea, and that even during the times of most bitter warfare between the inland or hill tribes and the coast tribes, those of the interior would bring down during the night choice plant foods from the mountain areas and place them in caches and return the following night and obtain the sea foods that had been placed in those depositories by the shore tribes. The individuals who carried these foods were never molested, not even during active warfare.[3]

According to Price, these islanders believed that they needed seafood at least every three months. In the highly stratified Tahitian society, the chiefs tended to eat fish every day, but the common people ate fish less frequently.

The livers, maw, roe and heads of fish, and the nutrient-dense yellow hepato-pancreas of shellfish were all important foods. The Maoris prepared a dish of the *kahawai* fish, during the season when the fish were fattest, by stuffing the cavity with all the organs except the gallbladder.[4] In Tahiti, shark livers were stuffed into shark stomachs and hung in the trees to ferment. Each liver yielded about a quart of oil, which the Tahitians consumed as a sacred food, necessary for virility and healthy reproduction.[5] According to Price, the men of the islands consumed the male reproductive organs of the shark,

---

* The coconut crab (*Birgus latro*), a species of terrestrial hermit crab, is the largest land-living arthropod in the world and can weigh up to nine pounds and grow to more than three feet long from leg to leg. Its distribution across the South Seas mirrors the distribution of the coconut palm. The indigenous people considered it a delicacy and an aphrodisiac. The only predator of the coconut crab is mankind; intensive hunting has threatened the species' survival on many of the islands.

while the women consumed the female reproductive organs.*

THE SOUTH PACIFIC hosts only two indigenous land mammals: the flying fox bat and insect-eating bat. But Polynesian colonists brought pigs, chickens and dogs to many of the islands. The predecessors of the Maoris brought the blue rat to New Zealand at least two thousand years ago. Until the arrival of Captain James Cook, who brought the pig, New Zealand had no other land mammal.†

On most South Sea Islands, pigs foraged in forest areas, where the islanders could easily hunt them; the natives—usually women—also raised them in enclosures. Pigs were a festival food, cooked in the typical earthen ovens. The part of the pig one received depended on one's social standing.

When Captain Cook arrived in Matavia Bay, Tahiti, in 1774, he noted that every hut had a pig or two.‡ It was a time of affluence, in contrast to the less prosperous conditions he had encountered during his first voyage. "Our very good friends the Natives," he wrote, "brought an abundance of pigs, fresh fruit and roots, including a present from the chiefs of a dozen hogs."

In Tahiti, the men primarily raised pigs to enhance their social prestige, using them as gifts or as the main dish of feasts. Prayers on important occasions demanded the sacrifice of a pig, the priests making the animal squeal before it was killed by strangulation so as to gain the attention of the gods. In Hawaii, pigs (and dogs) met their end by strangulation or by having their nostrils held shut in order to conserve the animal's blood.

In the journal Cook kept during his second visit to Tahiti, he provides a detailed account of how a pig was slaughtered and cooked. His Tahitian hosts strangled the pig to death, scalded the skin in the fire, and removed the hair by scrubbing the pig with

---

* Three towns in Papua New Guinea still engage in the practice of shark calling, which involves luring sharks from the deep and catching them using hand snares. To trap a shark, the caller submerges a noose made of braided cane attached to a wooden propeller float. When the shark swims through the noose up to its pectoral fins, the fisherman jerks up on the propeller's handle, which in turn tightens the noose around the shark. At this point, the shark struggles to break free, and the shark caller must resist the animal's force to keep it from escaping. Once the shark is exhausted, the fisherman can let the float bring it to the surface. At this point the caller stabs the shark in the eyes, clubs it to death, and brings it aboard his canoe.

† The lack of mammal predators allowed large birds like the moa and the kiwi to thrive. Hunting by the Maoris soon brought the moa to extinction. The kiwi is currently protected in nature preservation areas. As land animals were lacking, the Maoris especially prized bird fat, particularly that of the fatty mutton bird, which they preserved in special baskets, encased in its fat. Fat eels were also greatly prized.

‡ The South Sea Island pigs were small and docile enough to be kept as pets, although they mostly roamed freely in the brush where the islanders hunted them for sport. From the 1770s on, these native pigs were crossed with several larger European and Asian varieties. By the missionary period, the pigs had become aggressive and were uprooting gardens, which the Tahitians sought to prevent by fitting them with collars, or breaking their strongest teeth to stop them from gnawing their way in or out of enclosures.

sand. They then opened the belly, removed the fat, and laid it on a clean leaf. The entrails "were put into a basket and carried away so that I know not what became of them, but am certain they were not thrown away."* They then carefully drained the blood and put it "into a large leafe," presumably folded into the shape of a container.

The Hog was now washed clean both inside and out with fresh Water, Several Hot stones were put into his belly which was afterwards cram'd full with clean green leaves; by this time, or perhaps before, the Oven was sufficiently heated, what fire remain'd was taken away, together with some of the Hot stones, the rest were left in the bottom of the hole or Oven which was now covered with green leaves on which the hog was laid on his belly, the lard and fatt, after undergoing some washings with fresh Water was put in a vessel made just then of the bark of Plantain tree, two or three hot stones being put in along with the fat, it was tied up and put in the Oven by the hog as was the blood also prepared in the same manner, round the whole were laid to Bake Plantains, Bread fruit &c then the whole covered with green leaves on which were placed the remainder of the Hot stones and over them more leaves and then any sort of rubbage they could lay their hands upon and lastly finished the operation by well covering the whole with earth.

The interesting part of this description is the fact that the fat and blood were preserved and cooked along with the pig in such a way as to not lose any of either. When the hog was placed before them, so also was the fat and blood, which, according to Captain Cook, "they chiefly if not wholly dined off and said it was *mona-mona ta*, that is very good and we not only said but really thought the same by the Pork. The Hog weighed about fifty pound, some parts about the Ribs I thought rather over done, but the more thicker parts were excellent, and the Skin which by our way of dressing is generally either hard or tough had by this method a flavor superior to any thing I ever tasted. I have now only to add that during the whole process nothing could be done with more cleanliness."[6]

In principle, women were forbidden to consume pig that the men had hunted and prepared, but they could partake of pig they had raised themselves (a rule that was apparently often broken). Dogs, turtles, albacore, shark, dolphin, whale and porpoise were also forbidden to women, at least in some areas such as Tahiti. Dogs were cooked in a manner similar to pigs, and reserved for men during special occasions; Europeans compared the taste to lamb.

---

* I have been unable to find any description of organ meat consumption in the South Seas, which probably reflects the fact that early observers did not ask the right questions, not considering organ meats important. However, in the Philippines, consumption of pig organ meat in stews and soups is commonplace.

Chicken and other fowl served as food for children and women. Native rats were eaten on some islands but not on others. So the South Seas diet contained abundant protein from land and sea; but carbohydrate foods were abundant as well.

LUSH GROWTH COVERS all of the South Sea islands, but surprisingly few native plants provide food. With the exception of mineral-rich seaweed, most of the food plants that have nourished the healthy islanders over the centuries were actually brought in by ancient colonists. These include sweet potatoes, yams, taro, breadfruit, banana and coconut—all cultivated in gardens throughout the South Seas. (Sugarcane, mangoes and custard apples grow wild on many islands, as do a variety of green vegetables.)

In fact, the inclusion of seafood and pork notwithstanding, the South Pacific diet is relatively high in carbohydrates compared to other native diets, these carbs coming chiefly from roots, tubers and fruit—foods allowed on the paleo diet—rather than grains and legumes. In fact, in Fiji, Hawaii and Tahiti, the word "food" refers to starchy foods like taro, yam, sweet potato or breadfruit, while a "meal" is a starchy food plus an accompanying item such as meat, fish or coconut.[7]

The islanders recognized the role of these carbohydrate foods in promoting weight gain, as they used them for deliberate fattening, especially in women and young people. Women often removed themselves from society to put on weight and lighten their skin—rather like a prolonged visit to a spa. Their end goal was not to become tan and slim, as is common today, but rather to reenter society pale and pudgy. Fruits, bananas and breadfruits mashed and mixed with water until semiliquid were the preferred fattening foods, fed by servants to indolent women who remained in the shade and as inactive as possible. Thus, lack of sun and exercise, plus a high-carb diet, was the recipe for fattening. Likewise, teenagers of both sexes were systematically fattened using the same method, lying indolent in dark sheds and consuming the high-carbohydrate foods brought to them. According to D. L. Oliver, author of *Ancient Tahitian Society*, after the fattening period, the fattened ones made a parade to the priest for a blessing, after which admiring bystanders would "rush forward with a lot of clatter and yelling and rip off the parti-colored girdles, leaving the fattened ones with only their breechclouts on."[8]

LIKE THE EARLY COLONISTS in the Americas and Australia, early visitors to the South Seas assumed that the islanders lived passively in an uncultivated Garden of Eden. As one early observer put it, "And what poetic fiction has painted of Eden, or Arcadia, is here realized, where the earth without tillage produces both food and cloathing, the trees loaded with the richest of fruit, the carpet of nature with the most odiferous flowers."[9] Writing as late as 1935, another observer assumed that the islanders did not engage in agriculture: "As every part of the Island produces food without the help of man, it may of this country be said that the curse of Eden has not reached it, no man having his bread to get by the sweat of his brow nor has he thorns in his path."[10]

According to an important 1999 article in *Ethnohistory* by archeologist Dana Lepofsky, "The notion of the Tahitian Garden of Eden so colored people's observations that acts of hard labor were diminished or overlooked. As a result, the details of the drudgery of Maohi [Tahitian] production are often missing from these early ethnohistoric accounts."[11]

Indeed, on the islands with a stratified social structure and large population, such as Hawaii, Tahiti and Tonga, intensive agriculture carried out by laborers was the norm. According to Lepofsky, these cultures were "characterized by a complex, hierarchical society in which rigidly defined strata permeated political, economic and social spheres. Production was primarily at the household level, but chiefs owned and/or controlled the land. Surplus production, controlled by the status elite, was used for their aggrandizement at feasts, war ventures, and other public events. Large quantities of food and goods were paid to the chiefs in the form of first-fruit rites and as levies imposed on the commoners by the chiefs."[12]

The Europeans admired the neatly tended, fenced gardens of the aristocracy, but assumed that the inland and hillside plantations of tree crops like coconuts and bananas were wild rather than cultivated. Intensive taro and yam production tended to occur inland from the coasts, in areas where the early European colonists neglected to visit. "No countrey can boast such delightfull walks as this," wrote a visitor in 1769. "The whole plains where the people live are coverd with groves of Breadfruit and cocoa nut trees without underwood; these are intersected in all directions by the paths which go from one house to the other, so the whole countrey is a shade than which nothing can be more gratefull in a climate where the sun has so powerfull an influence."[13]

Nursery gardens for kava and the highly valued paper mulberry (used in tapa, or bark cloth, production) were located within the aristocratic household compound and "consisted of permanent plots with raised beds that were regularly weeded and mulched, neatly planted, and fenced."[14] Tree crops of bananas, coconut and other fruit, especially breadfruit, grew in the elite gardens as well as in hillside orchards.

Swidden culture, where plots were cleared, often by fire, cultivated for a year or two, and then left fallow, were the norm for staple crops like yam and sweet potato. As with the Australian Aboriginals and Native Americans, use of fire to clear the brush was widespread. Taro requires moist soil and was planted in irrigated fields or cultivated in swamps.

Later, after dramatic declines in

population from infectious and venereal disease destroyed the class system and reduced the pressure to produce foods for the elite, the islanders became more casual about food production, forgetting the accompanying rituals that ensured a good harvest and abandoning many inland and hillside plantations.

THE COCONUT IS AN OILY FRUIT with many important uses. One of the earliest descriptions of the coconut comes from the Italian Antonio Pigafetta who, as a member of Magellan's expedition, visited the Philippines in March 1521: "Cocoanuts are the fruit of the palmtree. Just as we have bread, wine, oil, and milk, so those people get everything from that tree." Pigafetta described the production of palm wine from the sap and of cords "for binding their boats" from the coconut husk: "Under that husk there is a hard shell, much thicker than the shell of the walnut, which they burn and make therefrom a powder that is useful to them." He described the flesh of the coconut as having "a taste resembling almond," usually eaten raw or dried and made into "bread," and the clear, sweet "water" from the center. "When that water stands for a while after having been collected, it congeals and becomes like an apple." He marveled at the extraction of coconut oil "like butter," and the production of vinegar from the water and milk from the coconut flesh. He continued, "This kind of palm tree is like the palm that bears dates, but not so knotty. And of these trees will sustain a family of ten persons. But they do not draw the aforesaid wine always from one tree, but take it for a week from one, and so with the other, for otherwise the trees would dry up. And in this way they last one hundred years."[15]

Throughout the South Seas, the natives often mixed coconut with other foods, such as pounded taro root, to make a pudding. Islanders of Pukapuka consume a pudding called *mawu*, which takes over three days to prepare. Day one involves gathering, peeling and grating the taro. Day two focuses on gathering coconuts and making coconut cream. On the third day, the mixture of taro and coconut cream is wrapped in banana leaves and baked twice in an underground oven.[16]

A typical sauce combines soft immature coconut meat immersed in salt water with raw, even nearly rotten, crustaceans.[17]

Pacific Islanders also used coconut oil on the skin, even considering the practice a source of nourishment. Weston Price mentions with disapproval the fact that the missionaries obliged the natives to cover their bodies: "This regulation had greatly reduced the primitive practice of coating the surface of the body with coconut oil, which had the effect of absorbing the ultra-violet rays thus preventing injury from the tropical sun. This coating of oil enabled them to shed the rain, which was frequently torrential though of short duration. The irradiation of the coconut oil was considered by the natives to provide, in addition, an important source of nutrition. Their newly acquired wet garments became a serious menace to the comfort and health of the wearers."

Coconut oil presents a dilemma to modern investigators because it is a highly saturated fat; yet South Sea Islanders consuming native diets are remarkably free of chronic disease, including heart disease. In one important study, published in 1981, researchers compared two populations of Polynesians living on atolls near the equator, those of Tokala and those of Pukapuka.* Oily coconut and coconut oil provided the chief source of calories for both groups. Tokalauans obtained a much higher percentage of energy from coconut than the Pukapukans, 63 percent compared with 34 percent, so their intake of saturated fat was higher. The serum cholesterol levels were higher in Tokalauans than in Pukapukans, but vascular disease was uncommon in both populations. The researchers concluded, "There is no evidence of the high saturated fat intake having a harmful effect in these populations."[18] Thanks to the recent revelations about coconut oil's many benefits—from weight loss to protection against pathogens—it has found its way back into many diets deemed traditional, even the paleo diet.

YAMS VARY IN SIZE from that of a small potato to over 130 pounds! A staple food in the South Pacific for thousands of years, they keep a long time in storage,

making them a very valuable source of nourishment during the wet season, when other food is scarce. For eating, yams are typically peeled, boiled and mashed, or dried and ground into a powder that can be cooked into a porridge.

An important 1974 paper on yam cultivation in Guadalcanal, British Solomon Islands, describes the cultivation of yams in the interior of the island, and their exchange for fish, coconuts and salt water from the coast, and also for pigs, possums and dog's teeth. Numerous feasts and ceremonies call on local gods to assist with planting, cultivating and harvesting the yams. Ceremonies and rituals elicit the goodwill of the ancestors and the help of garden spirits to produce a good crop.[19]

Yams take nine months to mature, producing only one main crop per year. They require good soil and good drainage. A yam garden can produce one or two crops, and then requires a fallow period of at least five years. Lush vegetation soon covers the yam garden during the fallow period; tree type and other factors determine whether the soil is again ready for yams. "If the vegetation has reached a stage where visibility at eye level has increased—indicating good development of larger trees—the area may be cleared again." Skilled gardeners know when the soil is ready. "Nowadays it is lamented that no one is able to select suitable yam soils by smell as it is claimed some men could do in the past."

---

* Dog bones dating back to about 2000 BC have been found on Pukapuka.

As in so many indigenous cultures, burning is used to clear land for yam gardens. The typical size is a half acre, but some communal yam gardens are as large as ten acres, and small kitchen gardens are around one thousand square feet.

Gardens are laid out with parallel logs or sticks and expected to be beautiful. Spells, rituals and taboos pertain to every aspect of clearing, planting and harvesting. For example, in some parts of Guadalcanal, it is forbidden to enter the garden after weeding or to touch any yam vine. Work takes place in company and with singing. Holes for the yams are dug with specialized digging sticks. The completion of clearing, planting and harvesting are all occasions for feasts. Harvested yams are stored in yam huts, to which more customs and taboos are attached. Magic spells help preserve the yams and ceremonies accompany the filling and shutting of the yam hut. "All elderly people attest to the efficacy of past yam customs and say that because they are no longer used, disease is rife today."

Sweet potato cultivation is rapidly replacing the traditional yam gardens on Guadalcanal. Sweet potatoes are easier to grow, have less demanding soil requirements, produce more in units of ground and time, and require less work. And pigs have become a menace to the large community yam garden because they are not hunted as much anymore.

THE OTHER MAIN SOUTH PACIFIC staple was taro, especially in the Cook Islands, Fiji and Hawaii. The elephant-eared taro plant grows better than yams at higher elevations and cooler temperatures and also does well in wet, swampy soils.

Taro contains the toxin oxalic acid, so it requires special treatment. Taro roots must be peeled and cut, steeped in cold water overnight, then drained in order to render them safe to eat. The root is typically boiled, then eaten. Taro leaves are a delicacy, cooked with coconut milk and meat or fish. Communal meals prepared by women are virtually identical across Polynesia, consisting of fish and glutinous puddings of taro or manioc, all wrapped in forest leaves.

The Hawaiian Islands are home to poi, fermented taro. The Hawaiians cook the root as do other islanders, then dry and powder it, mix it with water and ferment it for several hours. Poi is slightly tart and has the consistency of heavy molasses or very heavy cream. Even today some Hawaiian families get together to make poi, a good excuse for feasting and playing cards.

THE PREDOMINANT TAHITIAN staple was breadfruit, baked whole in earth ovens, boiled and eaten in chunks, or mashed and mixed with other fruits or vegetables into puddings. According to one observer, breadfruit baked in earth ovens remained edible for several weeks.[20]

The Tahitians also preserved breadfruit by removing the rind and throwing the pulp into a heap. The mass fermented for several days in a pit lined with leaves and covered with earth and stone. The paste, called *mahi*, was eaten on its own or mixed with other ingredients. Often the fermented paste was combined with more breadfruit and other fruit, as described by an early European visitor: "Before him two servants were preparing his dessert, by beating up with water some bread-fruit and bananas, in a large wooden bowl, and mixing with it a quantity of the fermented sour paste of bread-fruit."

The impressive breadfruit tree* grew in parklike settings, creating a high canopy and producing an extreme abundance of fruit. Wrote D. L. Oliver, "The high, shady canopy and park-like settlement clearings provided by these picturesque trees charmed even the most hard bitten of the European visitors."[21] A fully-grown breadfruit weighs from two to five pounds, but can grow to weigh up to ten. When cooked, the taste of moderately ripe breadfruit is described as potato-like, or similar to freshly baked bread.

When the breadfruit was in season, the Tahitians engaged in mass bakings. At these times the whole populace ate gluttonously, the people "seldom quit the house," according to an early colonist, "and continue wrapped up in cloth: and it is surprising to see them in a month or so become so fair and fat, that they can scarcely breathe: the children afterwards grow amazingly."[22]

Gorging at feasts and at certain times of the year was common throughout the South Seas; such times of heavy eating were often preceded by a period of fasting or curtailed consumption, or followed by seasons of low food supply. Today breadfruit still serves as a staple food in many tropical cultures.

BY ALL ACCOUNTS, salt was plentiful in South Sea diets. The Hawaiians gathered salt crystals from the rocks by the sea, and preserved many types of fish with salt.

One common practice was the addition of salt water to food, or even the straight consumption of salt water, as found in this 1769 description of a Tahitian meal by colonist Sir Joseph Banks:

He setts commonly under the shade of the next tree or on the shady side of the house; a large quantity of leaves either of Bread fruit or Banana are neatly spread before him which serves instead of a table cloth, a basket is then set by him which contains his provisions and two cocoa nut shells, one full of fresh water the other of salt. He begins by washing his hands and mouth thoroughly with the fresh water which he repeats almost continually throughout the whole meal. He then takes part

---

* The breadfruit tree has many other uses. The trunk and larger branches provided timbers used in house construction, and was also used for canoe hulls. The inner bark provided the material for bark cloth, and the highly viscous resin was useful for closing canoe seams and trapping small birds. The broad leaves served to wrap foods and to cover ovens.

of his provision from the basket. Suppose (as it often did) it consisted of 2 or 3 bread fruits 1 or 2 small fish about as big as a perch in England, 14 or 15 ripe bananas or half as many apples: he takes half a breadfruit, peels of the rind and takes out the core with his nails; he then crams his mouth as full with it as it can possibly hold, and while he chews that unlapps the fish from the leaves in which they remain tied up since they were dressed and breaks one of…them into the salt water; the rest as well as the remains of the bread fruit lay before him upon the leaves. He generally gives a fish or part of one to some one of his dependents, many of whom set round him, and then takes up a very small piece of that that he has broke into the salt water in the ends of all the fingers of one hand and sucks it into his mouth to get with it as much salt water as possible, every now and then taking a small sup of it either out of the palm of his hand or the cocoa nut shell.[23]

Early visitors were amazed to see salt water fed to babies!

LIKE MANY EUROPEANS, Dr. Weston A. Price described the decimation of the healthy South Sea Islanders by infectious disease. He noted, for example, that the native population of the Marquesas, ravaged by smallpox, tuberculosis, and venereal disease, was reduced from over one hundred thousand to two thousand; during the 1930s, the population of Tahiti declined from about two hundred thousand to ten thousand.

Price noted that those islanders living on native foods suffered only 0.14 percent tooth decay, while those consuming the "foods of commerce" had at least 26 percent decayed teeth. Even remote islands produced a product that had value in the civilized world: dried coconut, or copra. In the early days, the islanders traded copra for sugar and white flour, with disastrous effects on their teeth. Long before dentists arrived to cope with the epidemic of caries, the islanders suffered from the dreadful pain of tooth decay. Abscessed teeth often led to suicide. "If one will picture a community of several thousand people with an average of 30 percent of all the teeth attacked by dental caries," wrote Price, "and not a single dentist or dental instrument available for assistance of the entire group, a slight realization is had of the mass suffering that has to be endured. Commerce and trade for profit blaze the way in breaking down isolation's barriers, far in advance of the development of health agencies and emergency relief unwittingly made necessary by the trade contact."[24]

The next generation suffered from changes in facial structure—narrower faces resulting in crowded teeth and other detrimental structural changes. Price visited a tuberculosis ward in Hawaii and noted that every patient there had dental deformities—the crowded teeth did not cause TB, of course, but Price surmised that the poor lung development that accompanied poor facial development made these young people susceptible to the often fatal disease.

Today, throughout the South Pacific, white bread, rice, cassava and crackers have largely replaced sweet potato, taro, yams and breadfruit. Canned meat, beer, sugar, soft drinks and snack foods are consumed in place of fish, shellfish, free-ranging poultry, and the fat and blood of pigs. The high-carbohydrate traditional diet of the islanders can only work when augmented with nutrient-dense animal foods, particularly foods that supply the fat-soluble vitamins A, D and K_2. If the islanders are using chemical-based sunscreen rather than coconut oil, another source of nourishment is lost.

Today, modern islanders suffer from many chronic illnesses, especially obesity and diabetes. Health officials blame the decline on Spam ("Spam at the Heart of South Pacific Obesity Crisis," said one headline[25]) and turkey tails imported from the United States, and mutton flaps imported from New Zealand, popular foods that most resemble native meat products and that seem to be the *least* likely to cause health problems. Fiji banned the importation of mutton flaps in 2000 and Samoa banned imports of turkey tails in 2007, but health officials have yet to call for a ban on soft drinks and sugary snack foods.

The decline in health accelerated during the 1960s, as described in a touching letter written to the Weston A. Price Foundation:

As a child I had an experience similar to that of Weston Price. My family spent six weeks each summer traveling to different parts of the world. Our favorite was the Pacific Islands, so I was there four times, from 1958 to 1968. In that space of time, we noticed dramatic changes in the children on the islands. My father was a gynecologist (infertility specialist) and my mother was an anthropologist/sociologist, so we noticed these things! On the last visit, when our cruise ship arrived, the crew told us we had to wait to disembark because the Sara Lee coffee cakes got off first. They told us they would be sold out of the stores within twenty-four hours.

On our first visit, the children were round-faced, with wide beautiful smiles and gleaming even teeth. They always smiled, laughed and ran around playing. By the last visit, they looked like poor Americans with pinched faces, darkened uneven teeth and sullen expressions. There was more picking on one another than playing. The South Pacific was no longer paradise. During that time, the French completely transformed Papeete, Tahiti, for their nuclear program and American Samoa was likewise changed. Even in Hawaii the same thing was evident.[26]

CHAPTER 5

Africa

The Land of Fermented Foods

D R. WESTON A. PRICE visited Africa in 1935. His journey into the interior began in Mombasa, Kenya, on the east coast of Africa, then progressed inland through Kenya to the Belgian Congo, then northward through the Belgian Congo, Sudan and Egypt.

Throughout his studies of isolated populations on native diets, Price recorded the contrast of native sturdiness and good health with the degeneration found in the local white populace, living off the "displacing foods of modern commerce" such as sugar, white flour, vegetable oils, canned foods and condensed milk. Nowhere was the contrast more evident than in Africa. In addition to their susceptibility to chronic diseases such as cancer, heart disease, intestinal problems and tooth decay, Europeans living in Africa showed little resistance to infectious diseases carried by mosquitoes, lice and flies. Price noted, "In all the districts, it was recognized and expected that the foreigners must plan to spend a portion

of every few years or every year outside that environment if they would keep well. Children born in that country to Europeans were generally expected to spend several of their growing years in Europe or America if they would build even relatively normal bodies."[1] As we shall see, the African resistance to disease observed by Dr. Price stemmed not only from high levels of vitamins and minerals in the native diet, but also from the widespread use of a variety of fermented foods.

In many areas of Africa, even today, milk and milk products provide a large portion of calories. Africa shares the practice of herding—cattle, sheep, goats, camels, water buffalo, horses, donkeys, yak and reindeer—with Europe and large areas of Asia; in all these locations, dependence on lactating herds confers an advantage in terms of health and food security. In Africa, according to Price, "It was most interesting to observe that in every instance these cattle people dominated the surrounding tribes. They were characterized by superb physical development, great bravery and a mental acumen that made it possible for them to dominate because of their superior intelligence."[2]

TRAVEL IN AFRICA was considered extremely dangerous in the 1930s. Price observed:

> Dysentery epidemics were so severe and frequent that we scarcely allowed ourselves to eat any food that had not been cooked or that we had not peeled ourselves. In general, it was necessary to boil all the drinking water. We dared not allow our bare feet to touch a floor of the ground for fear of jiggers which burrow into the skin of the feet. Scarcely ever when below 6,000 feet were we safe after sundown to step from behind mosquito netting or to go out without thorough protection against the malaria pests... Disease-carrying ticks...were often carriers of very severe fevers. We had to be most careful not to touch the hides with which the natives protected their bodies from the cold at night... There was grave danger from the lice that infected the hair of the hides. We dared not enter several districts because of the dreaded tsetse fly and the sleeping sickness it carries.[3]

Yet the indigenous Africans exhibited a very high tolerance to infectious disease including malaria carried by mosquitos, typhus and fevers transmitted by lice, and sleeping sickness borne by the tsetse fly.

Price also marveled at the low rates of tooth decay among those Africans consuming their native foods. In fact, he studied six tribes "in which there appeared to be not a single tooth attacked by dental caries nor a single malformed dental arch. Several other tribes were found with nearly complete immunity to dental caries. In thirteen tribes we did not meet a single individual with irregular teeth."[4] Yet none of these healthy groups were immune to the rapid onset of tooth decay and degenerative disease that followed the advent of modern industrial foods. Dental deformities are very obvious in modern photographs of African tribesmen.

Africa afforded Dr. Price the opportunity to compare primitive groups eating large amounts of animal foods with those following a more plant-based diet. The Maasai of Tanganyika (Tanzania), Chewya of Kenya, Muhima of Uganda, Watusi (Tutsi) of Rwanda, and the Nuer and Dinka tribes on the western side of the Nile in the Sudan were all cattle-keeping people. Their diets consisted largely of milk, meat, and blood (removed from living cattle) supplemented in some cases with fish and small amounts of grains, fruits and vegetables. These nutrient-dense diets provided large amounts of the fat-soluble vitamins Price discovered to be so necessary for proper development of the physical body and for freedom from disease. The Nuer especially valued the livers of animals, considered so sacred "that it may not be touched by human hands...It is eaten both raw and cooked."[5]

These tribes were noted for their fine physiques and great height—in some groups the women averaged over six feet tall, and many men reached almost seven feet. Examinations of their teeth revealed very few caries, usually less than 0.5 percent. Nowhere in Price's travels had he yet found groups that had no cavities at all, yet among the tribes of Africa that herded cattle and had access to fish, Dr. Price found six tribes that were completely free of dental decay. Furthermore, all members of these tribes exhibited straight, uncrowded teeth.[6]

Largely vegetarian Bantu tribes in central Africa, such as the Kikuyu and Wakamba, were agriculturists. Their diet consisted of sweet potatoes, corn, beans, bananas, millet and sorghum. They were less robust than their meat-eating neighbors in terms of physical size. Price found that vegetarian groups had some tooth decay—usually around 5 to 6 percent of all teeth, still small numbers compared to local Europeans living off store-bought foods. Even among these largely vegetarian tribes, however, dental occlusions were rare, as were degenerative diseases.

Many investigators have mistakenly claimed that Bantu groups consumed no animal products at all. However, some tribes kept a few cattle and goats, which supplied both milk and meat; they ate small animals such as frogs; and they put a high value on insects as food. Price noted that "The natives of Africa know that certain insects are very rich in special food values at certain seasons, also that their eggs are valuable foods. A fly that hatches in enormous quantities in Lake Victoria is gathered and used fresh and dried for storage. They also use ant eggs and ants."[*7] Other insects, such as bees, wasps, beetles, butterflies, moths, crickets, dragonflies and termites, were sought out and consumed with relish by tribes throughout Africa, a practice that continues in many parts of Africa today.[†8] These insects are rich in the same fat-soluble factors found in blood, organ meats, fish and butterfat.

Whether their diet was carnivorous or largely plant-based, the African groups that Price studied supplemented the diet of pregnant women and growing children with nutrient-dense foods—including liver, insects and deep-yellow butter from pastured cows—that ensured ease of reproduction and optimum growth. The Maasai and related herding tribes placed the time

* Ugandans eagerly await the annual grasshopper feast, which occurs in December. When the rains are heavy, tens of thousands of grasshoppers swarm into cities, where they are stripped of their legs and wings, then fried and eaten. In Kenya, locusts fried in butter make a delicious snack.

† For an interesting insect dish, and also a look at how thick mosquitos in Africa can be, try searching YouTube for "mosquito hamburger."

for marriage after they set fire to dry pastures preceding the rainy season, after which green grass came up for the cattle to graze. They also took pains to give every pregnant and lactating woman, and every growing child, a daily ration of blood drawn from their cattle.[9]

The healthiest group that Price studied was the Dinka, a Sudanese tribe on the western bank of the Nile.[10] They were not as tall as the Nuer groups, but Price considered them to have better proportions and to have greater strength. Like the Nuer tribes, the Dinka kept cattle, but also supplemented their diet with fish and cereal grains.* This is perhaps the greatest lesson of Price's African research—that a diet of whole foods, one that avoids the extremes of the carnivorous Maasai and the largely vegetarian Bantu, and incorporates nutrient-dense milk products, meat, organ meats, grains and seafood, ensures optimum physical development and health.

FOR AFRICAN TRIBES that did not keep cattle, getting enough fat, and even enough meat, was a challenge. Although Vilhjalmur Stefansson wrote about fat consumption among the Eskimos, he also devoted several pages of his book *Fat of the Land* to the subject of fat and meat consumption among the African tribes.

Stefansson quotes his colleague Dr. Harley, writing in 1944, who noted that:

> Meat hunger is striking and constant among the tribes I have contacted. Although meat of any kind was in great demand, the favorite cuts included brisket of beef with the fat and cartilages; hogs head, brains and fat; the liver of any animal; the hands and feet of monkeys, because of the fat content; and the skin and subcutaneous fat of a wart hog. Pig skin is never saved for rawhide and leather. It is too valuable as food, and is eaten after singeing off the hair, and prolonged boiling. Plump cow skin is similarly eaten. A lean cow skin will be saved for rawhide and leather.

"Wild meat in Liberia is seldom fat," wrote Dr. Harley. "Even the fat of wart hogs is mostly subcutaneous. Antelope are lean all the way through. Even domestic cattle are lean. Consequently, it is interesting to note that certain animals which normally store more fat than others are preferred for that reason. These included the giant rat, called 'possum'; the domestic dog, fattened by the Kpelle people especially for eating; the cow that has turned out to be sterile and so has never suckled a calf, but grown fat instead; porcupines; wart hogs; snakes; leopards in their

---

* Price reported that the Dinka consumed mostly fish and grains; however, the Dinka are a cattle-keeping people whose diet lacks milk and meat products only during the "lean" times preceding the rains and new growth of pasture.

prime, which are very plump and fat; and snakefish, prized because very fat."[11] The Africans knew the best sources of fat and specifically chose them over lean meat.

Dr. George Prentice, writing in 1923 in the *British Medical Journal*, noted that Africans "when they can get it, eat far more meat than the white people. There is no limit to the variety or the condition, and some might wonder whether there is a limit to the quantity. They are only vegetarians when there is nothing else to be had. Anything from a field mouse to an elephant is welcomed. The meat may still be warm when thrown on the ashes to cook, or it may be so old that the maggots have to be beaten out of it. Even the skin of a hippopotamus is stored away and cooked when other meat is scarce. It makes a dish something like a jelly. My native carpenter calls it 'glue.'"[12]

According to an observer in 1993, the Sudanese are always in search of fat. When a villager wants to buy an animal for slaughter, he or she looks for one major criterion—fat—which also determines the price of the animal. After killing the animal, they collect the fat, roast it to melt away most of it as suet or as a cosmetic preparation for anointing the body and the hair, and consume the remaining crunchy lipid and protein matter.[13]

An important source of fat in the African diet is palm oil, which, unlike modern seed oils, contains almost 50 percent saturated fat. The red unrefined oil is rich in carotenes; dissolved in an oil, these carotenes are more easily transformed into true vitamin A than the carotenes in fruits and vegetables.

THE INDIGENOUS FERMENTED Foods of the Sudan: A Study in African Food and Nutrition by Hamid A. Dirar, published in 1993, is hardly a bestselling book or page-turner for bedtime reading. Yet this compendium of fermented foods from Africa merits the same attention as *Nutrition and Physical Degeneration* by Dr. Weston A. Price. Dirar approaches his subject hat in hand, so to speak, with awe and appreciation for the indigenous foodways of Africa and concern about the effects of industrial food on the health of the African people.

Sudan—now divided into the northern Republic of Sudan and South Sudan—situated in the center of Africa, is a kind of mini Africa, sharing borders with nine other African countries and occupying a stretch along the Red Sea across from Saudi Arabia. Sudan has seen countless waves of immigrants over the centuries. Dirar notes that it hosts many races and cultures, "from the nearly naked to the veiled, from the Muslim to the Christian to the pagan." It contains approximately 372 tribes speaking as many as 250 languages and dialects.[14]

The dominant features of the two countries are the Blue and White Nile Rivers, which meet at Khartoum and then run north into Egypt, but more than forty other rivers and seasonal streams also traverse the Sudan. Rainfall ranges from zero to over thirty inches per year; the area contains many different types of soils and habitats, including desert, savanna, meadow and equatorial jungle.

Herodotus, Strabo, Pliny, Seneca and Diodorus all wrote about what is present-day Sudan, calling it Ethiopia or referring to the ancient Kingdom of Meroe, which dominated the region from about 800 BC to AD 350. The Kingdom of Meroe was famous for its iron industry and knowledge of metalworking. Agriculture and domestication of animals in the Sudan dates from ancient times; the people grew cereal grains* and raised cattle. Herodotus writes that the king of Meroe told visitors that his people ate milk and boiled meat and that most of them lived to 120 years of age. Strabo visited Sudan in 7 BC, reporting that its people lived on millet and barley and used grass, tender twigs, lotus and reed roots as food in addition to meat, blood, milk and cheese. Instead of olive oil, however, they consumed butter and tallow. An inscription dating from AD 350 refers to the consumption of grain and dried meat.[15]

What binds the long history and diverse people of the Sudan is the consumption of fermented foods—over eighty fermented foods nourish the inhabitants of this fascinating African microcosm. In fact, almost all foods in the traditional tribal diets are eaten in fermented form. In addition to meat, blood, grains and milk, fermented ingredients include organ meats, intestines, fat, bones, hooves, hides, bile juice, cow urine, fish, frogs, caterpillars, locusts and honey. Fermented plant foods include grapes and dates (for wine), all cereal grains, tubers, legume press cakes and wild leaves.

Many tribes strongly believe that the consumption of fermented foods protects them from disease and gives them a long life. "He who does not eat fermented foods should expect disease" is a Sudanese saying.[16] In particular, uncooked fermented foods and beverages rich in probiotic bacteria protect against infectious disease such as malaria.† Vitamin content and mineral availability increase during fermentation; fermentation also increases "shelf life" in the hot climate of the Sudan, and preserves food for times of shortage.

The Sudanese divide their many fermented foods into four categories: "staple" foods that provide a lot of calories, such as

---

* Grindstones and scrapers, indicating the processing of grains into porridges and bread, dating to 16,000 BC have been found along the Nile, thus putting the cultivation and use of grains well back into the "Paleolithic" era, which supposedly ended about 10,000 BC.

† The U.K.'s Department for International Development and the Bill & Melinda Gates Foundation will spend more than four billion dollars over five years from 2016 onward in an effort to end deaths caused by malaria. Current eradication efforts include toxic spraying for mosquitos and expensive medications that can have serious side effects. But what if an effective preventive measure for malaria has existed all along—before highly educated scientists tried to solve the problem without considering native wisdom? In Djibouti, the natives brew a partially lacto-fermented, partially alcoholic beverage from palm sap. "It is very nutritious, even for children," explains camel guide Houssain Mohamed Houssain. "You can put it in their sorghum cereal. It's full of vitamins. That way, they don't get malaria. The mosquitos bite them, but they don't get the disease."

grains and tubers; "sauces" or relishes that are eaten with the staple foods, most frequently milk and milk products, butter or ghee, but also sauces based on meat, organ meats, fish, vegetables, flavors and meat substitutes;* alcoholic beverages including beer made from grain, wine made from grapes or dates, and mead made from honey; and "special" foods for festivals and occasions such as weddings, male circumcisions, Ramadan and for traveling.[17] Many fermented foods are considered sacred, necessary for vibrant health; the one nonfermented food considered sacred is fresh milk.

Dirar argues for a cottage industry of fermented foods in Africa to improve nutrition of the poor and hungry, and criticizes the fact that fermented foods are denigrated or ignored by scientists and the elite. "Whatever their history and prehistory, fermented foods today hold a central position in the nutrition of the Sudanese. Their actual contribution to the well-being of man has never been assessed and they have been completely overlooked by the concerned agencies and individuals."[18]

SORHGUM IS THE STAPLE food of Sudan, consumed as a sourdough flatbread[†] or sour porridge, usually with a "sauce" of sour milk. Over thirty different fermented sorghum foods and beverages, the preparation of which can be complicated and sophisticated, nourish the Sudanese. Without fermentation, sorghum is unfit for human consumption, as it contains many antinutrients: tannins, phytic acid and enzyme inhibitors among them. The grain is usually fermented in water, but sometimes in sour milk.

In 1951, 90 percent of the Sudanese used sorghum as a staple. Today it is still a major African crop—and not only for food.[19] The stalks served for animal fodder, building materials, mats, thatches and fences for huts. Sorghum stalks are burned to make a product called *combu*, a potash[‡] used in food processing.[20]

In folk medicine, a type of sorghum is used to cure whooping cough (although the most widespread treatment in Africa is donkey milk). A medicine is made from sorghum roasted almost to charcoal and soaked in water; the steeping water is given to patients suffering from nausea and loss of appetite resulting from prolonged hunger. Sour sorghum paste applied to the neck serves as a cure for a

---

* This dichotomy is similar to that found in the South Seas, where "food" refers to the staple carbohydrate dish of yam, taro, sweet potato or breadfruit, always eaten with a "sauce" of meat, fish, coconut, plant foods or some combination thereof.

† To see the preparation of the typical Sudanese sorghum flatbread, visit http://globaltableadventure.com /recipe/recipe-sudanese-kisra-sorghum-crepes.

‡ Potash is a mined and manufactured salt that contains potassium in water-soluble form. The name derives from "pot ash," which refers to plant ashes soaked in water in a pot, the primary means of manufacturing the product before the industrial era. The word "potassium" is derived from "potash." In Africa, potash or *combu* is used in a number of fermented food preparations.

common sore throat. Smoked sour sorghum paste is a major ingredient in Sudanese cosmetics.[21]

There are many types of sorghum, including selected and hybrid varieties like milo and Sudan grass, used in other parts of the world and foisted on Africa as well. Some of these produce a whiter flatbread. But a variety called *feterita* is considered the best sorghum cultivar by Africans, used for fattening sheep, goats or cows for slaughter or for milk production. The Sudanese consider *feterita* as more nutritious than milo, and think its porridge is best for "fattening women."* Peasants prefer it to white-floured sorghum, and even if pressured to plant the hybrid and whiter cultivars, they still prefer the old-fashioned *feterita* for their own porridges and bread. The academic bias against *feterita* is unfounded, as the native variety tends to provide more energy and is characterized by a large variety of polyphenols.[22]

But today, according to Dirar, the Sudanese elite have turned their backs on sorghum altogether, promoting the consumption of wheat, especially as white bread, and relegating sorghum to the position of despised poor man's food. Dirar relates that one professor, upon hearing about a book that praised the use of sorghum, "felt very indignant and the next morning expressed his strong opposition to the idea of eating sorghum...as an unacceptable invitation 'to go back' after all 'the progress the Sudanese have made'—presumably as wheat eaters."[23] Wheat may confer prestige, but it is an inappropriate grain for cultivation in the arid Sudan, requiring more water and deeper plowing than sorghum.

A sour, opaque sorghum beer called *merissa* or *bouza*† is an indelible feature of the African heritage. Sorghum beer is an effervescent, pinkish-brown beverage with a sour flavor resembling yogurt, the consistency of a thin gruel, and of an opaque appearance. Most of it is homemade and consumed daily within the family circle, although a few factories in the Sudan and other African countries produce opaque beer of a lesser quality.

Brewing is a long process that first favors lactic-acid production and then alcohol production. The beverage is an acquired taste for Westerners, having a sour smell redolent of vomit. *Merissa* has an alcohol content of less than 3 percent (compared to 4 to 7 percent for clear beers), contains a large range of beneficial microorganisms, and is a rich source of easily assimilated B vitamins and the minerals copper, zinc,

---

* Porridge of sorghum and other grains helps African beauty pageant contestants achieve the ideal shape, with "a rounded, full-fleshed bottom, well-developed and in movement when the woman moves." Africans will tell you that skinny, bony models in America remind them of famine. In preparation for pageant day, African women aim to surpass two hundred pounds by eating bowls of porridge and other high-carbohydrate foods like plantains.

† One can only speculate whether the African word *bouza* and the English word "booze" have the same root.

calcium and potassium. Pellagra, a vitamin B_3-deficiency disease, is never found in persons consuming the usual amounts of sorghum beer. Since opaque beers are a fermented food, they are likely to serve as a source of vitamin K_2, although no one has tested them yet for this nutrient.

Sorghum beer or Bantu beer is a traditional beverage of the Bantu tribes, and similar beers are made in other countries, including Egypt, Ethiopia, Kenya and Zimbabwe. Kenyans enjoy three traditional opaque beers: *busaa* from maize, *chekwe* from finger millet, and *marwa* from bulrush millet.

The traditional village process begins by soaking the grain for one to two days; the grain is drained and allowed to germinate, then sun-dried and left to mature for several months. The matured grain is then steeped in water, boiled and cooled; pulverized malt is added and the brew is fermented for one day. On the second day, it is boiled again and returned to the brewing pot for more alcoholic fermentation. On days three and four, more pulverized uncooked malt is added; on day five, the beer is strained to remove husks and is then ready to drink.

Africans consider opaque beer a nourishing food rather than a beverage, even a sacred food with mystical powers. Two-day-old infants receive *merissa* from their mothers as a way to protect them from disease—a practice discouraged by missionaries. Lactating women consume opaque beer to increase milk production.

Many Africans believe opaque beers give extra strength to the blood and recommend it for anemic patients.

The colonialists dismissed the value of *merissa* and similar beverages, claiming that it made the people lazy, but in fact opaque beers are largely brewed for work and consumed in great quantities during working parties. Agricultural workers obtain 35 percent of their calorie intake from beer during periods of agricultural activity. Five pints per day is not unusual for a working man and daily beer consumption can be as high as ten pints. A traditional Sudanese saying on the building of an animal byre goes, "We, Nuer, cut the supports with beer, we cut the grass with beer, we build the walls with beer, and we erect the supports with porridge."[24]

Thin sour porridges serve as child-weaning foods in Africa, along with sour or fresh raw milk, ideally goat milk. Fresh butter is sold in some markets for feeding small babies. Another weaning food is a sauce containing fermented dry meat and dry okra powder. The mucilaginous okra in the sauce helps the child take in as much meat and thin porridge as possible. The Africans believe that porridge is not enough for the babies; they must also have milk and meat. Many African fermented meat and organ meat products are ideal for weaning foods, as they are dried and powdered and can be easily reconstituted for babies. Indeed, in Africa fermented foods are ideal for growing children; they provide better availability of nutrients, particularly iron, better protein digestibility, and antimicrobial properties. Studies show that the friendly bacteria they contain survive stomach acid and help colonize the gut. They provide a strong protection against diarrhea.[25]

Another food for children is small pieces of sour sorghum or millet dough boiled in butter.* Children eat these once or twice a week for three to five months each year. African mothers believe this food protects children against catching colds in the cool rainy season or in the winter.[26]

Maize, millet, cassava, teff, false banana, rice and black gram are other staple foods in Africa, all of which are ideally consumed in sour fermented form. Raw cassava contains many poisons and must be fermented to make it edible. The inhabitants of Congo consume bacteria-fermented cassava called *chikwangue*, similar to *lafun*, a fermented cassava paste produced in Nigeria. *Gari*, a fermented cassava food of Nigeria and West Africa, is eaten with bean flour or fish and has a decidedly sour taste. Fermented breads in Ethiopia include *dabbo*, a leavened bread made from wheat, fermented teff pancakes called *injera*, and *kocho*, a fermented food made from corn and the pulp of an Abyssinian banana plant. The fermented product is baked as bread or cooked as porridge. *Ogi*, fermented maize cake, is popular in Nigeria while the inhabitants of West Bengal make a yeast fermentation of millet called *thumba* in sections of bamboo.[27] In Ghana, the inhabitants soak peanuts, corn, millet and cassava, sometimes adding tamarind, a very sour fruit, for acidity.[28]

In the Sudan, *kawal*, a strong-smelling fermented leaf protein, is used as a protein substitute in times of famine.[29] Fermented oilseed press cake made from peanuts or sesame seeds is another popular fermented food. Fermented watermelon juice can serve as a substitute for water during dry periods.

AFRICAN FERMENTED MEAT products almost defy description—or belief! Hamid Dirar describes many unusual fermented animal foods, some of which have never appeared in the scientific literature before.

First on the list are a variety of milk products similar to buttermilk, yogurt and sour cheese. Fermented camel milk serves as a treatment for many diseases.

In Africa, meat is traditionally eaten from freshly slaughtered healthy animals,† especially for festivals, but is also

---

* The purpose of adding the dough to boiling butter is to clarify the butter and produce ghee.

† Many African groups enjoy their freshly slaughtered meat raw. Eating raw meat was—and still is—especially common in Ethiopia, where early explorers noted the consumption of raw meat cut from the flank or dewlap of living cattle; they also described a dish of raw tripe and liver cut into small pieces, seasoned with the contents of the gallbladder, and the "half-digested green matter found in the intestines of the animal."

preserved by sun-drying, smoking, salting or a combination of these techniques, usually after an initial fermentation. The Sudan has more than ten different fermented meat products, the main one being *shermout*, fermented and sun-dried meat, similar to a jerky, but which includes the meat fat. Powdered *shermout* is a frequent ingredient in sauces, soups and stews, in spite of the fact that the dried fat gives it a putrid flavor—a taste that appeals to Africans raised on it, much like the taste of strong cheese appeals to Westerners.[30]

According to Dirar, consumption of decaying animal carcasses was—and still is—common among hunters. One early colonist reported that the meat of crocodiles and hippopotami was devoured by the Nuer even in an advanced state of decomposition.[31]

A product called *miriss*, made from pure fat, is "probably the most foul-smelling fermented food in the country," reports Dirar. Even so, it is a common product for sale in marketplaces. Made with the caul covering the outer surface of the stomach of a ram or ewe, sometimes mixed with the small intestines (emptied of their contents), it is pounded to a paste, mixed with potash, and fermented for two to six days. (*Miriss* can also be made with bone marrow.) Caul fat *miriss* is a white, smelly paste with the consistency of mayonnaise and keeps at room temperature for nearly a year.[32]

The Sudanese traditionally prepare small intestines by emptying them of their contents and letting them ferment for about three days. Potash powder is added to the mix. They spread the intestines in the sun to dry, then cut them up and sell them in small bundles in the marketplace. When powdered, the ingredient can be added to a relish or sauce.[33]

Intestine balls are made by emptying the components of the alimentary track from the rumen to the rectum by pressing and squeezing. The intestines are then washed, chopped into long strips and sundried. Long strips made from other organs such as the liver, spleen, lungs, heart and kidneys are also hung in the sun to dry; during this process, they undergo partial fermentation. In about five days all the meat is dry enough to be pounded together. Powdered potash, a little salt and some water are added to the meat meal, and a paste is prepared by hand-mixing and kneading. The stiff paste is molded into rounds the size of tennis balls, then slightly flattened and allowed to dry in the sun for eight more days. The fermented intestine disks supposedly keep for months. Like the other fermented meat products, they can be powdered and added to sauces.[34]

The colon of sheep or goat stuffed with the animal's chopped small intestines and caul fat is tied up and hung in a safe place to ferment and desiccate. A common practice is to smoke this "sausage" by hanging it in the smokiest part of the house.* Smoke prevents infestation by insects, cures the surface of the sausage, adds flavor, and contributes to the safety of the product. The product resembles summer sausage or Lebanon bologna. It is usually cooked, but slices can be pounded to a powder and added to sauces.[35]

Bones, with their attendant fat, marrow, tendons and meat scrapings, are chopped, fermented, crushed into a paste, mixed with potash, and then fermented a second time. The bone paste provides yet another ingredient for sauces and can also be sundried in large balls. The Sudanese refer to these fermented bone balls as the "food of kings"! Similar products exist in other parts of Africa. The calcium-rich bones are not wasted![36]

A dish reminiscent of the *beatee* prepared by the American Indians is *um-tibay*, prepared by removing and emptying the alimentary tract of a slaughtered gazelle. The intestines, heart, kidneys, liver, spleen and all the bones except the neck bones are chopped into small bits and stuffed into the rumen. The "sausage" is tied up and allowed to ferment for about three days, then buried in the hot sands and embers of a fire and left to cook slowly overnight. The Sudanese eat the product fresh from the fire or use it to make sauces, or even as a flavoring. The sausage can also be cut into strips and sun-dried.[37]

Beirta is a festival food. The process begins with the slaughter of a fat billy goat; the lungs, kidney, liver, spleen, heart and caul fat are chopped and mixed in a pot, along with about four pounds of chopped muscle meat and a pint of fresh milk. The mixture ferments in the covered pot for four days. After the addition of a dash of salt, the mixture ferments for another three days. The finished product has a strong odor and a faintly sour taste; when stored in its fermentation pot, *beirta* does not spoil due to its high fat content. However, it is customarily used to prepare sauce for wedding feasts. Whereas a rich man can slaughter as many animals as he wants for a feast, a poor man can feed all his guests with the fermented *beirta* added to a sauce. Freshly slaughtered, one billy goat provides enough food for ten people; fermented, it can feed one hundred. The Africans argue, "How can you feed a hundred persons on the meat of only one he-goat if you do not ferment it?"[38]

Other traditional fermented foods include rabbit and whole game, caterpillars, locusts, frogs, gallbladder and bile juice, and cow urine, which is fermented for up to nine months.

Fermentation of skin, hides and hooves is still common. Today in the cities and

---

* One story describes a Peace Corps worker in sub-Saharan Africa who convinced the tribesmen to cook their food outside their huts, rather than inside as was their practice. An increase in malaria soon followed, as the smoke kept malaria-carrying mosquitos out of the huts. The tribesmen soon returned to the wise cooking practices of their ancestors. High levels of vitamin A in traditional diets provide powerful protection for lungs constantly exposed to smoke.

towns of the Sudan, boiled calf, cow, camel and lamb hooves (excluding the hard caps) are consumed by many as a delicacy. The slimy soup has a reputation as a food for bachelors.[39]

Fermented hide makes a tasty snack. Fresh hides are buried in mud for a few days to undergo fermentation, or buried in wet ashes, then cut into thin strips and dried in the sun. Powdered fermented hide is used as an ingredient for sauces as well.[40]

While Africa does not have a reputation for the production of many fermented fish products—that distinction goes to Asia—they are indeed produced in many areas, especially to preserve a seasonal fish harvest. Fish are mostly preserved by smoking, air-drying and salting, but sometimes they are fermented, especially in the Sudan. The Nuer may become entirely dependent on fish during lean months of the year immediately preceding the rainy season. Sudan boasts four major fermented fish products, as well as a fermented roe similar to a product made in Italy and Greece. One food is made of the whole intact fish. Fermented fish sauce has a horrible odor, but many consider the taste superb. Another product is a paste made from whole fermented oily fish.[41]

The lungfish emerges from the mud when the land is drying out. Fermentation in large pots preserves the bountiful harvest. The thrifty Africans recover and consume the nutrient-dense oil that rises to the top of the pot.[42]

Another fermented food consumed throughout Africa, and universally ignored by most researchers, is a paste made from dried shrimp and hot peppers. This strong, spicy condiment is a rich source of fat-soluble vitamins, especially vitamin D.

In many areas of Africa, consumption of animal protein is low; but the animal foods that are consumed—fermented organ meats and whole fish, shrimp paste, frogs, small game and insects—are extremely high in fat-soluble vitamins, which ensure that all the protein consumed is efficiently assimilated. For this reason, even in areas with low consumption of animal foods, excellent physical structure and good health predominate.*

MORE THAN FORTY YEARS after Weston Price's epic visit to Africa, Drs. Edward Williams and Peter Williams wrote of their experience treating Ugandans at the Kuluva Hospital in the West Nile district of Uganda.[43] By the late 1970s, the nomadic cattle-herding tribes had largely disappeared from the region. The inhabitants who remained were peasant

---

* Another widespread African practice is pica or geophagy—the consumption of clay, dirt or even soft stones for the minerals they contain—especially among pregnant women and growing children. Edible clay and even dirt cakes made with clay, butter or margarine, and salt and pepper can be purchased from street vendors and outdoor markets throughout Africa. Fat-soluble vitamins ensure the assimilation of minerals in dirt and clay.

agriculturists, a mixture of Nilotic tribes, whose diet consisted of grain (usually millet), cassava flour, lentils, peanuts, green vegetables such as spinach and cabbage, and bananas, supplemented with small amounts of milk, meat and fish. Williams and Williams made no mention of the widespread practice of insect consumption—a common mistake among modern investigators. Millet was "processed at the homestead." Tea had become a favorite drink and sugar was very popular, with the average daily adult intake reported to be at least 100 grams (almost seven tablespoons). Peanut oil and cottonseed oil were recent additions to the diet, replacing the more nutritious palm oil and sesame oil. Both cigarettes and alcohol were available, but used only in small quantities.

The doctors associated the local emergence of diabetes with sugar consumption. They found that high blood pressure had become more common and could usually be reduced by cutting back on sugar. Dental caries had become more frequent. But other diseases and health conditions—ischemic heart disease, constipation, hemorrhoids, varicose veins, appendicitis, thyroid problems, ulcers, arthritis, anemia and kidney stones—remained rare. The doctors believed that the native foodstuffs still protected local populations against the incursion of refined foods.

In an article on the Africans of Zimbabwe, author Dr. Michael Gelfand reported that by 1980, Western foods such as white bread, refined sugar, jam and tea had become popular.[44] These were usually eaten between the main meals, which still consisted of native foods, including stiff maize porridge, vegetable relish and some meat or fowl. Diabetes had increased but other diseases remained relatively rare. The exception was high blood pressure, which Gelfand discovered to be quite common when he began his medical practice in the 1940s. He observed that hypertension in a Zimbabwean did not seem to predispose him to coronary heart disease. Obesity was rare in Zimbabwe—whereas it was endemic among more Westernized Africans living in South Africa.

Drs. Williams, Williams, and Gelfand noted the fact that the likely culprit in the slow emergence of dental caries and diabetes was not animal fat, but refined sugar. Nevertheless, their articles form part of a collection whose editors are firmly committed to the lipid hypotheses, namely that animal products and saturated fat, not sugar, are the main contributors to the Western plagues of atherosclerosis, diabetes, hypertension and obesity. While Dr. Price's *Nutrition and Physical Degeneration* moldered in obscurity, *Western Diseases: Their Emergence and Prevention*, edited by H. C. Trowell and D. P Burkitt, received widespread attention. Price noted that all healthy African groups had good sources of animal fat, and that the healthiest groups did not consume plant foods in excess; Burkitt and Trowell, however, postulated that the increase in Western diseases among Africans is due to a reduced consumption of plant foods containing dietary fiber. The 1970s work of George Mann is conspicuously absent from *Western Diseases*. Mann studied the Maasai tribes and came to the politically incorrect conclusion that their high-fat diet did not predispose them to heart disease.[*][45]

But Burkitt and Trowell were firmly committed to the U.S. government's dietary goals, namely the replacement of animal products with grains, as a way to "prevent cancer and heart disease" and "forestall world hunger."

Based on Burkitt's work in Africa, he concluded that many Western diseases that were rare in Africa were the result of lack of fiber in the diet. He subsequently wrote a book, *Don't Forget Fibre in Your Diet*, which became an international bestseller.[†] He also argued that the natural squatting position for defecation protects the natives of Africa and Asia from gastrointestinal diseases and conditions like hemorrhoids.

In his lectures, Burkitt was fond of pointing out that the typical African stool specimen was large and soft, and that stool transit times were rapid compared to the puny hard fecal deposits and slow transit times of hapless Europeans. Burkitt's writings on dietary fiber led to calls for increased amounts of whole grains in the American diet in order to prevent colon cancer and other diseases of the intestinal tract. "Dietary fiber" soon became a household buzzword, and America embraced the oat bran fad.[‡]

What Burkitt failed to consider was the fact that grains in the traditional African diet—"processed at the homestead"—are universally fermented, making them easy to digest and contributing to the health of intestinal flora; this is the most likely explanation for the easy, soft stools that Burkitt so admired in the Africans. In fact, after soaking and fermenting them in water, the Africans generally

[*] More recently, Dr. Timothy Johns of McGill University determined that 66 percent of calories in the traditional Maasai diet come from fat, primarily saturated fat, with a cholesterol intake of more than 2,000 milligrams per day. He attributed low cholesterol levels in the Maasai to their high fitness level, consumption of various plants rich in antioxidants, high calcium intake, relatively low caloric intake, and "unknown" genetic factors. No researcher seems willing to accept the premise that the low cholesterol levels among the Maasai are due to their high consumption of stable saturated fat, rich in fat-soluble vitamins.

[†] Although one study showed that people who eat very low levels of fiber—less than 10 grams per day—had an 18 percent higher risk of colorectal cancer, the more general idea that colon cancer is a fiber-deficiency disease is now considered incorrect by some cancer researchers.

[‡] Oat bran, which is high in phytic acid, can cause numerous problems with digestion and assimilation, leading to mineral deficiencies, irritable bowel syndrome, and autoimmune disorders such as Crohn's disease. Case control studies indicate that consumption of cereal fiber can be linked with *detrimental* effects on colon cancer formation.

wet-mill the grains and pass them through a sieve. The hulls or leavings in the sieve are discarded—in other words, *the Africans throw away the bran.**

Several researchers have noted that along with sugar, tea and white flour, vegetable oils made from peanuts, cottonseed or soy have made inroads into the African diet. What these oils replace is highly saturated palm oil, which has been a staple in Africa for millennia. This means that overall consumption of saturated fat in Africa has declined, not increased. Like vitamin D, saturated fats play a role in protecting the intestinal tract from cancer and other diseases, and in preventing osteoporosis.

Burkitt claimed that salt is new to the African diet; in the same volume, however, Gelfand asserted that salt has been in common use by Africans for a long period of time. Price and others, have noted that in parts of Africa where salt is scarce, the natives burn sodium-rich marsh grasses and add them to their food. Milk and blood are naturally salty, as are dried shrimp and fish products that find their way inland from coastal areas; the ubiquitous fermented shrimp pastes are extremely salty.

DR. WESTON A. PRICE encountered many Africans who wondered about the causes of the decline in health that accompanied modernization; but few made the connection with their consumption of refined and processed foods, often introduced by the missionaries.

Many traditional African foods are for sale at the Oyingbo African International Market in Hyattsville, Maryland—shrimp pastes, fermented millet flour, palm oil, dried shrimp and fish, peanuts, vegetables, liver and calves' feet. But most of the shelf space is filled up with new-fangled foods—Bisquick, Wesson oil, Cheerios, margarine, sugar, white bread, cookies, pasta and soft drinks. Only recent African immigrants—the ones with the fine physiques and beautiful straight teeth—buy the traditional items. Younger Africans, and those who were born here, have opted for the displacing foods of modern commerce…and it shows. Modern medicine may palliate the numerous health problems that accompany such physical degeneration, but only a return to traditional foods and preparation techniques can ensure optimal health for future generations of Africans, both in America and on their home continent. Even if they have lost their taste for the strange, stinky foods of their ancestors, they can still achieve good health with the right choices of nutrient-dense and fermented foods.

---

* This is especially important for millet, the bran of which contains potent antithyroid compounds.

CHAPTER 6

Asia

Variety and Monotony

MANY HAVE WONDERED why Dr. Weston A. Price did not include Asian countries like China and Japan in his monumental cultural studies; and what he would have discovered had he done so. In answer to the first question, the major nations of the East did not fit his criteria in the 1930s—that of isolated, nonindustrialized groups whose foodstuffs were entirely indigenous, with limited foods coming in from the outside. China and Japan, while still relatively "traditional" in that time period, had a long history of trade with other nations; and both had a considerable amount of industry, even in the production of food.

However, Price would certainly have found it worthwhile to study the peoples of both nations and their neighbors, especially in light of recent controversy over high rates of degenerative disease among Western nations and the notion that China and Japan, with their low-fat, largely vegetarian diets, are relatively free of such problems. Indeed, popular books such as *The China Study* have portrayed the nations of Asia as regions in which a fiber-rich diet based on grains and vegetables offers substantial protection against cancer, heart disease and osteoporosis. Americans, they argue, should reduce consumption of meat, milk and animal fats and follow the Asian model.

CHINA IS A VAST COUNTRY with a wide diversity of ethnic groups and eating habits—and large differences between the lifestyles of rich and poor. In general, however, the Chinese recognize the relationship of diet to good health and believe that the ideal diet is one that stresses diversity and balance. Ancient texts focus on the importance of the five flavors (pungent, sour, sweet, bitter and salty); the five grains (wheat, glutinous millet, millet, rice and beans); the five tree fruits (peaches, plums, apricots, chestnuts and dates); the five vegetables (mallows, coarse greens, scallions, onions and leeks); and the five domestic animals (fowl, sheep, beef, horses and pigs).[1] Chinese tradition values meat, although not in excess, for its strengthening properties.

Chinese restaurant meals today—both in China and in the United States—are rich in animal foods, but for most of China's history, the majority of Chinese people could not afford to include much in the way of meat or fish in their diets. Herein lies the great paradox of Chinese foodways. While a fundamental feature of Chinese diets today, and back in the 1930s, was the inclusion of a wide diversity of food items—everything from pickled ant eggs to dog hams—most Chinese, especially in rural areas, traditionally consumed a diet that was limited to just a few repeated foods. A 1946 survey of rural China indicated that 88 percent of the diet consisted of cereals and legumes, with only 5 percent vegetables, 3 percent meat and fish and 4 percent fats.[2]

Animal foods in the Chinese diet, while beyond the reach of many, are characterized by great diversity. The Chinese prefer omnivorous scavenging animals such as pig and chicken to beef and lamb, although beef and lamb—and more meat in general—were traditionally consumed by the northern Chinese, a population admired for their size and strength.

If the cowboy serves as the quintessential symbol of American food culture, the Chinese equivalent is the duck-herd—the peasant farmer guiding a line of ducks with a cane.* Today, in this era of newfound prosperity, restaurants in China featuring duck are full!

Whatever the animal, the Chinese traditionally ate—and still eat—every part of it—organs, feet, tail and tongue. Packages of duck's tongues are available even in Chinese markets in America, and shoppers in Chinese Walmarts can find chicken feet, live frogs, pig faces, whole dried fish, shark heads and sheep offal.[3] Goose, pigeon, turkey, dog, frog, monkey and snake are available in Chinese open-air markets often sold live, for the Chinese put a great store on freshness. Even rat figures in accounts of traditional cuisine, and the aristocracy considered bear paw a great delicacy. Mouse testicles are popular for helping childless couples become pregnant,[4] and a fast-food chain in Beijing called Baked Pig Face serves whole pig's heads.[†5]

---

* For an example of extreme duck herding, watch the video at www.youtube.com/watch?v=0cI5Kp4CWpc.

† "Weird" Asian foods that show up on Internet sites include tarantula; "drunken" shrimp (live shrimp in a pool of strong liquor, consumed decapitated and still wiggling); fertilized eggs containing developed chicks; white ant eggs; tuna eyes; fish sperm; raw horse meat; bee larvae; bird's nest soup (the swiftlet bird makes its nest almost entirely out of its own saliva); century eggs (preserved in alkaline clay or alkaline solution); sheep penis on a stick; dried seahorses; chicken soup containing rooster penises; snake meat; shark fin soup; turtle jelly; "three squeaks" (newly born mice wrapped in seaweed); monkey brain; jellied duck blood; rat kebabs; and snake wine (wine with a snake in the bottle, presumably consumed when the imbiber has finished the bottle of wine and is sufficiently drunk). Food sold at the 2008 Olympic Games in China included starfish fried in shark oil, sea urchins, grilled snake, dog liver, goat lungs, mixed cow and horse stew, cicadas, dung beetles, silkworms, scorpions, lizard legs, dog brain soup, iguana tails and seahorses.

Insects such as flies, gnats, earthworms, bees, cicadas, beetles, crickets, silkworm cocoons, waterbugs, locusts and stinkbugs all appear in Chinese cuisine, both as food and as medicine. The Chinese also cultivate caterpillars that have become infected with a fungus that roots in the caterpillar's neck and grows upward to a height of six to eight inches. When both die, they become dry, hard and brown and are used as an ingredient in broth. Insects are a valuable source of protein and fat-soluble vitamins in the Chinese diet, especially that of the poor, but their use and importance are generally overlooked by researchers.[6]

Until recently, cooking fats included rendered duck fat or pig fat, along with small amounts of sesame oil. Traditionally vendors set up their stone grinders in the street and sold the oil immediately after extraction, so that it was fresh and healthful. Today most cooking oil is extracted in factories from rapeseed, soybeans, peanuts and cottonseed—processing that creates many toxic breakdown products.

Eggs are highly valued as brain food throughout Asia. One study found that mothers in the province of Chongqing followed a period of special feeding for the first four weeks after their baby's birth. During this period they consumed up to ten eggs per day, along with large amounts of chicken and pork.[7] The Chinese consume eggs preserved or fresh, often scrambled with vegetables and other ingredients. In the northern areas, a breakfast dish is prepared by placing a raw egg in a bowl and pouring hot soy milk over it. The mixture is eaten with a flat pancake. Sometimes a raw egg is mixed with hot rice and soy sauce.

RICE IS CHINA'S MOST IMPORTANT grain, consumed at all three meals in southern regions. Cultivation of domestic rice in China dates back eight thousand to thirteen thousand years, a practice that supplanted the use of wild rice varieties found in sites that date to the end of the Paleolithic era.[8] These findings are consistent with what we have seen in other continents—the use of wild grains as a Paleolithic food.

A 1939 survey found that adult males in the region ate almost five hundred pounds of rice per year. In recent years, rice consumption in China as a percentage of calories has declined slightly, while consumption of meat and wheat have increased.[*][9]

Surprisingly, for the whole of China, consumption of rice lags behind consumption of wheat and sorghum. Millet and wheat production dominate the more arid regions of northern China—with millet consumed principally in the form of a fluffy porridge, and wheat made into

* Rice consumption is declining throughout Asia. In 1965 in Korea, rice constituted 47 percent of total caloric intake, but had decreased to 35 percent by 1995. Likewise, in Japan in 1965, rice constituted 43 percent of total caloric intake, but had decreased to 23 percent by 1995.

noodles and bread, although in the poorest regions, wheat feeds the populace as a rough porridge. Barley, sorghum, corn, buckwheat, rye and oats constitute minor crops in China, but the total of them all adds substantially to the amount of carbohydrate food consumed by the populace.

In the distant past, rice and wheat nourished the population as whole grains or whole meal, probably after a long, slow steaming in the case of rice, or a fermentative soaking procedure in the case of wheat. Noodle production involved a period of stretching and sun-drying that amounted to a partial fermentation. Today these grains are consumed as white polished rice and white wheat flour, shorn of their valuable vitamins and minerals. But millet and the other minor grains are still consumed in whole form, as porridges, gruels or cakes. Congee, a watery porridge made from rice or other grains, is a common food, either eaten plain or with other ingredients such as meat, fish, vegetables or flavoring.

Since the end of the seventeenth century, those of the more prosperous classes have used hand grinders to remove the bran from rice, consuming the partially refined rice and giving the bran to animals, while the unpolished brown rice remained a food for the poor. Only since the advent of modern milling techniques has completely refined rice become the food for everyone.[10]

Surprisingly, we find fewer indications of fermentation of rice for food in the past than we do for other grains. A sour bread prepared from fermented rice is common in the Philippines. In China, special fermentation techniques for grains are mostly applied to wheat. A common food in northern China is *meiminchin*—wheat gluten inoculated with mold and fermented in molds for several weeks, then fermented longer after the addition of salt.[11]

In general the Chinese do not add salt to food during cooking—rice is prepared without salt, for example—but because it is used in the production of condiments and pickled vegetables, Chinese food has a salty taste, and overall salt consumption is high. Most salt is produced by the evaporation of seawater in the coastal areas so that, unlike industrially processed salt in America, it provides a rich source of natural iodine.[12] Until recently, a large black market in salt thrived in China.[13]

SOY FOODS ARE WIDELY used in China as an adjunct to—not a replacement for—animal foods. The Chinese have perfected numerous ways of fermenting soy in order to neutralize phytic acid (which blocks absorption of minerals like zinc and calcium), enzyme inhibitors (which disrupt digestion), hemagglutinin (a clot-promoting substance that causes red blood cells to clump together), and goitrogens (which inhibit thyroid function). Soy contains high levels of phytoestrogens, which can cause endocrine disruption if eaten in more than small amounts—and these estrogenlike compounds remain even after a long period of fermentation. For this reason, soy provides only a limited number of calories in Asian cuisines. Soy consumption in China in the 1930s was estimated at about 10 grams per day (two teaspoons) or 1.5 percent of total calories, compared to 65 percent of calories from pork (meat and fat).[*][14] Soy consumption is likely higher today due to the incursion of Western processed foods, most of which contain soy in the form of soy oil or soy protein.

Traditional preparation of soy milk begins with soaking until the beans become soft. The softened beans are ground into a mush on a stone grinder, using copious amounts of water. The mush is then put into a cloth bag and placed under a weight or heavy rock so that all the liquid is squeezed out. The resulting soy paste is then cooked in freshwater. Large amounts of scum that rise to the surface are carefully removed. To serve, raw egg or dried shrimp are placed in a bowl along with scallions, soy sauce, flavorings and vinegar, and the scalding soy milk is poured over. The vinegar causes the soy milk to curdle slightly. In traditional times, homemade soy milk was saved as a food for the elderly and nursing mothers in the belief that it stimulated breast milk, but was not used as a food for infants.[†][15]

Traditional tofu production in China combines fermented soybean paste with some interesting animal foods. Consider the following description in the memoir *Sounds of the River* by Da Chen, born in 1962:

Laid in the formation of a square were some of the typical Yellow Stone breakfast dishes called *muie* to accompany the rice porridge: salty baby sardines with shiny scales and popped eyes; tiny red fried peanuts, tiny because the red mountain soil compressed their growth, making them deformed and compact with flavor; and thread-thin slices of jolly blind jellyfish, the kind that swam along the warm coast with tiny little shrimps on their noses as seeing guides. Then there was the fermented tofu, so salty that I wondered where they got the salt from. As a child, I helped grind soybeans into pulp in a stone grinder and strain the pulp into

---

[*] Similarly, in the Japanese diet, 65 percent of calories come from fish. A 1975 book on nutrition published by the California Department of Health, *Nutrition During Pregnancy and Lactation*, lists soy foods as minor sources of protein in Japanese and Chinese diets. Major sources of protein listed were meat including organ meats, poultry, fish and eggs.

[†] Industrial methods for the production of soy milk leave out the all-important squeezing and skimming steps. The presoaking is shortened by using an alkaline solution. This process helps deactivate some of the enzyme inhibitors, but not the other antinutrients. The high pH value of the soaking solution results in a decrease in cystine content when the beverage is heated, thus lowering total protein availability and soy milk's usefulness as a protein source. Various refined sweeteners, preservatives and stabilizers go into the brew.

a pure, milky liquid. Mom then treated it with some recipe that transformed the mixture into the tenderest tofu. She sliced the tofu thinly and had the sun bake it into curled bricks, which she dumped into a jar filled to the brim with fish sauce. The jar was sealed with mud, and when the lid was finally lifted months later, I'd see cute little worms swimming in the salty brine…

Sun-baked and fermented tofu, eaten with nutrient-dense animal foods like sardines, jellyfish, fish sauce and worms, is a far cry from modern tofu consumed with broccoli, the various steps in its production and the accompanying foods each playing a role in neutralizing or compensating for the various antinutrients in soy.*

The real value of the soybean is that it serves as the basic ingredient in soy sauce and similar condiments, salty elixirs that give Asian food its unique character. The fermentation process for traditional soy takes six to eight months to complete. This long and careful procedure creates a mix of phenolic compounds, and naturally releases glutamic acid, that contribute to the unique taste and aroma of traditionally brewed soy sauce.[†][16]

An unsung dietary staple in China is mung bean starch, produced by an acidic bacterial fermentation that reduces the pH to about four and protects the starch granules from the spoilage and putrefaction that would occur in ground bean slurries.[17] The resultant starch is the principal ingredient in clear "cellophane" noodles.

Various types of vinegars, fermented sauces made from oysters or fish, ginger, garlic, ginseng and a wide variety of peppers and spices contribute to traditional Chinese cuisine; these, too, have largely given way to industrial preparations in which MSG allows manufacturers to cut corners and use only minimal amounts of basic ingredients.

Since antiquity, the Chinese have used a number of sweeteners including honey, rice or barley malt, palm sugar (jaggery), sorghum syrup and dehydrated sugarcane juice, but only in moderation in accordance with the guiding concept of balance. Much like the other cultures explored in this book, the modern Chinese have adopted many Western habits of high sugar consumption. A recent study found that Chinese children in Malaysia derived as much as 30 percent of their total caloric intake as sugar in the form of candy, cookies, soft drinks and other sweets.[18]

Chinese cuisine includes a large variety of vegetables, although the diet of the

---

* A 2007 television program called *A Tale of Tofu*, produced by *National Geographic*, reports that soy milk must be boiled for at least six hours to get rid of enzyme inhibitors and other "poisons" contained in the bean.

† The modern bioreactor method produces a product by rapid hydrolysis, rather than by complete fermentation, in the space of two days, and uses the enzyme glutamase as a reactor, so that the final product contains large amounts of the kind of unnatural free glutamic acid that is found in MSG.

poor can be limited to a very few, notably cabbage and various forms of radish. Sweet potato consumption is also high, especially among the poor.

Many vegetables are pickled by lactic-acid fermentation methods that provide vitamin C and valuable enzymes to a diet in which much of the other food is cooked. In his sixth-century BC *Book of the Odes*, Confucius stated, "having *yan-tsai* [salted vegetables], I can survive the winter..."

In traditional Chinese food culture, various fermentation methods accomplished the production of beers made from grains. These were opaque beverages, with a low alcohol content but rich in vitamins, minerals and enzymes, similar to opaque beers found in Africa.[19] These opaque beers have given way to modern, factory-produced, pasteurized beers. The Chinese produce dozens of types of wine and distilled alcoholic beverages from rice.* The national drink, of course, is tea. In Manchuria, fermentation of sweetened tea results in the delightful drink called kombucha, now trendy in the United States.

IN GENERAL, THE TRADITIONAL Chinese diet does not protect against cancer. The overall rate of cancer in China is comparable to that of Western nations. The Chinese have fewer cancers of the colon, lung and breast, but far greater levels of esophageal, stomach and liver cancer.[†20] Heart disease mortality is greater in the United States, but the Chinese have more reported strokes.[21] While the Chinese have made great strides in reducing the incidence of infectious disease and rates of infant mortality, these still remain major public health problems, especially in areas that are either crowded or remote. Tuberculosis and parasite infections remain common.

Of particular concern is the high rate of intellectual disability—over ten million cases in China, including hundreds of thousands with overt cretinism, especially in the central regions.[22] This is blamed on a lack of iodine, and the United Nations has called for a World Bank–financed campaign to iodize salt in China. This will help the Chinese government eliminate the thriving black market in salt, but as naturally made Chinese salt already contains iodine, it is not likely to solve the problem. Another explanation is the blinding poverty of the region, where each village sports a population of intellectually disabled individuals whose families can afford to eat nothing more than wheat porridge.

In the 1980s, a group of researchers from Cornell University carried out a massive dietary survey—the so-called China Study—covering all twenty-five of

---

* Production of rice wine in Asia goes back many centuries. The Chinese and Japanese do not use malt to transform starches into alcohol, but mold that has grown on wet cooked rice.

† One theory blames these internal cancers on the ubiquitous use of talc in rice.

China's provinces, in an effort to determine food consumption and disease patterns. This study is often cited as proof that plant-based diets are healthier than those based on animal foods like meat and milk. Study director T. Colin Campbell claims that the Cornell findings suggest "that a diet high in animal products produces disease, and a diet high in grains, vegetables and other plant matter produces health."*[23] But the Cornell survey data, when carefully studied, does not support such claims.†[24]

What the Cornell data show is that meat intake in China was highest in the western border region and very low in a number of impoverished areas centering on Sian. They found that meat eaters had lower triglycerides and less cirrhosis of the liver—and that they took more snuff—but otherwise found no strong correlation, either negative or positive, with meat eating and any disease.

Some surprising and contradictory China Study findings were associated with egg consumption, with averages of about 15 grams per day in the northernmost parts of China, about 12 grams per day in the Shanghai region, and amounts bordering on zero in the impoverished area around Sian in central China. (An egg weighs about 50 to 60 grams.) However, another study found per capita egg consumption of 50 to 80 grams per day in the northern part of China,[25] which suggests that the participants in the Cornell Study were not truly representative of the Chinese population. The China Study found a positive association of egg consumption with the consumption of meat, beer, soy sauce, sea vegetables, sugar and "other oils" and a strong correlation with university education and employment in industry. Egg eaters had more cancers of the brain, lung and bowel, perhaps because egg consumption was highest in the polluted Shanghai region. They had less cirrhosis of the liver, fewer peptic ulcers and lower triglycerides. Egg consumption appeared to confer high protection against pulmonary diseases such as tuberculosis. There was no significant correlation of egg consumption with heart disease.

Fish consumption ranged from about 120 grams per day in seacoast areas to zero in remote inland regions. Fish consumption was positively associated with consumption of sugar, "other oils," beer,

---

* For excellent analyses debunking Campbell's claims about his China Study, see articles by Chris Masterjohn, PhD, at www.westonaprice.org/book-reviews/the-china-study-by-t-colin-campbell, www.westonaprice.org/book-reviews/the-china-study-by-t-colin-campbell, and www.westonaprice.org/our-blogs/denise-mingers-refutation-of-campbells-china-study-generates-continued-debate.

† In this computer age, it is surprising—even shocking—that the original data of Cornell's China Study is not available on the Internet. The original report is a large book found only in university libraries—too large to copy the pages easily, although in the late 1990s, I was able to copy sections of relevant pages and tape them together. The report contains pages and pages of data that Campbell said "awaits interpretation" by others. The problem is that it is very hard for others to access the original data.

liquor, meat and rice and negatively associated with consumption of salt, wheat and legumes. Fish eaters had more incidences of diabetes, nasal cancer and liver cancer, but less tuberculous, infectious disease, and rheumatism. Fish eaters had lower triglycerides. The data showed no significant correlation, either positive or negative, of fish eating with coronary heart disease, but did indicate a negative correlation of fish eating with pipe smoking.

Milk consumption was zero in the vast majority of the provinces. However, in the western border region, milk consumption averaged about one quart per person per day. (Whether this figure includes fermented milk products is not specified.) The rate of coronary heart disease in the western border region was about half that of Jiangxain and Longxian, where no milk products are consumed and where fat intake is under 10 percent of total calories. Milk consumption showed no strong correlation, either negative or positive, with any disease, but there was a high correlation of milk drinking with taking snuff.

Likewise, the percentage of caloric intake from fats, as determined by a three-day diet survey, showed no strong correlation, either positive or negative, with any disease. Fat intake ranged from 45 percent in the remote regions on the western border to as low as 6 percent in the impoverished Songxian district. Not surprisingly, people who drank milk and ate meat had the highest levels of dietary fat intake. Investigators lumped fats and oils together

in the dietary recall questionnaire so that no conclusions could be drawn about the effects of animal fats such as lard and duck fat versus the effects of vegetable oils such as sesame, soy, cottonseed, canola and peanut; nor did the researchers look at consumption of organ meats or insects and concentrated animal foods like shrimp paste, all of which provide important fat-soluble vitamins in the Chinese diet. They did, however, find that the high-fat group tended to take snuff while people on low-fat diets smoked pipes.

In his introduction to the research results, study director T. Colin Campbell claims considerable contemporary evidence supporting the hypothesis "that the lowest risk for cancer is generated by the consumption of a variety of fresh plant products."[26] Yet the Cornell researchers found that the consumption of green vegetables, which ranged from almost 700 grams per day in Jingxing to zero on the western border, showed no correlation, either positive of negative, with any disease. Dietary fiber intake seemed to protect against esophageal cancer, but was positively correlated with higher levels of tuberculosis, neurological disorders and nasal cancer—perhaps because there was a strong correlation between total fiber intake and pipe smoking. Fiber intake did not confer any significant protection against heart disease or most cancers, including cancer of the bowel.

All these correlations—and they are only correlations—make clear that the

China Study does not provide us with much useful data, except perhaps on tobacco habits. This "study" is actually a survey, one that includes too many geographic and lifestyle variables to allow any conclusions as to cause and effect. Yet today, advocates of a plant-based diet invariably cite the China Study as conclusive proof that eating lots of plants and avoiding animal foods is the recipe for good health.

Given the current emphasis on soy foods, it is puzzling that the Cornell China Study researchers did not single out soy foods for study as a separate food item. Instead soy foods are lumped together with other pulses in the category of legumes. Legume consumption varied from 0 to 58 grams per day, with a mean of about 12 grams (less than one tablespoon). Assuming that two-thirds of legume consumption is soy, then the maximum consumption is about 40 grams (about three tablespoons) per day with an average consumption of about 9 grams (about two teaspoons). However, the Cornell study found that consumption of legumes was not strongly correlated with the prevention of any degenerative disease, results that cannot be extrapolated to the extravagant health claims of soy promoters, who advocate industrially processed soy products in amounts far greater than those found in the typical Chinese diet.[*] (Actually, the most important legume in the Chinese diet is not the soybean but the mung bean, which germinates into beautiful crunchy sprouts and also serves as the chief ingredient in cellophane noodles, made from mung bean starch.[†])

The Cornell researchers found a relatively strong correlation between salt consumption with esophageal cancer and hypertension. Salt eaters had higher triglycerides, but no significantly higher rates of stroke or coronary heart disease. Salt eaters ate less fish and consumed less liquor that those with lower dietary levels of salt.

The Cornell project did not take data on the amount and extent of osteoporosis in China, so it is difficult to assess claims that bone loss is rare among Asians. They did determine that dietary calcium was low in China.[‡] The many references in Chinese medicine to the use of broth for old people and pregnant women indicates that bone loss is indeed a problem. Dishes considered important for pregnant women include fish heads in broth, eggshells dissolved in vinegar, pork ribs cooked in a sweet-and-sour sauce made

---

[*] Writing in 1994, Mark Messina, author of *The Simple Soybean and Your Health*, recommended one cup of soy products per day in his "optimal" diet as a way to prevent cancer, heart disease and osteoporosis.

[†] Starch extracted by bacterial fermentation from yams, potatoes, cassava and sweet potatoes can also be used to make cellophane noodles.

[‡] The Cornell researchers also concluded that vitamin A content was low, but that may be because they did not ask questions about consumption of animal fats, organ meats, insects and other "weird" foods.

with vinegar, and pickled pig's feet prepared with vinegar and sugar. Pig's feet chopped into small pieces and cooked in rice vinegar for as long as twelve hours, then sealed in containers, are traditional gifts for pregnant women and nursing mothers. A 1978 survey of the Peking (now Beijing) area reported mild rickets in 20 percent of children under seven years of age, but rickets appear to be rare in southern China, where consumption of seafood is high.[27]

While the Cornell study, for all the millions spent on it, does not tell us much about the various effects of food on the etiology of disease in China, it does present some intriguing findings about tobacco habits. Those who consumed more animal protein were more likely to take snuff, while those who consumed more plant foods tended to be pipe smokers. Snuff takers had a higher caloric intake than pipe smokers, but total caloric intake had no strong correlations, either negative or positive, with any disease.[*] In other words, the China Study does not tell us much at all about the Chinese diet.

Proponents of plant-based low-fat diets have argued that the Chinese cannot afford to devote more land to animal husbandry. Consider, however, the fact that the Chinese grasslands, concentrated in the semiarid lands of the north and west, cover nearly 40 percent of China, an area *three times* that

under cultivation. Such lands do not support crop production but are highly suited for grazing purposes—for the production of meat and milk—and many Chinese have proposed efforts in this direction. During the 1980s, the Beijing Food Research Institute opposed any increase in beef or dairy production, opting instead for increased cultivation of valuable agricultural lands in soybeans in order to provide factory-produced, mineral-blocking, protein-poor soy-based foods as a substitute for meat to the populace.

Traditionally, the Chinese kept cattle mainly for draft purposes. However, in the early 1990s, economic reform aroused farmer enthusiasm for beef production; the rapid development of the beef cattle farming, slaughtering and processing industries soon followed. The cattle farming industry has adopted the free-range rather than the confinement model. Beef production rose from just over one million tons in 1990 to almost seven million tons. Today, China is the world's third-largest beef producer after the United States and Brazil! The increasingly prosperous Chinese nation prefers to nourish itself on beef, not soybeans.[28]

More beef is a good thing for the Chinese; the real threat is the influx of processed vegetable oils—newspaper articles on supermarkets in China show row upon row of industrial seed oils in plastic

---

[*] Researchers found an intriguing indication that hand-rolled cigarettes *protected* against cancer while manufactured cigarettes were associated with increased rates of cancer, albeit very weakly.

bottles, which the Chinese will embrace in response to Western propaganda against cholesterol and saturated fat in China's traditional cooking fats rendered from ducks and pigs.

JAPAN IS PRESENTED TO the American public as a nation benefitting from all the dietary paradigms deemed politically correct. Their diet is low in fat, high in carbohydrates from plant foods, devoid of dairy and rich in soy foods, we are told, and for this reason the Japanese enjoy the longest life span in the world, with much lower rates of heart disease, osteoporosis, and breast and prostate cancers than the United States.

These are partial truths, and the relationship between diet and disease in Japan is more complex than we are led to believe. Close examination of the traditional Japanese diet proves that, although very different from the Western diet, Japanese cuisine embodies all the principles of nourishing traditional foodways: it is rich in fat-soluble vitamins from seafood and organ meats and in minerals from fish broth and seaweed, and contains plenty of lacto-fermented foods. Japanese preparation techniques eliminate most of the antinutrients in grains and legumes. As long as the Japanese get enough to eat, their diet is a healthy diet in many surprising ways.

As in many parts of China, rice is the main carbohydrate food in Japan, consumed with every meal. For the poor, it is the chief source of calories. However,

the real basis of the Japanese diet is not rice but fish, consumed at more than 150 pounds per person per year[29]—almost one-half pound per person per day. This is about the same amount by weight as rice, but in terms of calories, fish provides a greater amount for most Japanese.

Fish consumed in Japan come from waters surrounding the island nation and from around the world. Japan imports millions of dollars' worth of shrimp, salmon, trout and tuna every year. The Japanese also enjoy carp farmed in inland waters.

The Japanese usually consume fish fresh—even delivered directly to their doors by fishmongers—but they also eat fish in salted, dried and pickled forms. Fresh fish is grilled or baked and also eaten raw as sashimi. Generally there are two fish courses at each meal, one of cold fish and one of hot.

A typical Japanese fish dish is *hoshizakana*, fish that has been marinated for twenty hours in a mixture of soy sauce and sweet white wine, then hung up to dry for one day. It is then baked and served plain, without any sauce.[30]

The Japanese value soups made of fish, including the organs and bones, as strengthening foods and good for anemia. Carp soup is the traditional food for women after childbirth. The soup, cooked for four to eight hours, contains whole carp, including the head, bones, eyes and all the organs except the gallbladder, along with barley miso and burdock root. After the birth of her child, the new mother consumes this nutrient-dense dish for four days in a row, or even longer if she has difficulty producing milk.[31]

The Japanese also eat many other animal foods including beef, pork, chicken, duck and eel. Beef consumption has climbed in recent years, some of it locally raised but much of it imported. The famous Kobe beef is tender and full of fat. The Japanese even import large quantities of beef offal.[32] Consumption of beef liver, tripe and other organ meats is commonplace. Various organ meats are on the menu at specialty restaurants. Eel served at restaurants is often accompanied with a soup containing eel innards.

Beef, pork, and chicken are usually grilled and served with a sauce that contains soy sauce along with other ingredients such as mirin (a sweet wine), sake (alcoholic rice wine), vinegar, or sugar.

Almost without exception, Japanese sauces and marinades are based on soy sauce. But it would be a mistake to call soy a "staple" in the Japanese diet, in the way that fish and rice are staples. Dietary surveys indicate that the Japanese consume an average of about one-fourth cup of soy products per day, including the ubiquitous soy sauce.[33] Other soy foods include tofu, a precipitated product, and fermented soy foods such as miso, tempeh and *natto*. Until recently, these foods were produced at home or by artisans and added in small amounts to soups or used as seasonings. *Natto* has such a strong smell that restaurants serving it have separate *natto*-eating sections so that non-*natto* eaters can be spared the overpowering odor. *Natto* is a rich source of vitamin K_2—one of the few sources in the Japanese diet.

The Japanese recognize the fact that mature soybeans need careful processing to remove naturally occurring toxins.* When they eat beans that are simply cooked, they use small red ones called azuki (or adzuki) beans. A dish of cooked rice and red beans serves for festive occasions, such as weddings and births. Red beans are also an ingredient in sweet cakes.

Japan is not a milk-drinking nation, so they say, but the statistics prove otherwise. Average consumption of dairy foods in Japan is about 186 pounds per person per year, more than the total for fish.[34] This is only one-third the amount consumed in the United States, but it is not negligible. Dairy products used in Japan include milk, yogurt, butter and ice cream. Japan has a small dairy industry but also imports milk products from Australia and New Zealand.

In general, the Japanese do not like sugary desserts. But they enjoy pounded rice (mochi) covered with sweet bean paste. Another dessert is mashed sweet potato or chestnuts covered with breading.

Noodles made with wheat flour, egg

---

* Immature soybeans cooked in salt water, called edamame, are a popular snack in Japan. The antinutrients, including isoflavones, are lower in the immature beans, but not entirely absent.

yolks and salt are an important feature in the Japanese diet; rice, mung beans, sweet potato or buckwheat may substitute for wheat. Noodles accompany chicken or duck, sometimes lobster, and often in broth.

A great variety of vegetables and fruits are on display in the shops and markets. Favorites include daikon radish, eggplant, bamboo shoots and many types of mushrooms. Most vegetables are consumed cooked, not raw. Instead of salads, boiled spinach or watercress is served cold, seasoned with soy sauce.

The Japanese diet may seem monotonous to Westerners, but the Japanese actually put a great emphasis on variety. In nutrition classes, Japanese children learn to eat thirty different foods a day, and to aim for one hundred different foods each week.[35]

A fundamental component of the Japanese diet is fish broth, made in a variety of ways. Japanese chefs take pride in developing an individual style with broths. Fish soup made from *arajiru*, the discarded portions of the fish such as the head and bones, is a common traditional breakfast food. (The breakfast eater uses chopsticks to deftly remove the meat from the head, especially the meat behind the eye, which is extremely rich in vitamin A.) Usually, however, fish stock is made with dried sardines (*niboshi*) or dried bonito flakes or powder (*katsuobushi*). In the old days, housewives purchased bonito as a block of dried fish. The block was shaved into flakes with a "shaving box," a wooden box with a thin slot lined with a blade. The shavings would fall into a drawer inside the box. When the desired amount of shavings filled the box, the capable cook pulled out the drawer and dumped the contents into a pot of boiling water. Sometimes broken-up chicken bones go into the stockpot as well. The addition of vegetables, chicken, pork, tofu or eggs transforms the broth into soup.

Dried kelp (*kombu*) and dried shiitake mushrooms are frequent ingredients in nourishing Japanese broths. The mushrooms are placed in a pot of water and removed just before the water comes to a boil, then replaced by dried sardines or bonito flakes.

Egg consumption in Japan is higher than in America (forty pounds per person per year, versus thirty-four in the United States).[36] The Japanese consider eggs a brain food.* Eggs are consumed as omelets and custards and in soups. They are also an important ingredient in noodles and batters.

Another brain food in the Japanese diet is seaweed, which is added to soups, served as a vegetable, and used for wrapping sushi. Agar-agar, a gelatinlike

---

* My late colleague Mary Enig knew a Japanese woman whose husband was killed during World War II. She had an infant son, and throughout the years following the war, she gradually sold off all her furniture to provide her boy with one egg per day "so that he could go to college." The boy grew up to be an intelligent child and, in fact, did go to college in the postwar years.

product used extensively in Japan, is derived from seaweed. Seaweed provides an abundance of minerals, particularly iodine, which is so vital for normal thyroid function—which, in turn, is vital for normal brain function. Most likely, it is the presence of adequate iodine in the traditional Japanese diet that makes it possible for the Japanese to consume goitrogenic (thyroid-depressing) soy products on a daily basis without adverse effects.

The Japanese have traditionally used a variety of fats and oils in their cooking. In the past, delicious tempura—vegetables and fish dipped in batter and then deep-fried—went into a vat of hot sesame oil, rapeseed oil, whale oil, or rendered lard or beef tallow. Today, the Japanese are more likely to fry in cheap commercial vegetable oils, but lard is available at grocery stores in squeezable bottles, and beef fat and lard grease the skillets in the better restaurants. Use of shortening and margarine is rare.

Since World War II, the pattern of lipid intake in Japan has changed markedly. A threefold increase in the intake of saturated and monounsaturated fatty acids is a reflection of increased prosperity, which has allowed the Japanese to enjoy foods more interesting than fish heads and rice. Unfortunately, with the advent of cheap vegetable oils and processed foods, the Japanese diet has seen an increase in omega-6 fatty acids and a reduction of omega-3 fatty acids—just as we have in the United States. In a milestone review published in 1997,[37] Japanese investigators blamed the increase in cancer, heart disease, inflammatory disease such as asthma and allergies and even behavioral problems in Japan not on increases in saturated fat but on increases in omega-6 vegetable oil. According to the researchers, "Decreasing the n-6/n-3 ratio of foods is recommended for the suppression of ageing, carcinogenesis and atherosclerosis. This is because n-3 fatty acids suppress but n-6 fatty acids stimulate ischaemia/inflammation which causes increased free radical injuries. We suggest that a relative n-3 deficiency as evidenced by the very high n-6/n-3 ratios of plasma lipids might be affecting the behavioral patterns of a significant part of the younger generations in industrialized countries." The Japanese are willing to acknowledge the adverse effects of vegetable oils, but in America, the blame still goes to saturated fats.

Fermented vegetables in the form of pickles accompany all traditional Japanese meals. They range from pickled cabbage to eggplant to daikon radish. Pickled foods are an important adjunct to a diet that includes raw fish because they help protect against intestinal worms, which can be a frequent problem in Japan. One folk custom is to consume pickled daikon radish with sushi and sashimi to "neutralize toxins." Daikon radish is one of the best vegetables for supporting the growth of protective lactobacilli.

A typical recipe for pickling lettuce, cucumber and turnip calls for sprinkling the chopped or sliced vegetables with salt and allowing them to stand for about two days.[38] This combination is eaten as a separate course with rice. Pickled melon, prepared by covering melon slices with sake and mirin and sprinkling them with salt, stands for five days before serving as the last course of a meal.

An interesting fermented fish product called *kusaya* comes from the island of Izu. Mackerel and similar fish are soaked in a brine or "*kusaya* gravy," which was used over and over again because salt was a rare material. After soaking, the fish was dried. In the unused period, the "gravy" was kept alive by adding just one fish fillet. *Kusaya* is distinguished from other dried fish by its strong, unique, peculiar odor. "If you broil *kusaya* in your house, the odor will not leave for three months," say the Japanese.[39]

The typical Japanese dish of sushi originated with *funazushi*, a type of round shellfish from Lake Biwa in the Shiga prefecture of Japan. The shellfish was cleaned, salted, washed and fermented for four to twelve months. During fermentation, *funazushi* develops several kinds of organic acids such as lactic acid, acetic acid, propionic acid and butyric acid, all of which contribute to its distinctive sour taste and peculiar odor. The pickled crustacean was sliced and served on rice. In former times, those who could enjoy *funazushi* received recognition as gourmets. Once an important dish in the area around Lake Biwa, the catch of shellfish is decreasing year by year due to water pollution, introduced species and shoreline destruction, thus making *funazushi* a rare and expensive food.

The main fermented drink in Japan is a rice drink called *amazake*, prepared by boiling a block of malted rice until it becomes soft and drinkable. Salt and sugar are added to taste. In the winter, *amazake* is available from vending machines.*

All meals in Japan are served with a weak green tea, made with one teaspoon of tea to six teacups of water. Black tea, coffee and milk are also common beverages. Whole milk is available to schoolchildren and is recognized as a healthy food, one that helps Japanese children grow taller than their ancestors.

The Japanese have interesting ideas about beverages. On a hot day, most Japanese people, especially older Japanese, prefer hot green tea to anything cold. They say they want something the same temperature as their body, or that something cold will make them sweat more. In wintertime, they often add ginger to warm drinks, as ginger is said to be a warming food. The Japanese believe that drinking water is likely to make you fat![40]

---

* Surprisingly, this fermented milk drink is sold in Japanese vending machines right next to Coke or Pepsi. Unfortunately, the first ingredient listed is sugar.

Beer is a common beverage, and also recognized as one that causes weight gain. Sumo wrestlers, who can weigh as much as five hundred pounds, put on weight by consuming large quantities of beer, as well as lots of rice and a nourishing stew called *chankonabe*.

While the Japanese diet is held up as the paradigm of natural eating, Japan is also home to the world's quintessential imitation flavor: monosodium glutamate (MSG). Originally extracted from seaweed, MSG activates glutamate* receptors on the tongue and tricks the body into thinking it has eaten meat. Today most of the world's MSG is produced through a chemical process by Ajinomoto, a Japanese company, and is no longer derived from natural sources.

MSG is used to make cheap soy sauces, thus driving out artisanal producers who traditionally took great care and up to three years to produce the delicious fermented elixir. Factory-produced soy sauce can be turned out in the space of three days and contains, besides neurotoxic MSG, many carcinogens.

MSG was the main flavor for Japanese rice rations during World War II, and it is said that Americans who loved the taste of these rations helped introduce the flavoring into the United States. Today it flavors almost all processed foods, including those manufactured in Japan. Yet health-conscious Japanese recognize the dangers and search for the label "No MSG" on more expensive noodles and processed foods.

Many Japanese also recognize the dangers of McDonald's and other fast foods that are making inroads in Japan, and they deliberately adhere to traditional foodways. Some home cooks still make all traditional foods by hand, from *amazake* to miso. Typical of foods still produced by traditionalists and artisans are various preparations of the famous umeboshi plum. The plum trees grow in the region of Mito, in Ibaraki Prefecture, where a park is home to two thousand plum trees, attracting three million visitors per year. Each year thousands of Japanese women gather the famous *umeboshi* plums to make all sorts of delights, including salty pickled plums. Well-aged pickled *umeboshi* plums are a great delicacy— some of them are fermented for as long as thirty years!†

The manner in which the Japanese present their food is always attractive and distinctive, usually with handsome serving dishes and a great sense of proportion

---

* Glutamic acid is an essential amino acid that comes as part of animal proteins and is also present in certain plant foods, such as wheat, soy and seaweed. In this form, glutamic acid is not generally harmful, but essential to health. However, in MSG and related products, the glutamic acid is in "free" unbound form, and it is this form that causes problems such as insomnia, headaches, neurological disease and achy muscles and joints in many people.

† Other plum varieties are also used for salted pickled plums.

and harmony, and often with elaborate ceremony. On ceremonial occasions and at banquets, a number of bowls and dishes are set before guests so they may have a wide choice. Leftovers are carefully packed in decorated boxes and presented to guests when they leave.

Even lunch boxes—called bento boxes—are an art form in Japan, containing beautifully arranged foods such as large shrimp, rice rolled in seaweed, fish and pieces of fruit. One company in Japan prepares as many as fifty thousand of these lunch boxes per day.[41] Many Japanese mothers get up very early to make lunch boxes containing neatly arranged portions of fish, meat, rice balls, pickles and fruit for their children and husbands.

The Japanese suffered greatly before and during World War II. There were many food shortages, particularly of fats and animal foods. Tuberculosis was common. Many Japanese lived almost entirely on rice during the war.

It was during the postwar years that the American researcher Ancel Keys wrote his famous Seven Countries Study in which he included groups from the Japanese districts of Tanushimaru and Ushibuka. He noted that the Japanese in these two regions had very low levels of serum cholesterol, consumed a diet extremely low in saturated fat and cholesterol, and had low rates of coronary heart disease. It was primarily this Japanese data that allowed Keys and others to conclude that

consumption of saturated fat and cholesterol caused heart disease.

Critics have pointed out that Keys omitted from his study many areas of the world where consumption of animal foods is high and deaths from heart attack are low, including France—the so-called French paradox. But there is also a Japanese paradox. In 1989, Japanese scientists returned to the same two districts that Keys had studied. In an article titled "Lessons for Science from the Seven Countries Study,"[42] they noted that per capita consumption of rice had declined, while consumption of fats, oils, meats, poultry, dairy products and fruit had all increased. Between 1958 and 1989, protein intake rose from 11 percent of calories to about 15 percent and fat intake rose from a scanty 5 percent to over 20 percent. Mean cholesterol levels increased from 150 mg/dl in 1958 to 188 mg/dl (still low) in 1989. During the period, mean body mass gradually increased, with the percentage of the population that was overweight rising from 8 to about 13. High blood pressure became more common, while the percentage of smokers decreased from 69 in 1958 to 55 in 1989.

During the postwar period of increased animal consumption, the Japanese average height increased three inches and the age-adjusted death rate from all causes *declined* from 17.6 to 7.4 per 1,000 per year. Although the rates of hypertension increased, stroke mortality *declined* markedly. Deaths from cancer also *went down* in spite of the consumption of animal foods.

The researchers also noted—and here is the paradox—that the rate of myocardial infarction (heart attack) and sudden death did not change during this period, in spite of the fact that the Japanese weighed more, had higher blood pressure and higher cholesterol levels, and ate more fat, beef and dairy foods.

Misconceptions about the state of health in Japan abound. It is true that the Japanese have lower rates of cancer than the United States, although they are by no means cancer-free.[43] Japanese have low rates of lung cancer (even though they smoke far more than Americans) and low rates of breast, prostate, reproductive, colon and rectal cancers compared to the United States, which is attributed to the fact that they consume more soy and less meat, fat and dairy than Americans. But cancer rates went down in Japan during the period when consumption of animal foods went up. And the Japanese actually consume far less soy than Americans, because even today, they do not consume much soybean oil or many foods containing isolated soy protein. In fact, the most likely explanation for high levels of breast and prostate cancer in the United States compared to Japan is the high levels of altered and damaged fats from industrially processed seed oils in American convenience foods.

Fresh fish, rich in vitamin A and omega-3 fatty acids, is one component of the Japanese diet that protects them against lung cancer. A study carried out at the Cancer Centre Hospital in Aichik Mapan looked at the diets of more than four thousand healthy people and another thousand with lung cancer.[44] They found that both men and women who ate large amounts of fresh fish were significantly less likely to develop lung cancer. A diet that included salted or dried fish in place of fresh fish did not confer the same protective qualities.

The Japanese suffer from very high rates of stomach cancer, and relatively high rates of cancers of the pancreas, liver and esophagus, the so-called "Asian types" of cancer. There are many explanations for this trend, none of them proven. As with the Chinese, the most common theory blames the use of highly salted foods such as soy sauce and salted pickled vegetables. But other dietary components are equally suspect, including high levels of irritating talc present in white rice and carcinogens in modern processed soy sauce. A final explanation—one not accepted by mainstream science—is the widespread use of microwave ovens by modernized Japanese. Japan was the first country to adopt the microwave, which seemed to many a safer and more sensible way to cook food in tiny Japanese kitchens than the old-fashioned gas burner or stove.[45]

Japan has many lessons to teach us about

the risk of generalization in scientific studies. All claims about heart disease in Japan should be viewed with skepticism because the Japanese consider it shameful to die of heart disease but honorable to die of stroke.[46] Predictably, deaths reported on Japanese death certificates as due to stroke are much higher than deaths reported as due to a heart attack.

Japanese women do not suffer from hot flashes, we are told, but some investigators believe that hot flashes are "underreported," due to the shyness of Japanese women. Soy food promotion material states that "there is no word for hot flashes in Japan" without acknowledging the fact that there is no word for hot flashes in English, either. We use two words to describe the condition, and it is likely that Japanese women use some sort of euphemism.

Another claim is that the Japanese do not suffer from osteoporosis. But according to a 1998 study carried out by the Tokyo Institute of Gerontology,[47] Japanese women have much higher rates of osteoporosis than American women—one in three versus one in eleven. Furthermore, they found that bone mass deterioration begins much earlier in Japanese women, at age twenty versus age thirty-four in the United States.

According to the statistics, the Japanese have the longest life span in the world. Built into those numbers is a very low rate of infant mortality compared to the United States. Japan was one of the first countries to practice widespread birth control; the Japanese deliberately keep their families small. Great care and attention is lavished on children, starting with the mother's diet during pregnancy, and outright poverty in Japan is rare. When the high infant mortality rate in America is discounted, American men have life spans equal to those of Japanese men and American women live a little longer than Japanese women.[48]

In his doctoral thesis about coronary heart disease in Japanese emigrants, British physician Dr. Michael Marmot described another Japanese paradox.[49] Dr. Marmot discovered that when the Japanese in Hawaii maintained their cultural traditions, they were protected against heart attacks, even though their cholesterol increased as much as in Japanese emigrants who adopted a Western lifestyle and who died from heart attacks almost as often as did native-born Americans. The most striking aspect of Dr. Marmot's findings was the fact that emigrants who became accustomed to the American way of life, but preferred low-fat Japanese food, had heart disease *twice* as often as those who maintained Japanese traditions but preferred high-fat American food.

Dr. Marmot proposed the theory that certain factors in the traditional Japanese culture protected the Japanese from heart attacks *in spite of* a high-fat diet. He noted that the Japanese place great emphasis on group cohesion, group achievement and social stability. Members of the stable Japanese society enjoy support from other members of their society and thus are protected from the "emotional and social stress" that Marmot believed to be an important contributing factor to heart attacks. The Japanese traditions of togetherness contrast dramatically with the typical American emphasis on social and geographic mobility, individualism and striving ambition, said Dr. Marmot.

But is life less stressful among the traditional Japanese? "Group cohesion" and "group achievement" can also translate into unrelenting pressure and stress. Is the traditional Japanese family man, striving to perform and bring honor to his family, under less pressure than the Westernized Japanese bloke who has decided to chuck it all and hang out on the beach? And is the Japanese American living under America's wide-open skies, where opportunity abounds, under more pressure than his relatives in Japan, where opportunities are fewer and where crowding is commonplace? The Japanese people, including schoolchildren, work long hours, travel miles to school and work, and often have only one day a week free. The pressure on children to do well in school is intense, and the suicide rate among Japanese young people is among the highest in the world.

What Dr. Marmot's study really tells us is that increased animal fat in the Japanese diet protects them from heart disease *in spite of* their stressful lifestyle, not the reverse. High rates of heart disease among Americans should be blamed on processed foods based on industrial seed oils, not animal fats and a high-stress lifestyle.

Researchers espousing the dogma that saturated fats cause disease have consistently ignored evidence showing that saturated fats actually protect against heart disease and cancer. The many studies of the Japanese also ignore two very important sources of saturated fat in their diet.

One of these sources is Spam, the canned pork product provided to American soldiers during World War II. Americans may have loved the taste of Japanese rice rations, but the Japanese loved our rations even more. Spam provided exactly those dietary components that had been missing through the years of poverty and privation—animal protein and fat. In a nation with a history of resistance to foreign influence, Spam immediately became popular as a snack food. *Spam musubi* consists of a slice of Spam soaked in soy sauce on top of a bed of rice and wrapped in seaweed—a convenient morsel resembling sushi. *Spam musubi* sells at local convenience stores, including 7-Eleven stores, in Hawaii. In fact, Spam consumption in Hawaii is higher than total Spam consumption in all the other forty-nine states *combined* due to its popularity among Japanese Americans.

The other source of saturated fat in the Japanese diet is, surprisingly, white rice, a refined carbohydrate that the body efficiently turns into saturated fat. As long as the diet is rich in fat-soluble vitamins from fish and organ meats, and minerals from broth and seaweed, white rice can be consumed without adverse effects. In fact, for the Japanese eating a traditional diet, it is beneficial, providing the substrate for saturated fats that the diet may lack. Macrobiotic proponents claim that the traditional Japanese diet was based on whole brown rice, not refined white rice. It is said that the first samurai ate brown rice while the rest of the nobility ate white rice. Then the samurai slowly "softened" and started eating white rice. But the true explanation for the use of white rice may be somewhat different. Brown rice that is not soaked and fermented, as was done traditionally in India, may block mineral absorption and cause intestinal problems. The Japanese prefer the taste and texture of white rice, and this preference may reflect a profound intuition that when rice is consumed on a daily basis, it should be refined, not whole, unless a long and careful preparation is observed.

The challenge for the Japanese, like the challenge for all countries in the process of modernization, is to resist the temptations of processed foods. But Japan faces an additional challenge, and that is to resist the advice of meddling American health researchers who are telling them to eliminate vital components of their traditional diets—beef, pork, lard, tallow and even white rice. Better to pay attention to a few problematic additives such as MSG, talc in rice and impurities in salt, and to protect artisanal food production

from the cutthroat policies of the food processing industry. And one more piece of advice to the Japanese: throw out the microwave.

THE FOOD OF KOREA holds special interest in today's climate of political correctness, for while Korean cuisine is heavily influenced by China, it differs in one important respect—a reliance on beef as the main source of meat. Pork is the main meat of China, and fish serves as the preferred meat in traditional Japanese cuisine; Koreans eat plenty of seafood and pork, as well as some chicken, but the distinguishing characteristic of this Asian diet is the frequent use of beef. Consumption of beef is more common among the affluent who typically eat beef several times per week; the less-well-to-do consume more pork.

Beef consumption and preparation in Korea reflects a historical Mongol influence. A popular beef dish in Korea is one of the fattiest cuts—beef short ribs—prepared with a spicy sauce; or thinly sliced flank steak or brisket, marinated in a sauce made from toasted sesame oil, garlic, onion, sugar, pepper and soy sauce and broiled on a small charcoal grill. Skewered beef, ground beef, boiled beef and salted beef feature prominently in Korean cookbooks—along with recipes for offal including liver, tongue and tripe. A popular hors d'oeuvre or snack is dried beef, similar to beef jerky. Thinly sliced beef is marinated in a spicy sauce made from soy sauce, garlic, ginger and toasted sesame oil and dried in the sun or in a very low-temperature oven. Beef is also frequently eaten raw.

Since 1970, consumption of live-stock products such as meat in Korea has increased almost fivefold, while consumption of rice has declined. Korean farmers raise over two million head of Korean native cattle per year, mostly on small farms owning just a few steers. As beef consumption has increased with recent prosperity, so have imports; today less than half of all Korean beef comes from domestic cattle; much of the rest comes from the United States.[50]

Whatever the animal, the Koreans eat every part of it. Eating chicken means eating the meat, skin, gizzard, liver and feet—chicken feet roasted in spicy sauce is a popular side dish to accompany alcoholic beverages. All parts of the pig are used, including head, intestines, liver, kidney and other internal organs. The Koreans enjoy their pork steamed, stewed, boiled and smoked—they especially enjoy grilled fatty pork belly. Korean stews can include just about any kind of meat or organ meat, even blood sausage and Spam.

Another important source of protein in Korea is dog meat—even as late as 2006, dog meat was the fourth most commonly consumed meat in South Korea.[51] Korean tradition views dog meat as a kind of health tonic rather than a dietary staple.

Koreans enjoy seafood of every type, including shrimp, oysters, squid, crab, clams, abalone, snapper, cod, perch and whiting. Fish and shellfish are steamed or eaten raw. Nutrient-rich shrimp sauce, made of tiny preserved shrimp cured in salty brine, serves as a flavoring, and small dried shrimp are added to many dishes.

Eggs find their way into the Korean diet as egg custard, egg batters and egg pancakes, and not separately as a breakfast food. In fact, Koreans eat the same foods for breakfast, lunch and dinner.

With postwar prosperity, Koreans have increased their consumption of both fish and flesh. By the late 1990s, meat consumption in Korea was 88 pounds per year and fish consumption 110 pounds per year—that translates to over one-half pound of animal protein per day. At the same time, rice consumption has declined while consumption of bread and noodles has increased.[52]

In the pre-modern era, barley and millet were the main staple grains of Korea, along with wheat, sorghum and buckwheat. Rice is not indigenous to Korea but was introduced from China during the Three Kingdoms period (57 BC to AD 668); as imported rice was expensive, most Koreans stretched it with other grains—consuming rice with barley and rice with beans. The Koreans have preferred white rice since its introduction. Rice serves as the main ingredient in cakes and beverages as well as cooked down into congee or gruel.

Typically, Koreans prepare rice by soaking it overnight—a practice we have not seen in other Asian countries. The next day, the rice is brought to a boil, cooked for about a half hour, and then gently steamed for several hours. Rice shows up in various types of rice cakes, which are colored white, green and pink, or mixed with nuts and other seeds, and sold as convenience foods. "Five-grain rice," a combination of glutinous rice, black beans, sweet beans, sorghum and millet, often replaces plain rice at family meals. Additional carbohydrates are provided by potatoes and sweet potatoes; noodles made from wheat, buckwheat, sweet potatoes, mung beans or rice; or from various types of dumplings and cakes.

Traditionally the Koreans fermented, roasted or malted grains before turning them into dumplings and noodles— Korean markets carry wheat malt flour, barley malt flour, fermented soybean flour, roasted five-grain powder and potato starch, all of which are easier to digest than flours made with whole grains and legumes that have not been properly prepared to neutralize phytic acid and other antinutrients.

Soybeans play a minor but important role in Korean cooking, as soy sauce, as tofu or bean paste added to soups as a thickener or mixed with eggs. Mung beans are an overlooked staple, ground and made into a porridge, as an ingredient in pancakes, or fermented to extract the starch for cellophane noodles. These are consumed with a variety of ingredients including vegetables and blood sausage.

The Koreans eat vegetables with every meal, including radish, cabbage, cucumber, potato, sweet potato, spinach, bean sprouts, scallions, chiles, seaweed, zucchini, mushrooms, lotus root and lots and lots of garlic. A unique feature of Korean cuisine is its emphasis on wild roots, wild mushrooms and fern shoots, gathered from the forests and mountainous areas. Koreans also frequently consume seaweed, particularly kelp, which is an excellent source of iodine and trace minerals.

Enzyme-rich fermented foods accompany every meal, principally as kimchi, a spicy condiment made from cabbage, radish, cucumber and fermented fish or shrimp sauce. In the summer, Koreans still make kimchi every day. In the autumn, the whole family joins in to make winter kimchi, which is stored in large earthenware jars and buried in the ground so that just the mouth of the jar protrudes above the surface. South Koreans eat an average of forty pounds of kimchi per year.

Korea boosts a bewildering variety of fermented condiments such as pickled cucumbers, garlic, fish, crab, squid, anchovies, jellyfish, shrimp and many flavorful fermented sauces and pastes made from fish, shrimp, red beans and soybeans. These combine with typical seasonings, including red and black pepper, cordifolia (an herb of the mallow family), mustard, schisandra,* garlic, onion, ginger, leek, scallion and delicious toasted sesame oil, with its unique smoky taste.

Sesame oil is the chief oil used in Korean cooking, although meat fats are used for cooking noodles. Wild sesame oil, also called perilla oil, rich in omega-3 fatty acids, is not used for cooking but consumed by the spoonful as a health food, or mixed with raw egg.

On the whole, Korean cuisine is low in fat compared to that of China. Chinese food is characterized by the stir-fry technique and the use of rich sauces. The Japanese eat many things raw or deep-fried, but most Korean dishes are grilled or prepared as stews.

Medicinal foods include ginseng, chicken, black goat, abalone, eel, carp, beef bone soups, pig kidneys and dog. A soup of beef broth with added kelp and rice is considered an important dish for pregnant women.

As we have seen in the South Seas and in Africa, the centerpiece of any Korean meal is the staple carbohydrate food, such as rice or other grains; everything else is a side dish (called *banchan*)† or a soup or stew (which are not *banchan*).

A distinguishing feature of Korean cuisine is the use of bone broth. Most meals begin with soup based on a mineral-rich broth made from long-simmered beef bones, sometimes with the head and intestines included in the pot. Korean stores carry powdered bone and fish powders to facilitate the process of making broth. Dried anchovies along with kelp form the basis of a common fish stock. The addition of vegetables including radishes, cabbage and mushrooms, as well as meat, tofu, seafood, rice, noodles and spices turn broth into a soup.

Banquet chicken broth from the period of Korean kings (lasting until the end of the nineteenth century) calls for five chickens, five abalones, ten sea cucumbers, twenty eggs, half a bellflower root, mushrooms, two cups black pepper, two peeled pine nuts, starch, soy sauce and vinegar.

Korea is famous for *seolleongtang*, a broth made of beef bones to which slices of beef brisket, rice and noodles are added. *Seolleongtang* may be eaten at the beginning of a meal, but it also serves as a popular snack food, eaten morning, noon and night, and available at numerous mom-and-pop-style cafés—the Korean equivalent of McDonald's, the difference being that the fast food of Korea, produced by traditional methods, is actually good for you!

In general, Korea is not a tea-drinking nation. In the old days, the water in China

* *Schisandra chinensis* (also known as magnolia vine, Chinese magnolia vine, or chinensis) provides the "five-flavor-fruit," berries that taste salty, sweet, sour, pungent (spicy), and bitter.

† A different kind of side dish is *anju*, which might be described as macho hors d'oeuvres to go with alcohol. These include steamed squid, peanuts, shellfish, octopus, pork belly, and chicken feet marinated in fermented shrimp sauce.

and Japan required boiling in order to make it fit to drink—and tea was added to make the hot water palatable. Korea, however, was blessed with pure mineral water that did not require boiling, so widespread tea drinking did not take hold. Today, ginseng is often used as a base for herbal drinks, and as a hot drink. Other hot drinks feature roasted barley, cinnamon or lemons. A variety of punches made from peaches, strawberries, cherries, lemons, pomegranate seeds and persimmons can be found in Korean cookbooks. One popular beverage is sweetened and fermented rice water. Korean alcoholic beverages include a weak medicinal wine brewed from rice, and a stronger distilled beverage made from grain. Often flowers or fruits are added to these brews to produce plum-ginger wine, magnolia wine, hundred-flower wine and chrysanthemum wine.

An opaque Korean "beer" called *makgeolli* or *takju* reminds us of similar beverages from Africa. Also called "farmers' alcohol," the milky, sweet beverage is made from rice and has an alcohol content of 6 to 7 percent. Production involves using mold grown on wet rice as a starter, rather than malting, and fermenting the mashed rice for about a week. In addition to alcohol, *takju* contains enzymes, lactobacilli, lactic acid, amino acids and B vitamins. Folk medicine in Korea values this opaque beer for boosting metabolism, relieving fatigue and improving the complexion.

Despite the impact of the West on South Korea, and its embrace of industrialization, traditional Korean cuisine has changed relatively little. Like the French, the Koreans take food very seriously. Koreans believe that the happiness of a family depends on the quality of food served in the household. For Koreans who have emigrated to the United States, the ties to their native diet are less strong. While Korean markets in the United States are filled with a huge variety of Korean foods, from fresh seafood to fermented condiments, they also sell bread, cakes and pastries made with white flour and industrial seed oils. Candies made with sugar and high-fructose corn syrup take up far more shelf space than traditional sweets based on grains, seeds and honey or malt syrup.

The challenge for Koreans in their homeland will be to remain faithful to their traditional diets, while increasing the amount of animal foods, particularly animal fats, available to the poor, and reducing carcinogens in their environment and food supply. The great challenge for Koreans in America will be to resist adding sugary, devitalized foods to their healthy traditional cuisine.

THE FOODS OF THAILAND do not fit the low-fat, high-fiber, largely vegetarian paradigm said to protect us against disease. There's no denying that the delicious, spicy cuisine of Thailand is rich in saturated fat from coconut oil and lard, relatively low in fiber, and features many and varied animal foods. Yet a 1962 comparison of autopsy reports on a group from Bangkok with a group from the United States found that coronary occlusion or myocardial infarction was eight times more frequent in the United States, diabetes was ten times more frequent, and high blood pressure about four times more frequent.[53] Even more intriguing is the fact that Thailand has a very low rate of cancer compared to other countries around the world; in 1996, Thailand rated fiftieth in frequency of cancer compared to other nations.[54] Today, Thailand is not even listed among the fifty nations where cancer rates are the highest.[55] Here is yet another paradox—like the French paradox or the Japanese paradox—that the "experts" would rather ignore than explain.

"Thai cooking is an art form," writes Pinyo Srisawat in *The Elegant Taste of Thailand*,[56] and as anyone who has frequented a Thai restaurant knows, a particularly delicious art form. Mouth-watering curries and soups made from chicken or fish broth, creamy with whole coconut milk, offer the palate a variety of delicious spices and flavors, including coriander, anise, cumin, nutmeg, lemongrass, chile, ginger, turmeric, basil, mint, garlic and lime. Seafood is plentiful in the Thai diet, including fresh saltwater and freshwater fish, mackerel, shrimp, crab and eels, along with salted fish and dried fish. Fermented fish sauce and shrimp paste are popular seasonings. Pork and beef are consumed by those who can afford them, often raw or pickled. Other animal foods less likely to feature on restaurant menus, but consumed in the villages, include duck and chicken and their eggs, water buffalo, and more unusual items like snails, caterpillars, lizards, frogs, rats, snakes, squirrels and other small animals.

Plant foods include eggplant, onions, cabbage, baby corn, mushrooms, kale, mustard greens, radish, celery, cucumber, lettuce, several varieties of vegetable gourd, water chestnuts and swamp cabbage, which grows in ditches and rice paddies. Fruits include plums, tamarinds and bananas. Two plant foods are particularly associated with Thai cuisine. One is the kaffir lime (*Citrus hystrix*), with a distinctive wrinkled skin. The rind and leaves give a wonderful flavor to soups and curries. The other is bitter melon (*Momordica charantia*), of which there are several varieties. Bitter melon looks like a lime-green elongated cucumber with a furrowed, convoluted rind. The pulp is very bitter—an acquired taste for Americans—but the Thais are fond of it and believe it has potent healing qualities.*

Soy foods play a minor role in Thai

---

* A small variety of *M. charantia* grows wild in the southern United States, where some rural African Americans used it as a potent medicine, calling it *cerasee*.

cooking. Bean curd is a common ingredient in soups, while fermented soybeans, soybean paste and soy sauces serve as flavorings. The Thai consume other legumes in larger quantities, such as black beans and mung beans, either sprouted or as an ingredient in sweets. Yard-long beans and winged beans serve as vegetables.

Overall, the traditional Thai diet uses sweeteners sparingly. Unrefined cane sugar or palm sugar go into desserts made from coconut, fermented glutinous rice and bean pastes.

Thai dishes are always served with rice. In fact, the generic term for anything served with rice is "not rice." Long-grain, nonglutinous rice is favored in the central and southern parts of Thailand, while sticky or glutinous rice is the mainstay in the northern and northeastern regions of the country. With few exceptions, the Thais use polished white rice. Fermented glutinous rice flour features in noodles, cakes and other products.

In the early 1950s, as a kind of practice session for the larger China study (which began in 1983), a group of investigators from Cornell University made a detailed survey of food habits in Bang Chan, a village in the rice-growing region twenty miles northeast of Bangkok.[57] According to their surveys, about four-fifths of calories came from rice in prosperous households as well as those less well-off. A few families still consumed home-milled rice, a method that removed most, but not all, of the bran and other nutrients. The vast majority, however, took their rice to a local machine mill which returned the product to them in the form of thoroughly refined white rice. Although the machine mills are relatively new to Thailand, the practice of hand-milling or home pounding seems to date from ancient times, and was carried out even though it involved a good deal of work. If brown rice was ever used in Thai cooking, the memory of this custom is buried in antiquity. The bran or polishings from hand-milled rice go to chickens and other livestock, and were never consumed by humans. In fact, one peasant explained to the investigators from Cornell that the reason he continued to hand mill, when machine milling was readily available, was that if he took his rice to the local mill, the miller would keep the polishings for himself, and rice bran made excellent chicken feed!

According to the Cornell study, common protein foods for the villagers of Bang Chan included fish—mostly freshwater fish raised in ponds—some pork and eggs. The researchers admitted that the villagers used lard for frying. Chicken and other fowl were foods for feast days. The meat of water buffalo was available when a buffalo became too old to work, and dried beef paste was also used as a flavoring in cooking. The Cornell researchers did not discuss what was done with the internal suet and slab of back fat from the older buffalos that were butchered. The amounts can be considerable—one animal may yield well over one hundred pounds of valuable suet and tallow. We never learn what happens to the voluminous organs and intestine of the culled cow, but it is reasonable to assume they were not thrown away.

Other animal foods enjoyed by the villagers included turtles, snails, eels, frogs, cobras and other snakes. Field rats, available all year long, were roasted. In general, the villagers prepared their own fermented shrimp paste and sauce. Many families grew herbs and bananas in kitchen gardens, but few vegetables. Instead they gathered swamp cabbage from the canals, or purchased vegetables.

Given the emphasis on white rice in the Thai diet, it was not surprising to find that one of the country's chief health problems, particularly among the poorer families in the villages, was beriberi, a vitamin B–deficiency disease. The Cornell investigators were obliged to note that those families who did not suffer from the disease ate more animal foods, particularly beef, which they could afford to purchase. Ironically, those families with few chickens ate more eggs because those with numerous fowl sold their eggs in the market.

The Cornell investigators noted that overall intake of protein, vitamins and minerals among all but the poorest villagers seemed adequate, with the exception of calcium, although there were few signs of calcium deficiency except for short stature. Probably calcium levels were higher than those measured in staple foods, due to the use of bone broths in soups and unshelled shrimp in shrimp paste.

The other major health problem in Thailand is that posed by parasites and other pathogens in drinking water, and overall conditions deemed unsanitary. The Cornell investigators noted that "untreated water was the customary beverage with meals. Ordinarily no distinction was made in the source of drinking water for children and adults, although boiled water was given to mothers and infants to drink during the post-partum rest period."

The investigators noted that during the monsoon season, rain caught in tubs provided water for drinking and washing. Stored rainwater may be relatively clean, but overall conditions make germ-conscious Westerners squirm. During the rainy season, high water flooded the ground in Bang Chan but "caused time-consuming inconvenience only in the earth-floored cottages where it was necessary to keep the rice stores and chickens dry, move the cookstove, and either build plank walks or cook standing ankle deep in water."

When the supply of rainwater ran out, villagers drank water from the canals, rice paddies and fishponds. In general, there were no sewage plants or garbage collection systems in the villages—all garbage and human and animal waste went into the fields and waterways. Given the fact that until recently, most Thai people—and their livestock—consumed water that can only be described as filthy, and that both animal and plant foods serve as hosts to numerous parasites and pathogens,[58] it seems miraculous that the entire nation did not succumbed to food- and water-borne illnesses. On the contrary, most Western tourists express amazement at the sight of healthy, smiling children swimming in the murky waters of Bangkok's canals.

The answer lies in the protective factors inherent in the traditional Thai diet. Pickled garlic, onion and peppers, consumed frequently as condiments, inhibit the development of parasite eggs.[59] The practice of fermenting pork and other meats kills the larvae of the trichinosis organism.[60] Native maklua berries are an effective treatment for hookworm.[61]

But the most protective factor in the Thai diet—and one most ignored by investigators back in 1950—is the lauric acid found in coconut products. Coconut oil contains almost 50 percent of this twelve-carbon saturated fat, which the body turns into monolaurin, a substance that efficiently kills parasites, yeasts, viruses and pathogenic bacteria in the gut.

Coconut oil provides additional benefits: it strengthens the immune system; it promotes optimal development of the brain and nervous system; it protects against cancer and heart disease; and it promotes healthy bones. Finally, coconut oil seems to be the best fat for ensuring the proper uptake of omega-3 fatty acids into the tissues.[62] This may explain the beautiful, velvety skin tone of the Thai people. Tiny dried shrimp sautéed in coconut oil and formed into a cake is typical of Thai dishes that are both delicious and nutritious—rich in vitamin D,

calcium, high quality protein, omega-3 fatty acids and protective saturated fats.

The Cornell investigators claimed that the Thai diet was low in fat—about 15 percent of calories was the consensus among "experts." Most of this fat was saturated coconut oil or relatively saturated lard. Poor families used watered-down coconut milk for curries, and lard very sparingly. But more affluent families ate pork and beef frequently, made their daily curry with luscious thick creamy whole coconut milk, and used coconut oil or lard for cooking.

It can be argued that even among poor families, fat consumption was higher than the accepted 15 percent figure. The Cornell investigators made their own determinations of the amount of fat supplied by coconut milk, because "use of figures now available in food value tables, for coconut milks as prepared in Bang Chan, would lead to gross overestimate of caloric value and fat content of the diets." In other words, the researchers changed the fat value of coconut milk in order to get the low 15 percent total fat demanded by the "experts." What an amazing confession!

In an effort to improve the health of Thai villagers, medical workers over the years have encouraged the boiling of water, consumption of whole rice or rice polishings, and the use of industrial polyunsaturated oils—known to depress the immune system—instead of healthy coconut oil and lard. It is probably impossible to install Western-type sewage systems in the soggy Thai rice lands, and also unwise in that such systems would deprive the land of valuable manuring. A more rational—and certainly more effective—approach would encourage protective traditional foodways and higher prices for cash crops, so that this nation of subsistence farmers could afford more fish, meat and coconut milk to balance their intake of rice.

It seems unlikely that the Thai will accept brown rice—and probably foolhardy as well, given that phytic acid in rice bran blocks calcium, already low in the Thai diet. Instead, millers could receive subsidies to return rice polishings to farmers, and farmers could be encouraged to eat more vitamin B-rich eggs from chickens given rice bran.

The body stores the carbohydrates from white rice as fat. Thus, white rice may be a vital factor in the diet if overall fat consumption is low. But with white rice as the basis of Thai cuisine, it is imperative that "not rice" foods be rich in nutrients from adequate amounts of animal foods grown on mineral rich soils, seafood and, above all, healthy, protective coconut oil.

ASIAN CUISINES FEATURE many exotic ingredients and strange animal foods that Westerners may find unacceptable. But the underlying principles mirror those of every other healthy traditional diet: the recognition of animal foods as important for health, a preference for foods rich in fat-soluble vitamins, and the use of bone broths and fermented foods. The one variance from the other diets we have looked at so far is the widespread use of white rice, rather than whole-grain rice that has been soaked or fermented. But as we have seen, in the context of a diet that is very rich in nutrients, the body can make this refined carbohydrate into the saturated fat that is otherwise lacking in the diet. For Westerners who blanch at the thought of eating all those weird, nutrient-dense foods, eating a lot of white rice may not be such a good idea.

CHAPTER 7

Europe

The Foods We Like to Eat

THE EARLIEST WRITTEN recipes date from around 1600 BCE in the form of Sumerian tablets from the Tigris and Euphrates river basin in present-day Iraq—about forty recipes contained in 350 lines of text.[1] Irrigation allowed the intensive cultivation of grains and other crops in the fertile alluvial soil that nourished this cradle of civilization; date palms flourished in the southern areas and livestock, mainly cattle and sheep, populated the grassy steppes.

The best-preserved tablet contains twenty-five brief recipes; of these, four are vegetable broths and twenty-one are meat stews made from fresh beef, organ meats (intestines, stomach, spleen), venison, gazelle, goat, lamb, mutton, salted meat, pigeon and francolin (a large game bird).

Some of the recipes have added blood, or call for marinating the meat in blood before cooking. All have added vegetables,

especially garlic, leeks and onion, and a variety of herbs, especially cumin and coriander. And, most important, all but one call for the addition of fat—that would be highly saturated lamb fat a practice still followed today in Iraq and other areas of the Middle East. As explained in a cookbook for Iraqi cuisine, "dissolved fat from sheep tail…was important not only for flavor but because it helped raise the boiling temperature, which allowed for a more tenderizing process for tough cuts of meat."[2] A second tablet gives seven recipes for various types of domestic birds and game, some of which are lined and topped with a bread crust, like a potpie!*

We also know from these ancient texts that the Sumerians prepared many types of sour bread and porridge, made sour milk products and cheese, and manufactured a vast array of beers from barley and other grains. Many of the stews

---

* Interestingly, all seven recipes call for parboiling the birds first, before simmering in fresh water. This preliminary step ensures that you get a clean broth, free of scum particles and unpleasant smells.

139

feature a kind of sweet-and-sour gravy containing vinegar and honey; fermented fish sauce, the universal seasoning, is another frequent ingredient. We find the same practices in Roman cooking, which features elaborate sauces flavored with a variety of herbs, vinegar, honey and fish sauce served at banquets for the rich.

Whether they were rich or poor, fat was no less important to the Greeks and Romans than it was to the Sumerians. The *Iliad* makes reference to fat bulls, fat goats and pork meat "rich with fat." From Book XIII we read, "Verily our kings that rule Lykia be no inglorious men, they that eat fat sheep, and drink the choice wine honey-sweet." Sea urchins, cockles, sturgeon, fattened peacocks, crocodiles, cicadas and grasshoppers—foods rich in fat-soluble vitamins—all had a place in the diet of ancient Greeks.[3]

In the Roman Empire, fat was an ingredient in the peasant's simple breakfast porridge, made from emmer (a type of wheat), salt, water and fat. The Roman soldier's rations consisted of bread or porridge, a lump of pork fat, cheese and sometimes salt-cured pork (prosciutto) or sausage (salami).[*4] The typical Roman citizen ate pork, seafood (including fish roe), poultry (including fatty goose and duck), lamb and cheese; beef was reserved for temple sacrifices and the banquets of the ruling classes. Vegetables like cabbage and greens were often preserved in large crocks, the prototypes of sauerkraut.[†]

We see similar practices today in Iran and other parts of the Middle East, where sheep's cheese, sour milk products and stews provide nourishment for all classes. A typical soup made from lamb's head is simmered until the meat is tender and can be stripped from the skull. The brains, eyes, tongue and cheek meat float to the top of the pot, to be skimmed off as the main dish, with the broth served separately.[5]

The influential eleventh-century Persian philosopher and scientist Avicenna (AD 980–1037), author of *The Book of Healing* and the five-volume *Canon of Medicine*, recognized the relationship between sound dietary practices and good health. Avicenna's seminal works lauded the virtues of nutrient-dense animal foods, including yogurt cultured from raw milk, bone broth, and meats and organ meats from veal, lamb and goat.[‡6]

Typical throughout the Middle East

---

* A medieval document, *The Four Seasons of the House of Cerruti*, recommends pork fat and lard for young boys, women and "anyone else who has soft flesh; by contrast, beef fat suits laborers, hoers, harvesters, and all those whose flesh is hard constitutionally or because rough living has conditioned it."

† The Roman writers Cato (in his *De Agri Cultura*) and Columella (in his *De Re Rustica*) mentioned preserving cabbages and turnips with salt.

‡ Avicenna observed that milk should come only from "animals that have been fed from the most nutritious plants in a wide area" and also noted that "boiling the milk will make it rancid for the temperament of human beings."

is a product called *kishk*, a mixture of sprouted cracked wheat, mixed with sour milk, allowed to ferment for several days, dried in the sun and then reduced to a powder. Added to boiling water, *kishk* and similar products make an instant soup; added to stews, *kishk* serves as a convenient thickening agent.

Until industrialization wrested food processing from the hands of the artisan, we find the same dietary principles throughout the Middle East, Russia and eastern and western Europe: a variety of meats and poultry, including the bones and organ meats, most often cooked in a cauldron to make a nourishing soup or stew; seafood including shellfish and fish of all types, often salted, smoked or preserved in fat;* grains made into sourdough bread or sour porridges; milk consumed fresh, soured or made into cheese; cured pork, pâtés, terrines and sausages containing organ meats; vitamin B–laden beers, some of which provided lactic acid and lactobacilli as well as alcohol; fermented vegetables like sauerkraut,

a source of digestive enzymes, friendly bacteria and vitamin C; and salt, widely available from the British Isles to the borders of Asia.†

This diet provided everything the body needed for good health when times were good; during periods of famine, war, and disease, the people—mostly the peasantry—suffered greatly. For example, excavations show that around the year 1000, the people of the British Isles were strong and well formed, with excellent teeth. After that, the health of everyone, even the nobility, declined. Archeologists can pinpoint waves of plague in skeletons that are shorter and more frail.[7] In times of famine, or even during the "hunger gap" before the next harvest, the peasants ground beans, peas, beechnuts, acorns, roots and even bark to supplement flour. The desperate gathered up poppies, hemp and darnel (a weed that harbors a toxic fungus) to make a kind of cake called "crazy bread," resulting in mass hallucinations and hysteria.

The Italian historian Piero Camporesi

---

* Salmon was so abundant in England in the Middle Ages that apprentice boys sometimes rioted in protest at the amount of salmon their employers fed them; subsequent legislation prevented employers from feeding salmon to their servants more than three times a week.

† "The Social Influence of Salt," published July 1963 in *Scientific American*, notes that in Europe, most salt was obtained from low-lying flatlands at the ocean's edge, where seawater flowed into natural or diked pans and then was evaporated by the action of the sun. Tracing old shorelines shows the level of the sea during various time periods. At the height of the ancient Greek and Phoenician civilizations, the sea level was more than three feet lower than it is today. For about a thousand years, salt-making in solar pans and peat marshes flourished in the Mediterranean, the Atlantic and the North Sea. But the seawater was rising. By AD 500, the ocean was more than six feet higher (three feet higher than it is today), a change that wiped out the salt pans. The covering of the salt pans corresponded with the Dark Age of Europe—it eliminated an important source of wealth and commerce and resulted in reduced health and intelligence of the population; only as the sea level became lower again and salt more available did Europe recover, about AD 1000. In the British Isles, salt was available from inland salt springs, so the effects of rising seas were mitigated.

gives the following description of peasant lives in Italy:

> The masses of the pre-industrial era—suffering from protein and vitamin deficiencies, poorly protected from the attacks of infectious diseases by precarious and inadequate diets, tormented by shingles (particularly widespread in the areas of rye consumption), subjected to sudden attacks of convulsions and epilepsy, the deliria of fevers, the festering of wounds, ulcers which ate away at the tissues, unrelenting gangrene and disgusting scrofula, the crazed patterns of "St Vitus's dance" and other choreographic epidemics, and the constant nightmare of worms and choleric diarrhoea—also suffered the harmful effects of "ignoble" breads, the toxic deliria of impure flour mixtures, and the stunning, demented stupidity and dullness of food poisoning.[8]

Yet when food was abundant, good health was the rule, even into the twentieth century. Dr. Weston A. Price, who began his studies in the early 1930s, made haste to visit any remaining examples of "primitive" European groups before they disappeared. In fact, he found only two isolated European populations: Swiss villagers living in the remote Lötschen Valley in the Alpine regions of the Vaud, and Gaelic islanders living off the coast of Scotland in the Outer Hebrides. By practicing "accumulated primitive wisdom" in regard to their local foods, both groups exhibited excellent health, immunity to tuberculosis, straight teeth and freedom from tooth decay.[9]

The isolated Swiss villagers grew tall and strong on a diet of raw dairy products—raw milk, raw butter, raw cream and raw cheese—from their cows and goats, which grazed on lush Alpine pastures, along with dense sourdough rye bread. Nothing came into their villages from the outside except salt; they ate meat about once a week, usually veal, including the organ meats. Bones went into the soup pot, along with seasonal vegetables from their gardens, but their dietary staples were dairy foods and grain, a fact that challenges the primary tenet of the paleo diet, namely that good health can be achieved only by avoiding dairy foods and grains.

The inhabitants of the Isle of Lewis in the Outer Hebrides raised no livestock on their windswept island, nor could they cultivate gardens or even trees. Instead they consumed seafood and shellfish of all types, including the heads, organ meats and oil. They lived in thatched cottages with no chimneys, but suffered no lung disease in spite of their smoky environment.

They also managed to grow oats in the thin soil by spreading the smoke-blackened thatch of their cottages onto their fields in the spring.* The other important plant food was seaweed. A typical dish, considered very important for growing children, was fish heads stuffed with oatmeal and chopped fish liver. Often, the fish heads were further "ripened" for two days or more, as the Scots considered fresh fish to be "harsh." For additional "high" flavor, the good Scots housewife rolled the fish heads in a cloth and stuffed them in the crevice of a stone wall.†

THE MENU FOR A MONDAY morning breakfast served in honor of King James I's visit to the northern English town of Preston in August of 1607 read as such: *Pullets; Boiled capon; Shoulder of mutton; Veal roast; Boiled chickens; Rabbits roast; Shoulder of mutton roast; Chine of beef roast; Pasty of venison; Turkey roast; Pig roast; Venison roast; Ducks boiled; Pullet; Red deer pye cold; Four capons roast; Poults [young chickens] roast; Pheasant; Herons; Mutton boiled; Wild boar pye; Jiggits of mutton boiled; Jiggits of mutton burred [buttered]; Gammon of bacon; Chicken pye; Burred [buttered] capon; Dried hog's cheek; Umble pye; Tart; Made dish.* Dinner the previous evening featured thirty dishes for the first course and twenty-seven in the second.

Travelers of less exalted station did not find such elaborate banquets at the end of their day's journey, but nevertheless expected a variety of meats for their evening meal. John Byng, a guest at the White Swan Inn at Middleham in 1792 made the following inscription in his diary: "I now felt a haste for dinner, and this is a description of it: Cold ham; A boiled fowl; Yorkshire pudding; Gooseberry pye; Loyn of mutton roast; Cheesecake."[10]

Further north, in Scottish manor houses, large breakfasts were the norm. The following description of an eighteenth-century Highland breakfast appears in the novel *The Expedition of Humphry Clinker* by Tobias Smollett: "One kit of boiled eggs; a second, full of butter; a third, full of cream; an entire cheese made of goat's milk; a large earthen pot, full of honey; the best part of a ham; a cold venison pasty; a bushel of oatmeal, made into thin cakes and bannocks; with a small wheaten loaf in the middle, for the strangers; a stone bottle full of whiskey; another of brandy, and a kilderkin [half a barrel] of ale."

The French geologist Barthélemy Faujas de Saint-Fond noted that a 1784 breakfast served at the house of Maclean of Torloisk on the Isle of Mull included "plates of smoked beef, cheese of the country and

---

* Dr. Price planted oats in several samples of soil from the Isle of Lewis, adding various types of fertilizer. Only the soil to which the black thatch had been added supported the growth of mature oats.

† The small shark called skate is very tough, but Lewis Islanders hung them up in the air, unsalted, until they became gamey. Visitors described the fermented skate as an acquired taste but "a most excellent breakfast."

English cheese, fresh eggs, salted herrings, butter, milk and cream; a sort of *bouillie* of oatmeal and water, in eating which, each spoonful is plunged into a basin of cream; milk worked up with the yolks of eggs, sugar, and rum; currant jelly, conserve of myrtle, a wild fruit that grows among the heath; tea, coffee, three kinds of bread (sea biscuits, oatmeal cakes, and very thin and fine barley cakes); and Jamaica rum."[11]

Starting with the Elizabethan era, a time of increased prosperity in Britain, animal foods of every description served as the basis of the British diet for all but the poorest, from game—including deer, beaver, boar, pheasant and heron—for the aristocrat to domestic animals—including beef, veal, lamb, mutton, pork, rabbit, chicken, pigeon, turkey, goose and duck—for the less privileged. The diet also included organ meats such as liver, kidneys, tongue, calf heads, sweetbreads, brains, heart, ears and feet. *The English Housewife*, written during the early part of the seventeenth century, contains recipes for "puddings of a calf's mugget [entrails]" and "roast cow's udder."[12] Umble pie, made from the entrails, or umbles, of deer, was a peasant food—the nobleman kept the muscle meats of the deer he hunted,* while the umbles went to his huntsman and servants. Tripe (cow's stomach) formed an important part of the diet, especially among the poor. Organ meats began to go out of fashion, particularly among the upper classes, during the Victorian era, but even today tripe is still sold in specialty shops in some parts of the British Isles.

Various sorts of puddings—black pudding, kidney pudding, marrow pudding, blood pudding, suet pudding and so on—also supplied nutrient-dense organ meats and fat to the English diet. These puddings came to the British Isles from the Romans, who made *ur*-puddings by stuffing minced meat, fat and organ meats along with blood, salt, spices and other ingredients into an animal's intestines.[†] Sometimes these puddings were then smoked. At some unknown date, the animal intestines were replaced with a pudding cloth and puddings came to be distinguished from sausages, smaller versions still encased in animal intestines.[‡] Later, sweet things like raisins found their way into these puddings, resulting finally in the Christmas pudding, containing sugar, breadcrumbs, dried fruits and suet. In some parts of the British Isles, these Christmas puddings still contained meat as late as the early 1800s.[13]

Of course, the most famous "pudding" of all is the Scottish haggis—still enjoyed

---

* Typically, venison hung in the lord's larder for six weeks before the cooks considered it ready for consumption.

† Homer's *Odyssey* mentions grilled goat stomach stuffed with blood and fat.

‡ Germany boasts almost fifteen hundred varieties of sausage.

today—made from finely minced organ meats mixed with oats and aged or fermented in a sheep's stomach, According to the 2001 English edition of the *Larousse Gastronomique*: "Although its description is not immediately appealing, haggis has an excellent nutty texture and delicious savoury flavor."[14]

Beef, pastured on lush Irish grass, predominated in Ireland. "Flesh they devour without bread," wrote an observer in 1570, and of course dairy products of many types. "They drink whey, milk and beef-broth."[15]

Seafood for fast days (which amounted to almost half the days of the year) included trout, turbot, sole, whitebait, carp, cod, mackerel, anchovies, cockles, mussels, oysters, eel and crab. Salmon was brought in fresh from the northwest of England to the London markets. According to the novelist Daniel Defoe, "This is performed with horses, which changing often go night and day without intermission, and, as they say, very much outgo the post, so that the fish come very sweet and good to London." Fresh shellfish were available in season in the largest towns, particularly near the seacoast. Oysters were a favorite snack food consumed at the Elizabethan theater. However, inhabitants of inland smaller towns had to content themselves with preserved seafood, such as pickled or salted oysters. Oysters, being cheap, were a favorite food of the poor. "Poverty and oysters always seem to go together," observes Sam Weller in Dickens's 1836 novel *The Pickwick Papers*.

Scots cuisine features a number of recipes for fish livers. According to F. Marion McNeill in her 1929 cookbook *The Scots Kitchen: Its Lore and Recipes*, "The livers, which must be perfectly fresh, make a rich and nourishing stuffing. (Cod liver is richest in oil.) In Shetland, where they are much used, a special utensil called a pannabrad…is used for melting fish livers, and the oil obtained is stored for winter use."[16]

Dairy products added richness to the diet and, unlike meat and fish, were available to those on the lowest rungs of the social ladder. Until the twentieth century, most peasant families owned a cow, or a cow and a goat. "Why, sir, alas, my cow is a commonwealth to me," says a rustic character in the Elizabethan play *A Looking Glass for London and England*, "for first, sir, she allows me, my wife and son, for to banquet ourselves withal: butter, cheese, whey, curds, cream, sod [boiled] milk, raw milk, sour milk, sweet milk and buttermilk."[17] Eggs were used liberally in omelets, puddings and pastries.

Without refrigeration and cookstoves, food storage and preparation presented challenges to families and innkeepers alike. Fortunately, the salt needed for preservation was plentiful in England. Cattle were brought into the market towns in September and October. The beef was salted and then hung up and preserved by smoking. Pork was likewise both salted and smoked to make bacon and ham. For poorer families, these were practically the only meats available during the winter months. Fish such as cod was also preserved by salting or, in the case of salmon, by pickling in salt brine, and transported in tubs to the larger markets. Another preservation method was "potting," in which shrimp and smaller fish such as trout were placed in small containers and covered with butter or other fat mixed with spices.*[18]

Dinners in the houses of the gentry could be elaborate affairs, with roast meats and "made" dishes—elaborate concoctions featuring dozens of ingredients, including a variety of spices. Chefs for the great lords often used a *cullis*, a stock made from large quantities of meat and bone cooked in water over a long period to extract all the goodness, after which the meat and bones were discarded, leaving a rich broth that served for sauces and "made dishes."[19]

But most English households lacked ovens and utensils necessary for complicated dishes. Food preparation was achieved by slow boiling in pots hung over the hearth fire; the Christmas turkey or goose required carrying to the baker's for roasting. This meant that soups formed the mainstay of peasant diet, prepared by boiling bones, meat, organ meats and vegetables in a pot over the fire. Soups were known either as "running" or "standing" pottages. A running pottage, or broth, was a thin soup containing bits

of meat, vegetables and herbs in season. A standing pottage was thickened with bread crumbs or grain until it was similar in consistency to a present-day mousse.[20] Sausages could be cooked on a grill or in a skillet—or even speared with a stick and held over the fire. Preparation of haggis-like pudding—purchased from the butcher—was a simple matter of seething it in a pot over the hearth fire, resulting in a dish that was satisfying, nutritious and easy to prepare—a kind of Shakespearean takeout.

As for grains, rye, barley and oats were staple crops, made into coarse gruels or cakes. Oats and other grains were prepared as porridges or "frumenty" by soaking in warm water for twenty-four hours. Butter or cream along with honey or sugar made them palatable.[21] A Welsh recipe for *llymru* reads as follows: "Mix oatmeal with sufficient buttermilk and water to make a liquid consistency. Leave for 2 nights then rinse through a hair sieve. Let it stand and pour off the surface water. Simmer for 40 minutes and keep stirring. Serve with sweet milk."[22]

Oats and barley were also made into cakes, often cooked on a griddle. Before baking soda made its appearance in the middle of the nineteenth century, such cakes would have been prepared using a sourdough starter, and allowed plenty

---

* Further north, the Icelanders preserved shark by burying it in the ground for several months. Restaurants in Iceland still serve rotten shark, known as *hákarl*.

of time to rise. In the north, dough made from oats was "clapped and driven out as thin as paper on a round board, then transferred to a round iron plate of like size and baked over the coals." Such "clapbread" was crisp and wafer-thin, like modern-day crackers, the perfect accompaniment for butter and cheese.

The Scots prided themselves on kiln-dried oats. According to the 1920 article "Gastrologue," which appeared in *The Scotsman Magazine*, "A good miller knows just what samples of grain to select, just how long the process of drying in the kiln requires, just how to set the stones for the correct shelling and grinding of the cleaned and dried oats. The method of kiln-drying is somewhat more arduous than the modern method of mechanical drying, but it is to the kiln that we owe the delectable flavor of the best oatmeal."*[23]

Farmers who grew their own oats but sent them to the local mill to be threshed, winnowed and ground into meal also received in return a bag of *sids*—the inner husks of the oats to which some of the nutritious kernel would adhere. From these *sids* an ancient Celtic dish called *sowens* was made.

The *sids* were soaked in water for several days until they were well soured. The liquid was then poured off and reserved, and the *sids* squeezed to extract the last bits of goodness and then discarded. The reserved liquid would sit for another two days, collecting as sediment at the bottom of the vessel. F. Marion McNeill noted that *sids* "contains practically all the nutritious properties of the oatmeal in its most easily digested form. When required for use, pour off all of the clear liquid (*swats*) and put some of the sediment (*sowens*) into a saucepan, allowing a gill [five ounces] for each person, with two gills of water and salt to taste. Bring to the boil, stirring continuously, and cook gently for ten minutes or longer, until thick and creamy. Serve like porridge, in wooden bowls or deep plates, with cream or rich milk."[24]

In the British Isles, wheat was the grain for breadmaking among the upper classes and in the large towns. White bread made from refined flour was available from medieval times and held in high prestige. While the lower classes ate dark coarse bread, usually made with rye and often with ground peas or other pulses mixed into the dough, the upper classes regarded black and brown breads with

---

* One physician from the Shetlands, writing in the 1930s, attributed the good health of older inhabitants to the hand-milling of oats: "Children's teeth seem to decay early, quite a contrast from former times. While it is rare to find a child of school age with a good set of teeth, it is quite the rule to see old men and women with almost perfect sets. In connection with this, it will be noted that the old folk were brought up first on their mothers' milk and later on the produce of their land, home-grown oats ground into meal in the hand-mills, plenty of milk, and fresh fish. Now there is far too much fine, clean oatmeal and wheat flour used, too much tea." Not mentioned is all the sugar put into the tea.

aversion.[25] White flour was also used for making pastries of various sorts—both those that enclosed meat dishes such as umble pie or chicken pasties, and those that served as a basis for dessert tarts and pies. Pastry dough was prepared by mixing butter, lard or suet with "fine white flour." As long as the diet provides plentiful vitamins and minerals, small amounts of white flour do not pose an impediment to good health; but when white flour predominates, as it did among the British upper classes and as it does in Westernized countries today, the consequences can be tragic.

Fermented grains were the key ingredient in various sorts of ales and lagers—either made at home or in alehouses that existed in almost every town. These beers served as an excellent source of nutrients including B vitamins, minerals and enzymes. Small beer, which contained only a small amount of alcohol but large amounts of lactic acid and beneficial enzymes (and reminiscent of the low-alcohol lacto-fermented grain beers we have seen in Africa), was traditionally consumed in the morning, accompanying a heavy breakfast of fish or cold meat, bacon and eggs.[26] Strong beers, with their high alcohol content, were recognized as providing "comfort for the poor." During a visit to Manchester in 1618, the poet John Taylor recorded a total of nine different ales served at the same meal. Eight of them were herbal ales, flavored with hyssop, wormwood, rosemary, betony and scurvy grass. Wines from France and Spain were imported to England and found their way to almost every region, but they were beyond the means of most.

Farm families drank milk, buttermilk, whey or small beer. Even as late as Victorian times, farm families and laborers drank small beer at every meal.[27] Whey, in particular, was recognized as a digestive aid and thirst quencher, and was thought to be beneficial to the skin.[28] It was served at spas or baths—frequented by the well-to-do for "cures"—and often mixed with herbs, fruit or wine.*

In the north, both rural and city-dwelling Scots drank buttermilk in the summertime. It "was valued as both food and drink, and was held to cool the stomach in fever and to aid the cure of dysentery and other ailments."[29] In the *Book of the Old Edinburgh Club*, J. Jamieson recounts the popularity of buttermilk in the city:

In old Edinburgh, throughout the summer months, one might witness daily the picturesque sight of milkmaids on horseback riding into town with soordook [buttermilk] barrels strapped across the saddle behind them...It has

---

* The Whig political party gets its name from the old Scots word *quhig*, "the acetous liquid that subsides from sour cream." The term was first applied by Scottish Episcopalians (who were almost invariably Tories) to Presbyterians, and by Presbyterians of the Established Church to those of the dissenting bodies, presumably because they drank more whey than alcohol.

been estimated that at the end of the eighteenth century a thousand pounds a year was paid in Edinburgh during the months of June, July, August, and September for this very inexpensive beverage, which was sold for a penny the Scots pint (i.e. two Imperial quarts).*

Cookbooks up to the twentieth century attest to the availability of a wide variety of vegetables in Britain, including those of the allium family—onions, leeks, and garlic—plus root vegetables such as parsnips and beets, along with spinach, asparagus and artichokes. These were used in soups and stews rather than served plain. Most cookbooks list a salad made of lettuces and herbs. In general, the upper classes looked upon vegetables with disdain, as a lower-class food, to be eaten by the farmers who grew them.[30] Potatoes† and tomatoes, although introduced in the sixteenth century, did not gain acceptance until the Victorian era. Poorer families ate lots of porridge made from dried peas, as we know from the nursery rhyme: Pease porridge hot, pease porridge cold, pease porridge in the pot, nine days old.

As with meats, preservation of vegetables was a problem and most recipes books of the period contain a number of recipes for pickled vegetables—french beans, cucumbers, onions, cabbages, artichokes, mushrooms, asparagus, beet, cauliflower, radishes, herbs and even walnuts and grapes—prepared with a salt and vinegar brine, then protected from the air with a weighted cover or a layer of butter or tallow. A number of foodstuffs, including mushrooms, walnuts, cucumbers and oysters, were added to "catsup," originally a pickled fish sauce made from anchovies or other small fish, something like Worcestershire sauce. Writing in 1730, Dean Swift mentions catsup as one of several fermented foods favored by the English: "And for our homebred British cheer, Botargo [fish roe relish], catsup and cabiar [caviar]."

The British considered raw fruits "unwholesome." Medical books of the period warned that fresh fruits "filled the body with crude and waterish humours, that dispose the blood unto putrefaction."[31] Apples, pears, quince and berries were stewed or made into tarts, pies and other sweet "puddings."

Not all foodstuffs in wide use were locally produced. Since the Crusades, a variety of spices and other exotic foods enriched the diets of the upper classes and townspeople. In Shakespeare's *The*

---

* Scots immigrants brought their fondness for buttermilk to the southern United States; New Englanders, like the British who colonized the region, found buttermilk disgusting.

† Before the potato, cooked and mashed eggplant often served as a carbohydrate food at meals; taro root also provided carbohydrates, and was consumed by the early Romans in much the same way the potato is today. The Roman cookbook writer Apicius mentions several methods for preparing taro, including boiling, preparing with sauces, and cooking with meat or fowl. The inhabitants of Ikaria, Greece, credit taro for saving them from famine during World War II. They boil it until tender and serve it as a salad.

Winter's Tale, Perdita instructs the Clown to obtain foods for the sheep-shearing feast. Her shopping list includes rice, saffron, mace, dates, nutmegs, ginger and sugar. Almonds were another imported food, widely used, often made into almond milk, which served as a thickener for sauces on feast days when dairy products were forbidden.[32] Liberal amounts of sugar and spices went into piquant sauces, served with the ubiquitous cold meats, and in "made dishes" for the tables of the well-to-do.

Inhabitants of the British Isles enjoyed sweet desserts, sometimes made with honey but more often with sugar, which was available since the time of the Crusades.* In fact, it was the British demand for sugar, even more than spices, that fueled the era of exploration and colonization. *The English Housewife*, published in Shakespeare's day, calls for sugar in almost every dish— salads, omelets, fritters, pancakes, broth, boiled meat, stewed fish, roast meats, meat pies, and of course dessert pies, tarts and puddings.[33] Later it became unfashionable to use too much sugar in sauces and meat dishes, but the consumption of sugared foods continued to grow with the advent of confectioners and pastry shops in every town, and the popularity of a new custom—taking tea with sweet cakes in the afternoon. The widespread use of

sweet wines added to the amount of sugar in the diet—and often sugar was added to wines to make them sweeter.[34] Excess sugar was the cause of the proverbial English bad teeth. A visitor to England in 1598 said of the sixty-four-year-old Queen Elizabeth that her "teeth [were] black, a defect the English seem subject to from their too great use of sugar."[35]

Until the Victorian Age, the British diet contained many protective factors that offset the deleterious effects of sugar—most notably organ meats, raw dairy foods, eggs and butter, all rich in fat-soluble vitamins. Bone broths and whole grain products, including hearty ales, provided minerals in abundance and fermented foods provided enzymes. During the nineteenth century, these homespun foodstuffs gradually gave way to factory-produced, canned and pasteurized foods. Organ meats fell out of favor, and toast and tea replaced the hearty English breakfast of bacon, black pudding and eggs. In fact, tea became the national drink, replacing buttermilk, ale and whey at the morning meal.

The disruption of industrialization left many in extreme poverty. A survey taken in the 1840s revealed that most factory workers were limited in their choice of food to white bread (now cheap and available to the poor), cheese, butter,

---

* While sugar has featured in the British diet for over one thousand years, the stimulants coffee, tea, and chocolate did not arrive until the 1600s.

sugar, tea, salt and potatoes, with a small amount of bacon or other meat used for flavoring.[36] The decline in the use of traditional foods, accompanied by crowding and unsanitary conditions in the major cities, paralleled the rise of disease in the 1800s—cholera, tuberculosis, diphtheria, typhoid fever and typhus. Later in the century, fresh meat, vegetables and fruit became more available, but the trend toward the use of fabricated foods was exacerbated with the introduction of margarine as a substitute for butter and bouillon cubes as a substitute for the rich broths of earlier days.

Ironically, the nutrition of British Islanders improved during the Second World War and even into the early 1950s, when sugar was largely unavailable and food rationing ensured that every British child got cod liver oil, eggs and whole milk.* Nutrition pioneers such as Sir John Boyd Orr lobbied for more meat and whole-milk products in the British diet.

But by 1953, sugar was back with a vengeance, and in recent years, the English have fallen for claims about the "Prudent Diet," one in which vegetable oils are substituted for animal fats and the use of cholesterol-rich foods is minimized. The suet, lard, butter, eggs and

shellfish of Shakespeare's day are spurned as unhealthful; government campaigns discourage the consumption of liver as too high in cholesterol. These are the very foods that Dr. Weston A. Price discovered to be so necessary for attractive development, good health and successful reproduction. The diet of Merrie Olde England may not have been perfect, but it nourished a people who were energetic, curious, lusty, capable and strong. "Prudence," said the English poet William Blake, "is a rich, ugly old maid, courted by incapacity."

"THERE ARE AMONG the Russians many people aged eighty, one hundred, to one hundred twenty years old. They are not subject to illness as in these parts. Except for the emperor and some principal lords, they do not know about physicians. They even consider to be unclean several things which one uses in medicine. Among other things, they do not take pills voluntarily. As for enemas, they abhor them…If the common people are sick, they usually take a good draught of aqua vitae, place in it…a peeled clove of garlic, stir this and drink it. Then they go immediately into a hot house which is so hot as to be almost unendurable, and

---

* In many European countries during World War II, meat was rationed but organ meats were not, resulting in an improvement in nutrition in spite of the privations of the war. As reported in *Starvation in Europe* by Geoffrey H. Bourne, in German-occupied countries, people got a double ration for pigs' heads, pigs' feet, oxtail, brawn, lungs, hearts and goose liver sausage, and a quadruple ration for pigs' bones, sheep's or calf's heads, pigs' tails, marrow bones, tripe and bacon rind. One British journalist remembers getting stew made with brains for school lunch as late as the 1960s.

remain there until they have sweated an hour or two. They do the same for all sorts of maladies."

This excerpt is from the account of a French soldier of fortune, Jacques Margeret, who served Tsar Boris Godunov of Russia from 1600 to 1606. "'Tis almost a miracle to see how their bodies, accustomed to and hardened by cold, can endure so intense a heat, and how that, when they are not able to endure it any longer, they come out of the stoves, naked as the back of a man's hand, both men and women, and go into the cold water...and in winter how they wallow in the snow... The Muscovites are of a healthy and strong constitution, long lived and seldom sick; which when they are, their ordinary remedies, even in burning fevers, are only garlic and strong waters."

Like other European nations before the twentieth century, Russia fostered a highly sophisticated diet for the nobility while also supporting a simple and nutritious peasant cuisine. And, as in other areas of Europe, the famines of the Middle Ages remained as searing memories for the Russian peasant. When the grain harvest on which the Russian peasant depended failed, the suffering was intense. From the Russian *The Chronicle of Novgorod* (1017–1471), we read:

AD 1125...The same year there was a great storm with thunder and hail... it drowned droves of cattle in the Volkhov, and others they hardly saved alive.

AD 1127...And in the autumn the frost killed all the [grain] and the winter crop; and there was famine throughout the winter.

AD 1128...This year it was cruel; the people ate [linden] leaves, birch bark, pounded wood pulp mixed with husks and straw; some ate buttercups, moss, horse flesh; and thus many dropping down from hunger, their corpses were in the streets, in the market place, and on the roads, and everywhere...fathers and mothers would put their children into boats in gift to [foreign] merchants [to be slaves], or else put them to death.

When crops were good, the Russian peasant consumed close to two pounds of dense sourdough bread per day, especially that made from rye, but also from spelt, millet, barley, oats and buckwheat, as well as kasha or porridge from buckwheat and other grains. A sour grain product called *kissel*, virtually identical to *sowens* in Scotland, was made by soaking, fermenting and cooking grain or even grain leavings (and also dried peas) to produce a gelatinous liquid "concentrate" of the grain. The procedure for oat *kissel*, for example, involved drying whole oats carefully on the floor of a warm brick oven and then pounding the oats in a mortar to partially crush them. The oats were covered in hot water and left to sour in a warm place for a day and a half. The soured oats were then pushed through a sieve, and the thick oat "milk" collected and slowly cooked until it thickened further like a jelly. It was then poured onto a wide plate and left to cool, jelling even further. Russian folk wisdom considered this oat aspic especially good for children, the elderly and convalescents—nutritious and easy to digest. The soured oat remnants did not go to waste, but were stirred into flour, left for twenty-four hours to further sour, and baked into flatbreads called *lepyoshki*.[37]

The other mainstay of the Russian diet was soup, and in particular *shchi*, a soup made from green cabbage in the summer and soured cabbage or sorrel in the winter, often made with a rich meat broth. Two other basic soups were *borshch** (or borscht) and *ukha*. Today, there are literally hundreds of *borshch* recipes, some including sausages and other cuts of meat and even beans; some are vegetarian, but always containing beets and often enhanced with pickle brine. *Borshch* is traditionally served in a soup plate and garnished with sour cream.

Ukha is made from poaching whole fish in water with herbs and seasonings; the entire fish (including softened bones) with its broth serve as a meal. The Russian Orthodox church calls for fasting from meat about 250 days per year, including every Wednesday and Friday, and fifty days in Lent, so the Russians have been particularly creative when it comes to preparing the fish and crayfish that thrive in the country's many lakes, streams, rivers and ponds. A menu for a feast day in a nineteenth-century middle-class household featured fish in four dishes: mushroom and sturgeon marrow *pirog* (a dough case with filling); sturgeon head soup; potatoes with herring; and pike in yellow sauce. Accompanying dishes included cranberry *kissel*; plum soup with wine; potato cutlets with mushroom sauce; and stewed fruit compote.[38]

Dairy foods play an important part in the traditional Russian diet, consumed fresh, soured as clabbered milk (*prostokvasha*) and sour cream (*smetana*), or made into a simple peasant cheese. Another sour milk product, kefir, originally a product of the tribal peoples of the northern Caucasus region, became a popular Russian food later on, along with *kumis*, fermented mare's milk.†

Russians enjoy a healthy soft drink called *kvass*, a lightly fermented, slightly alcoholic beverage made from stale rye bread and sweetened with honey, fruit juices or raisins, still available from street vendors in cities and villages. Like the African low-alcohol beers, *kvass* is a rich source of B vitamins, amino acids and enzymes.

---

* *Borshch* originated in Ukraine and is popular throughout the Slavic world.

† In the seventeenth century, the Russian Orthodox church forbade the consumption of horse flesh and drinking of mare's milk as unclean, and *kumis* disappeared from the Russian diet. In recent years, however, it is enjoying a comeback.

Honey and birch sap also served as ingredients for various mildly alcoholic beverages. Of course, the quintessential Russian distilled alcoholic beverage is vodka made from rye grain, which first appeared in Moscow in the fifteenth century.

Fermented cabbage in the form of sauerkraut is another important Russian food.* In fact, many of the typical tastes in Russian cooking come from sauerkraut, pickled cucumbers and many other brined vegetables and fruits, which provide vitamin C during the winter months. In the warm months, the Russians enjoy a variety of fresh vegetables and herbs including radishes, parsley, dill, chervil, green onions and garlic. Wild-growing chicory, nettles, sorrel and purslane often go into the soup pot, and wild mushrooms from Russia's forests enhance many recipes.

The ingenious Russian oven,† which served as the focus of family life, determined the distinctive character of Russian cuisine. The oven had no burners, so all food, even soup, was cooked inside in the coals and ashes after the fire had died down: bread was cooked first and then other foods were put inside as the oven cooled. Nooks and shelves built into the sides of the oven served for souring foods at a steady warm temperature. Most food was cooked in earthenware containers that had rounded sides to maximize heat exposure.

Decades of revolution, war and famine forced the Russian people to abandon many dietary and agricultural traditions in the late nineteenth century. War and famine began in the late nineteenth century. But after the fall of communism in the 1990s, one of the first books to appear in the bookstores was the 1861 culinary classic *A Gift to Young Housewives* by Elena Molokhovets, a compendium of traditional Russian recipes condemned as decadent and bourgeois after the country's 1917 revolution. The renewed popularity of Molokhovets's masterpiece, along with an explosion of interest in artisan food, shows that traditional food is alive and well throughout the vast Russian nation.[39]

PASTA OR PASTRAMI? Will the real Mediterranean diet please stand up? According to modern diet gurus, the Mediterranean diet "is characterized by abundant plant foods (fruit, vegetables, breads, other forms of cereals, beans, nuts and seeds), fresh fruit as the typical daily dessert, olive oil as the principal source of fat, dairy products (principally cheese and

---

* The Mongols brought the art of fermentation to Russia from China.

† Weighing a ton or two, the Russian oven was the centerpiece of the peasant hut as well as the parlor of the city dweller. Made of clay, stone or brick, and sometimes covered with colorful tiles, it had an internal channel system that directed hot smoke through a series of chambers before it exited the dwelling. The structure burned fuel very efficiently, and a single firing was enough to prepare the oven for cooking all meals and heat the house for the entire day.

yogurt) and fish and poultry consumed in low to moderate amounts, zero to four eggs consumed weekly, red meat consumed in low amounts, and wine consumed in low to moderate amounts, normally with meals. This diet is low in saturated fat (less than or equal to 7–8% of energy) with total fat ranging from less than 25% to greater than 35% of energy throughout the region."[40]

This, according to the experts, is the "healthy traditional" European diet we should adopt to protect ourselves from chronic disease, especially heart disease. According to this theory, pasta is fine, but we should definitely avoid that quintessential Mediterranean food, pastrami.

The author of this dogma, and the first to describe the Mediterranean diet in these terms, was Ancel Keys. Keys was the architect of the lipid hypothesis, the premise that heart disease is caused by saturated fat from meat and dairy products, which he called "the major dietary villain."[41]

According to Keys, his introduction to the Mediterranean diet began in the early 1950s when he was a visiting professor at Oxford. In 1951, he chaired the first conference of the Food and Agriculture Organization of the United Nations at their headquarters in Rome.

"The conference talked only about nutritional deficiencies," wrote Keys. "When I asked about the diet and the new epidemic of coronary heart disease, Gino Bergami, Professor of Physiology at the University of Naples, said coronary heart disease was no problem in Naples."

Dr. Keys returned to Oxford where, as an underpaid visiting professor, he and his wife endured an unheated house and got by on food rations. He then had the brilliant idea of visiting sunny Naples to check out Professor Bergami's claim. Once there, he discovered the *trottorias* and dined on "simple pasta and plain pizza." Keys says he discovered that heart attacks were indeed rare in Naples, "except among the small class of rich people whose diet differed from that of the general population—they ate meat every day instead of every week or two." His wife amused herself by measuring serum cholesterol concentrations "and found them to be very low except among members of the Rotary Club." After this exacting research, Keys was able to conclude that "there seemed to be an association between the diet, serum cholesterol and coronary heart disease."

"The heart of what we now consider the Mediterranean diet is mainly vegetarian," he reported. "Pasta in many forms, leaves sprinkled with olive oil, all kinds of vegetables in season, and often cheese, all finished off with fruit and frequently washed down with wine."

At first, Dr. Keys found little support for his revolutionary theories. But he encountered a sympathetic listener in 1952 when he presented his views to a small audience in New York at Mount Sinai Hospital. Fred Epstein found Keys's data convincing and began spreading the message "with great effect over Europe and America."[42]

Keys then published his Seven Countries Study[43] in which he claimed a relationship between high rates of coronary heart disease and consumption of saturated fat in seven countries. He was able to do this by handpicking countries where both heart disease and consumption of saturated fats were high and by ignoring countries—such as France and Spain—with the same kind of diet but where heart disease was low.*[44]

Since Keys published his "research," the Mediterranean diet—at least, what is perceived to be the Mediterranean diet—has become government policy. The USDA has immortalized Keys's fond remembrance of *trottoria* fare from sunny Naples in the form of a food pyramid, based on lots of white bread and pasta topped with a generous layer of fruits and vegetables. This strangely garnished pizza slice then gets a splash of olive oil and cheese, an anchovy or two, a pinch of sugar, and voilà—the dietary solution to rampant chronic disease!

Chronic disease is still rampaging in spite of the food pyramid's worldwide acceptance, but Keys, at least, fared rather well. In 1993, after Fred Epstein gave the summary lecture at the international celebration of the Seven Countries Study in Fukuoka, Japan, and at the fourth annual Ancel Keys Lecture at the 1993 American Heart Association Convention, Keys was deluged with requests for interviews and advice. "In May 1993, a crew from an American magazine came to our home Minnelea in Minnesota, bringing a photographer from California to record the scene while I talked about the Mediterranean diet."

Dr. Keys no longer had to winter in Minnesota, but could escape to his second home in southern Italy. But his vacations to Naples included some sad moments, as he observed unfortunate changes in the Mediterranean diet: "The restaurants are increasingly popular but the food they serve is commonly far from the Mediterranean pattern...Everything has to be loaded with butter or margarine and ground meat. Serving only fruit for dessert is not common; ice cream or pie is customary. Whereas Italian restaurants brag about the healthy Mediterranean diet, they serve a travesty of it." Keys does not tell us whether his newfound prosperity, which allowed him to dine in white-tablecloth restaurants rather than sidewalk cafés, caused him to abandon his monkish

---

* The statistician Russell H. Smith had this to say about the Seven Countries Study: "The word 'landmark' has often been used...to describe Ancel Keys' Seven Countries study, commonly cited as proof that the American diet is atherogenic...the dietary assessment methodology was highly inconsistent across cohorts and thoroughly suspect. In addition, careful examination of the death rates and associations between diet and death rates reveal a massive set of inconsistencies and contradictions...It is almost inconceivable that the Seven Countries study was performed with such scientific abandon. It is also dumbfounding how the NHLBI/AHA alliance ignored such sloppiness in their many 'rave reviews' of the study...In summary, the diet-CHD relationship reported for the Seven Countries study cannot be taken seriously by the objective and critical scientist."

regimen of "leaves sprinkled with olive oil" and fresh fruit. It must have been distressing indeed to observe sophisticated Italians feasting on such travesties as pasta Alfredo, veal scallopini and prosciutto, especially to one who has taken the stringent vows of the dietary priesthood.*

But the life of the missionary is never easy. No, it is a lonesome road, filled with disappointment. Imagine the late-night soul-searching of Dr. Francisca Pérez-Llamas and his colleagues, who set out to study the consumption patterns of a group of adolescents in the region of Murcia, in southeastern Spain.[45] Were these Mediterranean teenagers consuming a "balanced diet," with plenty of vegetables and fruit? Not at all. The naughty youngsters consumed mostly sausage! "The results showed a very low consumption of vegetables, some deficiencies in the intake of the milk and fruits and an excessive intake of fats...while the intake of fish and pulses was insufficient in our study."

Alas, lamented Pérez-Llamas, "the study reveals that although Murcia is a typically Mediterranean region, the characteristics of the diet of Murcian adolescents are quite different in some respects from the typical alimentary habits of the Mediterranean diet."

Pérez-Llamas proposed to remedy these dietary sins with the modern version of the Spanish Inquisition: "nutritional advice was given to mothers and adolescents. The use of Spanish portions from the six basic food groups proved to be a very helpful method to popularize the principles of balanced diet in our population."

Another group of diet-priests, headed by Dr. Alberti-Fidanza, made a pilgrimage in 1994 to study elderly Italians in the rural areas of Crevalcore and Montegiorgio, two of the districts Keys had included in the Seven Countries Study.[46] But the older generation had fallen away! They no longer practiced the food puritanism that Keys claimed he observed three decades earlier. "In both areas, but particularly in Montegiorgio, these subjects have been abandoning the traditional Mediterranean diet," wrote Dr. Alberti-Fidanza.

The question that the believers haven't asked themselves is this: was the lean, so-called Mediterranean diet they observed after World War II the true Mediterranean diet? Or were they observing the tail end of deprivation engendered by half a decade of conflict? Were the inhabitants of Crevalcore and Montegiorgio abandoning the traditional Mediterranean diet, or were they taking it up again? And did Keys miss the sight of Italians enjoying rich food in the early 1950s because Italians had never

---

* Actually, Keys recommended the practice of renunciation for the general population but not for himself or those of his inner circle. The esteemed researcher Fred Kummerow, PhD, defender of eggs and butter in the human diet, once spied Keys and a colleague eating eggs and bacon at a conference for cardiologists. When Kummerow inquired whether Keys had changed his mind about dietary fats and cholesterol, Keys replied that such a restricted diet was "for others," not for himself.

done such a shameful thing, or was the visiting professor too poor at the time to afford anything more than plain pizza in a sidewalk café?

At the end of the nineteenth century, soon after the unification of Italy into one nation, Pellegrino Artusi wrote *Science in the Kitchen and the Art of Eating Well*,[47] a collection of traditional recipes from Tuscany and the "foodie" region of Emilia-Romagna, which became the second most bestselling book in Italy (the first being the Bible).*

In the book, Artusi points out that the most famous Italian products are animal-based, including four hundred types of traditional cheese, many of them raw, and hundreds of cured meat products. The book and its recipes defy the precepts of the Mediterranean diet. For example, one breakfast recipe calls for eggs, butter, anchovies, capers and tuna. Artusi emphasizes the use of animal fat and meat; in fact, the book is a feast of animal food. Artusi rates the different nutritive power of different kinds of meat, with beef at the top of the list. Regarding pasta, he warns children, the elderly and pregnant or lactating women against consuming pasta "because it would distract from the consumption of more nutrient-rich foods, as meat or fish," and cautions "people with tendency toward obesity" to refrain from consuming it "because every doctor knows that flour has no nutritive power and immediately turns into body fat."

Countess Morphy's *Recipes of All Nations*,[48] another important book, was published in 1935, almost two decades before Keys and others proclaimed the new diet religion to the suffering millions. Consider Morphy's description of the food in Sardinia: grains are certainly a part of their diet, consumed as bread, pasta or polenta, but in most interesting ways. "One of their favorite ways of cooking macaroni is to cook it in either lamb or pork fat...with small pieces of either lamb or pork, chopped tomatoes, chopped garlic and curd, mixed with a little water and salt and moistened with a little game stock, if this is obtainable." Gnocchi is flavored with saffron and "served with a tomato sauce, or with gravy and cheese made from ewe's milk." Bland polenta is enlivened with "chopped salt pork, small pieces of sausages and grated cheese." *Favata*, a fava bean stew, is made with "pieces of salt pork, cut in large chunks, ham bone, special homemade sausages, a handful of dried beans, wild fennel, and other herbs and a little water."

Nothing low-fat so far. But perhaps Keys and his entourage were right when they said that meat is eaten sparingly in the Mediterranean region. Read on. "The Sardinians are great meat eaters, but their methods of cooking various kinds

---

* A high school textbook, *History of Italian Literature*, notes that Artusi's book was responsible for the spread of "a common language" in the new Italian middle class. It remained the bible of Italian food until the 1980s, when the low-fat craze kicked in and Italians began eating large quantities of pasta and bread.

of meat are simple—almost primitive, in fact." Like most Italians, the Sardinians prefer young animals—lamb, kid or suckling pig—usually roasted in front of a wood fire. "The meat is finally browned by constant basting with hot fat..." The baby pigs "are so tender that even the skin, ears and all can be eaten."

The diet of Corsica "has in no way been subjected to any outside influence." No new catechism, no diet evangelists here. So Corsicans can enjoy the following without guilt: all manner of fish, including small lobster, cuttlefish and shellfish; anchovy paste made with the addition of figs; dried salt cod; beef browned in lard; strips of goat fillet, salted and sun-dried; chestnuts mixed with polenta and cream and served with different kinds of meat or black [blood] pudding.

You Eat What You Are,[49] a beautiful encyclopedia of traditional foods first published in 1979 and released in a revised edition in 1999, gives yet another view of Italian cuisine than the one proclaimed in the Gospel According to Ancel Keys. Author Thelma Barer-Stein notes that butter is the cooking fat of choice in northern Italy, lard in the middle region, and olive oil in the south. But pork is consumed throughout the entire peninsula, usually in the form of sausages—which anyone but an American visiting professor could discern are the sine qua nons of Italian cuisine. Salami, bologna, mortadella and *zamponi*—there would be no Italian cuisine without these. Sausage is

a way of making offal taste good—as in *pezzente*, an Italian specialty made from pork sinews, livers and lungs. Cooks use plenty of pancetta (Italian-style bacon) and children love crisp cracklings of pig skin called *ciccioli*, rich in vitamin D.

The Jewish population living in Italy made sausage and cold cuts, but they did not use pork. In her book *The Classic Cuisine of the Italian Jews*,[50] author Edda Servi Machlin remembers her father's *carne secca* (salt dried meat) and *salsicce de minao* (beef sausage): "Both dishes were renowned and appreciated among the Jewish communities all over Italy." These foods were made in late winter and hung in "an open north window" for four to six weeks to air-dry. Other specialties included *lingua salmistrata* (pickled beef tongue), the aroma of which would "resuscitate the dead," and *salame d'oca* (goose sausage). These cured meats were all fermented—and eaten raw.

About eggs, Machlin reported, "Eggs have always been among the most inexpensive of the highly nutritious foods. For us, they were not only a staple, but also a universal remedy for most ailments, real or imaginary, much as vitamins are for many people today. In order to be fully effective, eggs had to be ingested raw and very fresh—in fact, warm, directly from the chicken nest. So, naturally, every family had a small poultry yard in their orchard."

Italy produces as many kinds of cheese as France, including two of the very best:

Parmesan and Gorgonzola, both full fat and creamy rich. Italian cheese garnishes more than pizza. It is used in turnovers, vegetable dishes, salads and sandwiches. A favorite is mozzarella, cut into squares, dipped in batter and deep-fried.

Italians are masters at preparing every kind of meat—from sweetbreads to knucklebones. Lean meat gets a cream sauce or stuffing of ham and ricotta cheese.

Fish and shellfish of every variety appear in seafood platters, fish soups and fish stews. The diet dictocrats, flush with the success of their food pyramid, seem to have missed the ecstatic experience of calamari, dipped in batter, deep-fried and served heaped on platters—a healthy snack as long as traditional fats, not partially hydrogenated vegetable oils, are used in frying. In Naples, where Keys had heard that heart disease was rare, snacks of fresh seafood are as popular as pizzas and small containers of oysters can be eaten on the run.

Italians love their vegetables for sure, and that's because they know how to make them taste good. They know that salads taste better with a good dressing of aged vinegar and olive oil; and cooked vegetables blossom when anointed with butter, lard or cream.

Italians don't generally start the day with eggs but they make up for it later on. Eggs are used in rich sauces and custards, like zabaglione. Soups are often served with a poached egg.

And what about ice cream? Is this something new to the Italian diet—an American travesty? Not quite. "The first ice cream shops or *gelateria* opened in Tuscany in the 1500s, but the southern Italians are believed to be responsible for the popularity of ice cream in North America."[51] And no one uses ice cream with greater inventiveness than the Italians, from the *spumone* of Naples to *cassata*, a decorative ice cream cake, to *semifreddi*, a type of soft foamy ice cream that also comes in many flavors. It is true, however, that Italians sometimes consume ice cream with fresh fruit.

AS IS CLEAR TO ANYONE who has traveled to Italy or eaten in an Italian restaurant, the backsliding Italians have reverted to the food paganism of their ancestors—if they ever left it. So it appears that orthodox nutritionists have recently enshrined the Greek diet as the most virtuous of politically correct Mediterranean cuisines, described as consisting principally of olive oil, bread and tomatoes.

Rosemary Barron ran a cooking school on Crete from 1980 to 1984 and spent many months living there, as far back as 1963 when she participated in an archeological dig. In 1991 she published *Flavors of Greece*, which received an "Editor's Choice" award in the *New York Times* book section.

It is true, Barron reported, that the Greeks eat lots of bread. In the countryside, families still make bread using stoneground flour baked in wood-burning ovens. White bread is found in the stores but there still is a long and strong tradition of all sorts of brown breads, including a fermented "shepherd's" loaf made with wheat bran, oat bran and whole wheat flour. Much bread is "twice-baked" into rusks, normally consumed at breakfast.

Two reports indicate that the Greeks practiced soaking and fermented grains. One, from a Greek cookbook, describes soaking wheat grains overnight, then drying them in the sun before grinding and making them into pasta.[52] The other involves a product called *chodra*, made from grinding wheat stalks, mixing them with the whey from cheese, bringing to a simmer, then hanging the mixture in sacks to dehydrate—talk about making the most of an agricultural waste product!

Barron estimates that Cretans eat several pounds of cheese per week, providing about six hundred calories of fat per day, or 25 percent of calories in a 2,400-calorie diet, just from cheese alone. Since the fat in goat milk cheese is almost 70 percent saturated, one-half pound of cheese per day would supply about 18 percent of calories as saturated fat, more than twice as much of that "dietary villain" than allowed by the diet priests, and that's just from cheese.

Other sources of saturated fat include yogurt, milk and small amounts of butter used in pastries. Olive oil is the preferred fat for cooking and salads. It is used very generously, providing lots more fat calories, including some calories as saturated fat.

And there's also plenty of saturated fat from meat in the Cretan diet. Lamb or kid are foods for spring, and goat is a food for throughout the year. Pork is a frequent dish, either as chops or roast, and old hens and roosters are served up boiled. The most common meat of all is game in season—birds, rabbit and hare. Tiny birds grilled and wrapped in vine leaves are popular. Thin smoked sausages serve as appetizers and garnishes.

Egg consumption averages about ten per week, used as ingredients in omelets, cakes, savory dishes and avgolemono, an egg-lemon soup. Barron remembers her surprise on cracking her first Cretan egg—the yolk was bright orange, so bright that the scrambled eggs she made with it were also orange.

Cretans love unusual foods like snails and organ meats—kidneys, liver and spleen. Fish roe is a common appetizer, made into small cakes and fried in oil, or whipped into creamy *taramosalata* dip.

Those who live near the coast eat fresh seafood every day—including shellfish, sea urchins, octopus, squid and cuttlefish. Until recently, the only transport was by donkey, and there were no refrigerators. This meant that unless you lived by the sea, you rarely ate fresh seafood. Cretans had several methods for preserving fish by salting or smoking, and for creating odorous sauces from rotting fish. Smaller fish were placed in earthenware jars and covered with herbs and olive oil. Donkeys then carried these "fish up the path" to the interior.

All of these animal foods, including the

orange egg yolks, are excellent sources of vitamins A, D, and K_2, the fat-soluble vitamins Dr. Price discovered to be vital for attractive facial development and robust health. When foods rich in these fat-soluble activators are abandoned, subsequent generations have more narrow faces, more tooth decay and more disease. They are less good-looking and less strong. The presence of adequate amounts of fat-soluble vitamins in the Cretan diet is probably what protects populations throughout the Mediterranean from the large amount of bread or pasta and frequent use of sweets.

The main meal in most of Greece is lunch, eaten at home and consisting of a main course, usually a stew or casserole containing meat and organ meats, along with vegetables, salad, bread and cheese. Then everything shuts down until about five in the evening. Dinner is late by American standards, preceded by a few hours of *mezedes* (little nibbles) taken in a café, or at home with a drink. *Mezedes* might be bits of cucumber, tomato, cheese, olives, seafood or slices of sausage. In a typical village scene, the men sit in cafés for a couple of hours and the women sit outside their houses chatting. The men then come home to dinner at about ten in the evening. Desserts like ice cream and pastries are eaten in cafés during family outings and at home on feast days.

The European Union is a breeding ground for zealots of food puritanism, so the Greeks are under pressure to conform. No more long lunches and leisurely hors d'oeuvres hours. Greece has to follow the same hours as the rest of Europe—and eat the same foods, like standardized low-fat factory-made cheeses, white bread, lean meat packaged without the bone, commercial baked goods based on vegetable oils and soft drinks. These are the real travesty of the modern Mediterranean diet, not foods rich in animal fats, and this garbage is much easier to sell when doctors say that it's better for your health than the traditional foods of your ancestors.

"Unhappily," wrote Keys, "the current changes in Mediterranean countries tend to destroy the health virtues of the diet as we saw them forty years ago. Efforts are needed to reverse this change. Education is important. We should concentrate on the medical profession and the schools. It is not enough that doctors measure serum cholesterol and tell patients with high values to avoid butter and fatty meat. They also should emphasize prevention by targeting the general public."

This means more seminars, in villages by the sea. The second annual meeting, Keys reports, was held in Pioppi, a village on the Mediterranean coast, "about four kilometers from our home in Italy." Sponsored by the International Society and Federation of Cardiology, these retreats have attracted "some 800 doctors from 30 cities in 22 countries." Oh, what sacrifices are made in the name of science!

And what does this college of cardiologists eat when convened on their Italian retreat? Do the learned doctors confine themselves to plain pasta and lean meat? Do they nibble on lemons and leaves in the land of *spumone*?

The greatest of the seven deadly sins is not gluttony but pride, pride so blinding that it presumes to inflict one's own pathology of renunciation upon a whole population, starting with the children. "In these seminars," says Keys, "we stress the Mediterranean type of diet and its helpful role in controlling the concentration of serum cholesterol and reducing the associated risk of coronary heart disease...I believe it is important to bring the diet message to school children...Our challenge is to figure out how to make children tell their parents that they should eat as Mediterraneans do. At least, we should help children get rid of some nonsense ideas and convince them that meat and rich dairy products will not make the boys any stronger and the girls any prettier."[53]

CHAPTER 8

True Blue Zones

How Long-Lived People Really Eat

THE ARGUMENT AGAINST rich traditional foods goes like this: native peoples on their native diets, which were high in animal foods and animal fat, may have been attractive and healthy when they were young, but they did not live into old age. If you want to live a long life, we're admonished, you need to eat a diet that is low in fat, low in salt, high in plant foods, and rich in dietary fiber. In short, the penalty for a long life is adherence to the sad and unsatisfying diet foisted on us by government bodies and medical "experts" from the Western world.

The book that promulgates this point of view the most extensively is *The Blue Zones: Lessons for Living Longer from the People Who've Lived the Longest* by Dan Buettner. The bestseller is based on his work for the *National Geographic*. In it, Buettner opens a lot of creaky gates, walks up driveways with crunchy gravel, and visits a number of dimly lit bars to explore several "Blue Zones," areas known for

having a large number of centenarians—long-lived people who invariably have wrinkly smiles and live fairly isolated, physically active, low-stress lives.

As for the diet, Buettner gives you the bottom line in chapter 1, which includes the suggestion to eat six to nine servings of vegetables a day and to make sure your meat is lean. He advocates a diet of "moderation." Meat is okay if eaten in "European," not "American" portions. "Are you eating meat a couple of times a week, or are you eating it every day for two meals a day?" he asks. "Are you eating processed meats that are filled with fat? Or are you eating good cuts of fairly lean meat?"[1]

BUETTNER'S FIRST EXAMPLE of a Blue Zone is the mountainous Barbagia region in the province of Ogliastra on the island of Sardinia. A paper given at a longevity conference in 1999 found, for example, seven centenarians in a village of 2,500 people, ratios that were confirmed in later studies. In the United States, only about one male in 20,000 reaches the age of one hundred.

Barbagia is characterized by "rough pastureland" with "patches of hardwood forest and occasional vineyards." Like other Blue Zones, the region was relatively isolated until recent times. Buettner describes mountainous Barbagia as a place where life is difficult, and where kidnapping, stealing and vendettas are common. "A vendetta can last generations. A son of one family might get shot today for something his father did decades ago...If a boy catches you looking at his girl, expect to be confronted...everyone in Barbagia has a knife in his pocket."

Knife-wielding peasants carrying grudges seem to contradict the notion that life in Barbagia is stress-free...but we digress.

Back to the diet. "The Sardinian diet was lean and largely plant-based," Buettner insists, "with an emphasis on beans, whole wheat and garden vegetables, wine, goat milk and mastic oil."*

Buettner first visits the alert and chipper Giuseppe Mura, age 102, whose house "smells vaguely of sausages and red wine." Does the house smell of sausages because Mura eats sausages? We never find out. Here is a wonderful opportunity to ask a non-senile centenarian whether he has eaten foods like

sausages over the years—after all, it would be good to know whether our centenarian peasant has enjoyed "processed meats filled with fat" during his long life. Instead, Buettner follows a protocol developed by the National Institute on Aging, designed to "tease out" from the elders narratives about their early lives in response to "nonleading," "carefully crafted questions....Instead of asking a man what he ate when he was a child, the question would inquire, 'Can you think about things you do every day or have done most days of your life?'"

Buettner's meal at the house of Giuseppe Mura included wine and cured ham, followed by cups of hot coffee. But according to Buettner's carefully crafted questions, the centenarian's diet consisted largely of fava beans, pecorino cheese, bread and meat as he could afford it, which he rarely could.

Next, we visit a fit and active seventy-five-year-old named Tonino Tola, who was definitely not eating fava beans. "When I caught up with Tonino...he was slaughtering a cow in the shed behind this house, his arms elbow-deep in the animal's carcass...The cow would provide meat for two families for the season as well as gifts for several friends." What a great opportunity to tease out the parts of the cow that Tonino actually ate—did he eat the liver and kidneys that evening, before they

---

* From a brief Internet search, we learn that mastic oil comes from a tree that is a relative of the pistachio, which actually produces a resin called mastic, not an edible oil. Mastic has medicinal and industrial uses as an additive to perfumes, cosmetics, soap, body oils and body lotion. In ancient Egypt, mastic was used in embalming. But according to Buettner, in some parts of Sardinia, mastic oil squeezed from the nut serves as a substitute for olive oil.

could spoil? Did the tripe get consumed or did the impoverished folks of the Sardinian mountains throw it out? Did Tola prefer lean or fatty cuts? Did he boil up the head? We never find out.

Buettner says that Tola slaughters his cow in the fall "to make meat easier to preserve." How is that meat preserved? Another mystery left unsolved by carefully crafted questions. But it's a good bet that Tola preserves his beef in salt, especially as we later learn that meat is boiled on Sunday (the usual preparation for salted beef) and roasted during festivals (the usual preparation for freshly killed meat). Of course, if Tola preserves his meat in salt, that means he is consuming quite a bit of salt, a habit that is not supposed to result in a long life. But there's not a single mention of salt in the chapter—best to avoid the embarrassment of conflicting evidence.

The next fellow we meet drinks goat milk for breakfast and carries bread, cheese, wine, sheep milk and roasted lamb on journeys. No fava beans for him, either! Buettner admits that the shepherds of Sardinia consume a lot of sheep and goat milk products; in isolated Barbagia, these sheep- and goat-milk products are almost certainly raw. He notes that the centenarians seem to avoid bone loss and fractures and speculates that goat's milk and the mysterious mastic oil, along with bread and wine, may be Sardinia's "other two longevity elixirs." (Those Sardinian peasants do drink a lot of wine, maybe to

make their life of isolation and hard work tolerable.)

Better information about the Sardinian shepherd diet comes from a 2014 article, "Male Longevity in Sardinia," published in the *European Journal of Clinical Nutrition*.[2] Here we learn that the main activity in the Sardinian Blue Zone was animal husbandry, whereas on the rest of the island it was agriculture: "The major discrepancy between the lowland areas, where peasants were the majority of the population, and the mountain areas, essentially pastoral, was the relatively superior consumption of animal-derived foods in the latter." The shepherds also ate more animal fat and consumed very little vegetable oil. Carbohydrate consumption was also lower among the long-lived shepherds. Both shepherds and peasants did consume fairly high levels of "vegetable proteins," in the form of fava beans, white beans, lupini beans, chickpeas and lentils, although none of Buettner's informants seemed to eat much of any of these pulses. Seasonal vegetables came from their gardens; seasonal fruit (mainly grapes and figs), chestnuts and walnuts added variety to the diet.

The authors of the article asked good questions and came up with some fascinating details: "Two vitally important foods were widely consumed throughout the island, that is, sourdough-leavened bread and vegetable soup (minestrone) that contained fresh vegetables...in the mountain area (Ogliastra), that soup also included some tubers (potatoes) and pork stock." Also, "consumption of dairy products both from goats and sheep, was higher in the mountains [including] a sort of fresh sour cheese called *casu ajedu*, which was rich in *lactobacilli*."*

In fact, the Sardinian Blue Zone diet sounds similar to other traditional diets we have seen from around the world, containing raw milk, lactobacillus-rich sour cheese, sourdough bread and soup made from pork stock. The diet almost certainly contained organ meats—shepherds eking out a living do not throw the organ meats away.

Speaking of pork, the island of Sardinia is famous for the Sarda pig, raised mainly in the mountainous provinces of Ogliastra and Nuoro. Sarda pigs range freely in the mountainous areas, "which often including public land, where they feed on acorns, chestnuts and roots. Additional feed is given only in the summer, when natural sources of food are scarce. Pigmen train the pigs to come at their call to the usual feeding-place; feed is often given directly on the ground, or at the side of the road."[3]

This seems like a picturesque custom that Buettner would have heard about and that *National Geographic* would want to record, but one that would lead to uncomfortable questions, because pig meat is preserved by making it into sausage and ham, "processed meats that are filled with fat." A quick search of Sardinian pork products reveals that Sardinian

ham is fattier than prosciutto—with a one-inch-thick ribbon of fat around the edges. Did Buettner's first Blue Zone meal of ham give him qualms about writing a whole book promoting a low-fat diet as the secret to longevity? He doesn't say.

More research reveals photographs of whole lambs skewered and roasted over an open fire—these are for festivals, which apparently happen frequently in the Sardinian mountains. You will also find photographs of skewered, roasted intestines, another food that Buettner failed to tease out in his carefully crafted questions.

NEXT BUETTNER TURNS his attention to Okinawa, an island situated equidistant from Hong Kong and Tokyo. The average life span for women in Okinawa is eighty-four (compared to seventy-nine in America), and the island boasts a disproportionately high number of centenarians. Okinawans have low levels of chronic illness—osteoporosis, cancer, diabetes, atherosclerosis and stroke—compared to America, China and Japan, which allows them to continue to work, even in their advanced years. In spite of Okinawa's horrific role as the site of the last major battle—and one of the bloodiest—of World War II, Okinawa is a breezy, pleasant place, neither crowded nor polluted, with a strong sense of family and community, where the local people still grow a large portion of their vegetables in family gardens.

---

* Another typical Sardinian sheep-milk cheese is *casu marzu*, notable for containing maggots.

Buettner subtitles his chapter on the Okinawan Blue Zone "Sunshine, Spirituality, and Sweet Potatoes," but what he reveals in the very first paragraph is that the favorite Okinawan dish is Spam-and-vegetable stir-fry. Readers, please note: Spam is a processed meat that is full of fat.

From a USDA Foreign Agricultural Service report we learn that the "Annual average consumption of luncheon meat per person in the prefecture [of Okinawa] is about 14 cans (340 g per can)/year. It is even more impressive when you learn that Okinawa, with only 1.1 percent of the total Japanese population, is responsible for over 90 percent of the total luncheon meat consumption in Japan. The local menu using luncheon meat ranges widely from stir-fried vegetables to rice balls. 'SPAM omusubi'…is particularly popular." The Okinawans also eat more hamburger than people in Japan.[4]

In his visit to Sardinia, Buettner asked "nonleading questions, carefully crafted to tease out the lifestyle by eliciting a narrative." Unfortunately, such questions were not very useful for finding out the important details of a traditional diet. But Buettner uses a different approach for the centenarians of Okinawa: "a survey developed by the National Institute on Aging to systematically interview…Okinawans in search of common lifestyle characteristics. And I'd connect with scientists to find out how those characteristics connected to longevity."

The scientist he teams up with is Dr. Greg Plotnikoff. Dr. Plotnikoff has a decidedly vegetarian bent, having written a paper entitled "Nutritional Assessment in Vegetarians and Vegans: Questions Clinicians Should Ask," published in *Minnesota Medicine.*[5] On his website he recommends a ghastly sounding smoothie made of coconut milk, protein powder (from whey, rice, pea or hemp), sunflower lecithin, medium-chain triglyceride oil and liquid fish oil.

As Plotnikoff says to Buettner, "People don't realize how bad sugar and meat are for them over time." Okinawans, he says, eat mostly fresh vegetables, fewer salty pickles and less canned meat (hello—Spam is canned meat), and have good vitamin D status because they get plenty of sun.

Buettner does admit that in Okinawa, people eat almost every part of the pig—unlike the mainland Japanese, who get more protein from fish. But he insists that the Okinawans eat pork only for festivals. His conclusion about the Okinawan diet (presumably based on what he found from using the National Institute of Aging survey, although he doesn't say): "Older Okinawans have eaten a plant-based diet most of their lives. Their meals of stir-fried vegetables, sweet potatoes, and tofu are high in nutrients and low in calories.…While centenarian Okinawans do eat some pork, it is traditionally reserved only for infrequent ceremonial occasions and taken only in small amounts." He mentions bitter melon as a source of antioxidants and compounds that lower blood sugar.

Of course, life was hard during World War II. "We had famines, times when people starved to death," says one of Buettner's informants. "Even when times were good, all we ate was *imo* (sweet potato) for breakfast, lunch, and dinner." But they also ate fish and pork from the family pig, and it's obvious that this starvation diet was a temporary phenomenon and not a reason to eat a diet centered on sweet potatoes.

What have other surveys revealed about the diets of long-lived Okinawans? In 1992 scientists at the Department of Community Health, Tokyo Metropolitan Institute of Gerontology, Japan, published a paper[6] that examined the relationship of nutritional status to further life expectancy and health status in the Japanese elderly. It was based on three epidemiological studies. In the first, nutrient intakes in ninety-four Japanese centenarians investigated between 1972 and 1973 showed a higher proportion of animal protein to total proteins than in contemporary average Japanese. The second demonstrated that high intakes of milk (!) and fats and oils had favorable effects on ten-year survivorship in 422 urban residents aged sixty-nine to seventy-one. The survivors revealed a longitudinal increase in intakes of animal foods such as eggs, milk, fish and meat over the ten years. In the third study, nutrient intakes were compared between a sample from Okinawa Prefecture where life expectancies at birth and sixty-five were the longest in Japan, and a sample from Akita Prefecture (on the mainland) where the life expectancies were much shorter. It found that the proportion of energy from proteins and fats was *significantly higher* in Okinawa than in the Japanese mainland.

According to the paper, "The food intake pattern in Okinawa has been different from that in other regions of Japan. The people there have never been influenced by Buddhism. Hence, there has been no taboo regarding eating habits. Eating meat was not stigmatized, and consumption of pork and goat was historically high... The intake of meat was higher in Okinawa... On the other hand, the intake of fish was lower... Intake of NaCl was lower... Deep colored vegetables were taken more in Okinawa... These characteristics of dietary status are thought to be among the crucial factors which convey longevity and good health to the elderly in Okinawa Prefecture... *Unexpectedly, we did not find any vegetarians among the centenarians*" [emphasis added].

From another source,[7] we learn that:

Traditional foods of Okinawa are extremely varied, remarkably nutrient-dense as are all traditional foods and strictly moderated with the philosophy of *hara hachi bu* [eat until you are 80 percent full]. While the diet of Okinawa is, indeed, plant-based it is most certainly not "low fat" as has been posited by some writer-researchers about the native foods of Okinawa. Indeed, all those stir fries of bitter melon and fresh vegetables found in Okinawan bowls are fried in lard and seasoned with sesame oil. I remember fondly that a slab of salt pork graced every bowl of *udon* I slurped up while living on the island. Pig fat is not, as you can imagine, a low-fat food yet the Okinawans are fond of it. Much of the fat consumed is pastured as pigs are commonly raised at home in the gardens of Okinawan homes. Pork and lard, like avocado and olive oil, are a remarkably good source of monounsaturated fatty acid and, if that pig roots around on sunny days, it is also a remarkably good source of vitamin D.

The diet of Okinawa also includes considerably more animal products and meat—usually in the form of pork—than that of the mainland Japanese or even the Chinese. Goat and chicken play a lesser, but still important, role in Okinawan cuisine. Okinawans average about 100 grams or one modest portion of meat per person per day. Animal foods are important on Okinawa and, like all food, play a role in the population's general health, well-being and longevity. Fish plays an important role in the cooking of Okinawa as well. Seafoods eaten are various and numerous—with Okinawans averaging about 200 grams of fish per day.

Buettner implies that the Okinawans do not eat much fish, but in fact, they eat quite a lot, just not as much as Japanese mainlanders.

The Okinawan diet became a subject of interest after the publication of a 1996 article in *Health Magazine* about the work of gerontologist Kazuhiko Taira,[8] who described the Okinawan diet as "very healthy—and very, very greasy." The whole pig is eaten, he noted, everything from "tails to nails." Local menus offer boiled pig's feet, entrail soup and shredded ears. Pork is marinated in a mixture of soy sauce, ginger, kelp and small amounts of sugar, then sliced or chopped for stir-fry dishes. Okinawans eat about 100 grams of meat per day—compared to 70 grams in Japan and just over 20 grams in China—and at least an equal amount of fish, for a total of about 200 grams per day, compared to 280 grams per person per day of meat and fish in America. Lard—not vegetable oil—is used in cooking.

According to Taira, Okinawans also eat plenty of fibrous root crops such as taro and sweet potatoes. They consume rice and noodles, but not as the main components of the diet. They eat a variety of vegetables such as carrots, white radish, cabbage and greens, both fresh and pickled. Bland tofu is part of the diet, consumed in traditional ways, but on the whole Okinawan cuisine is spicy. Pork dishes are flavored with a mixture of ginger and brown sugar, chile oil and "the wicked bite of bitter melon."

Damage control soon followed in the form of the Okinawa Centenarian Study.[9] The study confirmed the longevity and good health of Okinawans and focused on genetic and family factors. However, in the press, the study was described as follows: "Okinawa, a chain of islands in southern Japan, has the highest concentration of centenarians. Uniformly these old folks have a vegetable-based, low-calorie, low-fat diet and exercise daily. They eat on average seven servings of vegetables and seven servings of grain per day, several servings of soy products, fish rich in omega-3 fatty acids, and little dairy or red meat."[10]

Bradley Willcox, D. Craig Willcox, and Makoto Suzuki repeat this description in their bestselling books *The Okinawa Program* and *The Okinawa Diet Plan*. The factors that confer longevity, they insist, include a politically correct low-calorie, plant-based, high-complex-carbohydrate diet, exercise and "attention to spirituality and friendships." The high content of monounsaturated fatty acids from lard in the Okinawan diet gets translated into a recommendation for politically correct canola oil.

The recipes in the Okinawa diet books feature a great deal of tofu, leading vegan author John Robbins, author of *Diet for a New America*, *May All Be Fed* and *The Food Revolution*, among others, to claim that the reason the Okinawans enjoy such longevity is because they eat two servings of soy foods per day, with soy constituting 12 percent of their calories. Numerous other vegan spokespeople soon repeated these figures like gospel in their articles, blogs, YouTube videos and Facebook posts.

As pointed out by Kaayla Daniel, author of *The Whole Soy Story*, "The amount of soy that Okinawans eat is not at all clear in these books. The authors say that the Okinawans eat '60 to 120 grams per day of soy protein,' which means, according to the books' context, soy foods eaten as a whole food protein source. But the authors also include a table that lists total legume consumption (including soy) in the amounts of about 75 grams per day for the years 1949 and 1993." Contradictions abound, with claims that Okinawans eat an average of three ounces of soy products per day, mostly tofu and miso on one page and two one-ounce servings of soy on another. "As for soy making up 12 percent of the Okinawan diet, Robbins pulled that figure from a pie chart in which the 12 percent piece represents flavonoid-rich foods, not soy alone. Will the correct figures please stand up?"[11]

What's clear is that the real Okinawan longevity diet is an embarrassment to modern diet gurus. The diet was and is greasy and good, with the largest proportion of calories coming from pork and pork fat, and many additional calories from fish; those who reach old age eat more animal protein and fat than those who don't. Maybe that's what gives the

Okinawans the attitudes that Buettner so admires, "an affable smugness" that makes it easy to "enjoy today's simple pleasures."

THE NICOYA PENINSULA is a fertile rectangle on the Pacific coast of Costa Rica. Since the arrival of the Spaniards, the region has hosted herds of beef and dairy cattle. Many tropical fruits thrive there, including citrus, mango and papaya.

The region has always teamed with animal life. Early sixteenth-century Spanish settlers reported that the Amerindians of Costa Rica consumed significant amounts of poultry, fish, eggs, turtles and many types of forest game. The Spaniards introduced cattle to the area in the late 1500s, and cattle-raising has remained an important practice since that time. The Spaniards also introduced pig farming to ensure a source of ham and lard. It is clear from all reports that the Nicoyans have never been vegetarians.

Until very recently, the Nicoya Peninsula has remained relatively isolated from Western influence, with many people raising vegetables and fruit in their own gardens. Their water is noted for its high levels of magnesium and calcium.

Costa Rica is one of the Blue Zones that Buettner visited in writing his book. He interviewed several centenarians and noted that people seemed "sharper and more active than anywhere else." He described a strong work ethic and sense of intergenerational family ties, even though the men are not noted for marital fidelity.

Corn and beans are definitely staples in the diet. The women still prepare the corn at home, soaking it in ash and lime water (*lime* referring here to calcium hydroxide, not the citrus fruit), the process of nixtimalization, which releases the niacin in the corn. "This creates the foundation of perhaps the best longevity diet the world has ever known," says Buettner. "This food combination [corn plus beans] is rich in complex carbohydrates, protein, calcium and niacin. Recent research shows that in diets high in maize can reduce bad cholesterol and augment good cholesterol."

"Like the people in most other Blue Zones," Buettner insists, "Nicoyans ate the emblematic low-calorie, low-fat, plant-based diet rich in legumes."

Just one little problem with this description: the corn and beans—and also eggs, meat, and fish—are cooked in lard. Buettner follows one Don Faustino as he shops for a Sunday meal. Don Faustino visits a butcher stall in the market, "handing two-liter plastic bottles to the butcher to fill with liquefied lard. Then the butcher sliced off two slabs of pork from a dangling pig carcass and wrapped them in newspapers."

A 2013 study[12] of the Nicoya region confirmed the longevity of Costa Rican males: "Reliable data show that the Nicoyan region of Costa Rica is a hot spot of high longevity...For a 60-year-old Nicoyan male, the probability of becoming centenarian is seven times that of a Japanese male, and his life expectancy is 2.2 years greater. This Nicoya advantage does not occur in females, is independent of socio-economic conditions...Nicoyans have lower levels of biomarkers of CV risk; they are also leaner, taller and suffer fewer disabilities."

Looking at the diets of the nonagenarians, the researchers in this study were more honest and more systematic than those of Buettner:

The data on frequency of food consumption...showed some significant but small differences in the diet of elderly Nicoyans compared to other Costa Ricans. Nicoya diets include significantly more plain, quotidian foods like rice, beans, beef, fish, chicken, light cheese and sodas; and significantly less of "fancy" foods like aged cheese, olive oil or mayonnaise, less salad ingredients (lettuce, avocado, carrot, tomato) and less processed and fast foods such as white bread, cookies and hamburgers. They also drink significantly less milk (an average 0.5 glass per day compared to 0.7 glass by other Costa Ricans). There are no differences in consumption of fresh fruits, eggs, sugar, pastries and potato chips...[Compared to other Costa Ricans] Nicoyans eat or drink more calories, carbohydrates, proteins (mostly of animal origin) and fibre. Although they do not differ in the consumption of total fat, their significantly *higher levels of saturated and trans fats* [emphasis added] probably come from the use of cheaper brands of oils.

Those "cheaper brands of oils" were either unprocessed lard (it's hard for modern researchers to use the L-word) or partially hydrogenated lard. Of course, the centenarians grew up on unprocessed lard—vegetable oils were not around in the early 1900s, at least not in isolated places like the Nicoyan Peninsula.

These are fascinating details—the long-lived people of Nicoya ate *more* animal protein, *more* fish, *more* meat and *more* saturated fat than inhabitants of other parts of Costa Rica. Still, there are other details we would like to know. Did they eat more organ meats? Are the centenarians still using lard today rather than vegetable oil? Seems like they drank less milk, but was the milk they drank straight from the cow, or processed milk from the grocery store? Did they make broth with bones?

Fortunately, Costa Rica resident Gina Baker made a point of interviewing Nicoyan centenarians in 2011 and again in 2016,[13] and provides some answers to our questions. "On my way to visit a one-hundred-and-nine-year-old woman in the village of Mansión," writes Baker, "I stopped at a house to ask for directions. The lady of the house, upon learning about my research, enthusiastically described a common local dish aptly named *sustancia* (the Spanish word for "substance") consisting of pork shanks cooked with liver, kidney, ears, cheek, brain and heart, spiced with cilantro, garlic, onions and bell pepper. She also described a soup eaten daily by pregnant and nursing women, containing black or red beans cooked with a bone, lard and a type of green plantain that is very rich in potassium and magnesium, eaten along with boiled eggs."

The granddaughter and son of one centenarian told Baker they "lived on meat and that everybody in the past loved meat and, in particular, fresh liver. Don Pedro hunted game, and when he or other hunters killed an animal, everybody fought over who got to eat the liver. Don Pedro also fished (he loved dried salted fish) and ate plenty of eggs and chicken. Don Pedro noted that children often went to look for shrimp and other seafood to eat. It was common to drink whey and sometimes make soup with it...Don Pedro and other older Nicoyans reported that pork, lard and chicken skin were the principal foods and fats traditionally consumed, while other menu items were perceived as 'extras.' Nicoyans used abundant lard and other animal fats for cooking."

According to Baker, "One hundred years ago, Costa Rica produced so much lard that the country exported it. Even in recent years, indigenous people came to the town of Turrialba...by bus to purchase every single part of the pigs, including all available fat the butchers render to make *chicharrón* (fried pieces of pork

belly or rind), a big treat to Costa Ricans. When families slaughtered one of their pigs, the animal yielded five gallons of lard, providing one month's worth of cooking fat for seven to eight people."

Baker also interviewed an extremely alert ninety-nine-year-old, Don Cristobal Nuñez, who was born in 1917. "Don Cristobal was a fisherman, just like the other male members of his family. He stated that he was raised on seafood, eggs, organ meats (including one of his favorites, a dish called *sofrito*, made from the brain and cheeks of a pig) and plenty of chicken soup. In Don Cristobal's day, people also viewed *sopa de jarrete* (beef shank soup) as an excellent means of strengthening children's bones. He added that he drank a glass of sour milk (fresh cow's milk left to sour overnight) every morning to 'refresh the liver'...He also remembered the exact year...when industrialized cottonseed oil arrived in his part of the world." That year was 1932. Thus it is clear that the centenarians of Costa Rica ate lard during their growing years and by all accounts continue to do so today.

Several oldsters reported that they had no white sugar as children, but occasionally used *tapa dulce*, a dark brown traditional sweetener made from evaporated sugarcane juice.

So for the centenarians of Costa Rica, yes to organ meats, continued use of lard, raw milk and bone broth. And all accounts of their diet indicate that they eat plenty of eggs—sometimes several eggs per day. None of the centenarians Baker talked to had ever suffered from joint pain or gastritis. But times are changing: these ailments affect virtually all modern-day Costa Ricans, including the centenarians' children and grand-children. Centenarians have noticed that their descendants are sickly and that food has changed. "Today's food has the appearance of food but not the substance of it," said one of Baker's informants.

And the centenarians are disappear-ing. Writes Baker: "Sadly, in my recent travels I found far fewer centenarians than I did five years ago. Everywhere I went, I was told that some centenarians had recently died. Before leaving the retire-ment home in Nicoya, I asked employee Danny Espinosa about the shrinking pop-ulation of local centenarians. He said, 'When I arrived here six years ago, the home had forty-five centenarians. Today, we have just two.'"

TOURISM IN THE GREEK ISLAND of Ikaria got a boost when scientists determined that Ikaria was a Blue Zone. According to an Ikarian tour guide web-site, "After extensive research on the island, acclaimed *New York Times* Best Seller author of *Blue Zones*, Dan Buettner and his team, discovered the secrets of longevity on Ikaria and declared it as one of only five other Blue Zones worldwide. A Blue Zone is defined as a place where the environment is conducive to old age and in Ikaria it was found that residents are

several times more likely to reach the age of ninety+ compared to normal. It's also notable that on Ikaria instances of cancer, cardiovascular disease and diabetes are significantly lower, and dementia is rare."[14]

The usual factors get credit for Ikaria's longevity: "Little or no stress, maintain-ing a home vegetable garden, looking out over the bright blue Aegean Sea, walking in nature, picking and eating fresh fruits, vegetables and nuts, drinking wine with your friends and family, sleeping well and taking a siesta (short afternoon nap) and eating according to the Ikarian Diet."

The Ikarian longevity diet is described as "rich in olive oil and vegetables, low in dairy (except goat's milk) and meat prod-ucts, and also included moderate amounts of alcohol. It emphasized homegrown potatoes, beans (garbanzo, black-eyed peas and lentils), wild greens and locally pro-duced goat milk and honey." Ikarians also drink a lot of coffee and wine, have low sugar consumption and consume an herbal mountain tea as a panacea for a variety of ailments. Overall, Buettner describes the Ikarian diet as plant-based with a "low intake of saturated fats from meat and dairy."

This description is similar to descrip-tions applied to other Blue Zones: Sar-dinia, Okinawa and Costa Rica. But as we have seen, the common factor is all these diets is generous consumption of lard and pork, and higher consumption of animal foods among those who reach great old age. And as with our other three examples, Buettner's descriptions of the meals he eats and the foods consumed are inconsistent with his low-fat conclusions.

For example, goat milk. Inconvenient fact: goat milk is a dairy food. The Ikarians consume a *lot* of goat milk and goat milk products, such as cheese and yogurt. This is *not* a diet that is low in dairy foods; it is a diet where dairy foods are consumed with almost every meal. And goat milk is higher in fat and higher in saturated fat than cow's milk. And remember this is *raw* goat milk (Buettner never mentions the R-word), with all its nutritional components intact—nature's perfect food, especially for the elderly.

Buettner notes that "everyone has access to a family garden and livestock." What kind of livestock is lurking in those family gardens? Certainly goats; probably chickens and geese; and also pigs. Buettner visits a couple named Thanasis and Eirini. "At Christmas and Easter," he says, "they would slaughter the family pig and enjoy small portions of larded pork for the next several months." That sounds like at least six months of the year. But wait, the couple seems to have several pigs: "During a tour of their property, Thanasis and Eirini introduced their pigs to me by name." So maybe they kill pigs on other occasions, not just for Christmas and Easter. And what is "larded pork"? Could that be homemade salami, speckled with hard white fat? This is one of those many details we wish he had supplied.

When articles about Ikaria appeared in the press—this Blue Zone was not included in Buettner's book but described in 2012 in a *New York Times Magazine*[15] article—I was puzzled that there was no mention of lamb—after all, Ikaria is in Greece. I emailed Buettner asking details about lamb consumption, but never got a reply. A quick survey of the Internet creates the impression that the Ikarians keep goats, rather than sheep.[16]

However, I did find a YouTube video of sheep in an Ikarian garden, which begins with the hushed statement, "This is where the Blue Zone team is staying…"[17] Of the sheep shown in the enclosure, the narrator says, "Sheep milk is strong and fatty." If the lamb shown in the video is male, he will soon end up on a platter as a Sunday roast. So the inn where Buettner was staying had sheep in the garden.

Since Ikaria has been declared a Blue Zone, there has, naturally, been a study about it, "Determinants of All-Cause Mortality and Incidence of Cardiovascular Disease (2009 to 2013) in Older Adults: The Ikaria Study of the Blue Zones," carried out by the First Cardiology Clinic, School of Medicine, University of Athens.[18] In the study, the researchers subjected 673 individuals older than sixty-five to a variety of tests and assessed dietary habits using a diet score called MedDietScore, "which assesses the level of adherence to the Mediterranean dietary pattern." The MedDietScore determines through a single dietary survey adherence to the so-called Mediterranean diet, namely "the weekly consumption of 9 food groups: non-refined cereals (whole grain bread and pasta, brown rice, etc.), fruit, vegetables, legumes, potatoes, fish, meat and meat products, poultry, full fat dairy products (like cheese, yoghurt, milk) as well as olive oil and alcohol intake."[19]

Here's how it works: for the consumption of items presumed to be close to the pattern (nonrefined cereals, fruits, vegetables, legumes, olive oil, fish and potatoes), scores of zero are assigned when someone reports no consumption and scores of one to five are assigned for rare to daily consumption. For the "bad" items (meat and meat products, poultry and full-fat dairy products), scores are assigned on a reverse scale. Thus, if you eat full-fat dairy every day, you get a zero, and if you never eat it, you get a five.

The main things they learned in the study: 1) the older you were, the more likely you were to die; and 2) the participants didn't adhere very well to the "Mediterranean diet." Out of a total of fifty-five points, adherence was about thirty-eight. According to the report, "None of the food groups or macronutrients intake was associated with the outcome." Surprisingly, "energy intake was inversely associated with mortality," meaning that those who ate the most calories lived the longest. Could it be that full-fat dairy and red meat—which add a lot of calories to the diet—are associated with a longer life?

Indeed, with all the hype about the amazing Ikarian plant-based diet, it has been difficult to determine just exactly how our garden-tending Greek nonagenarians actually eat. Fortunately, a letter from Greek native George Voryas to the Weston A. Price Foundation provides us with important details:[20]

Regarding…an NPR-aired report by Dan Buettner on longevity on the Greek island of Ikaria, it seems Buettner failed to take into account the demographics of the island, or was fed inaccurate information by locals, perhaps only intended for tourist consumption.

According to various sources, in the early twentieth century, Ikaria had a population of about twenty to twenty-five thousand, which declined steadily to the current level of six to eight thousand, due to emigration to mainland Greece, the United States and other destinations in the world. So, the one-third of today's residents on the island said to have reached ninety years of age, is about twenty-two hundred to twenty-seven hundred people. That's not one-third of the population of which they were part at the time they were born. Today's superannuated Ikarians on the island are at best only 2–2.7 percent of their generation. Is that an amazing longevity feat? I don't think it is much different from longevity figures for other parts of Greece and, probably, many other parts of the world.

Some of that generation have emigrated to the Greek mainland or abroad, some may still be alive elsewhere, and some may have died elsewhere, but there is no reliable, verifiable, comprehensive information about their longevity or about some identical lifestyle or a uniform nutrition regimen they maintained, regardless of where in the world they had moved. Was the nutrition of their generation better or worse than that of subsequent generations? It's hard to say, but there are historical and cultural indications that show it was not what the cholesterol-mythology "science" in the West has inventively defined in modern times as "The Mediterranean Diet."

First of all, it's important to note that there never was one Mediterranean diet anywhere in the Mediterranean. Nutrition was always dependent on local production and local consumption for numerous reasons, and it varied according to proximity to food sources. Some seaside villages ate more seafood, if isolated from pastures by topography. Mountain villages consumed more meat, because they had more grazing land and raised more livestock, so they also supplied some seaside areas, wherever accessible.

However, both mountain and seaside villages consumed healthy amounts of game in the fall and spring. There was much less shipping of perishable, fresh foodstuffs, because there was no refrigeration and because transportation was costly, time consuming and limited to only a few road-accessible locations.

Different areas had different sources for their essential nutritional cholesterol intake. Mountainous areas sustained flocks of a variety of free-grazing, fat sheep and goats. In fact, the Maltese goats were famous everywhere in the basin for producing the most and the fattest milk, while Anatolia sheep were prized for their plentiful storage of fat on their tails.

Without refrigeration, meat was preserved by cooking it well in kebab-size pieces and storing it in lightly salted, melted fat, which acted as a healthy, edible preservative. The meat was kept in big, wax-sealed, earthen jars in basements for at least several months at a time. The practice continued in many areas in the country even after the end of World War II. Mountain villagers also provided the nearby plains and seaside populations with dairy products and mountain game, such as wild boar in the mainland, lots of rabbits traditionally cooked with onions in wine flavored with bay leaves, and an occasional *dorkada*, a small antelope in northern Greece, or a wild goat or *kri-kri* on Crete.

Seaside villages had more poultry roaming freely in their backyards and plenty of wild fowl. They trapped whole flocks of quail with big fishing nets spread on the ground or anchored on tree trunks; they caught smaller birds with homemade adhesive pads or *xoverges*, tied to tree branches, and used individual snares, called *thilies*, and shotguns for the large number of wild geese moving south from the Balkan peninsula and Asia Minor toward the big islands like Cyprus and Crete and to North Africa.

In many islands and some mainland residential areas, people also raised flocks of pigeons and still do, not only for communications and competitions, but also for food. Much of the folk architecture of many Aegean islands traditionally includes highly decorative multiple pigeon pens on top of residences. Old Greek cookbooks have various recipes for cooking these delicacies in wine and olive oil, thyme or oregano, or even salting them for year-round consumption, just like fish. Most of the salt was washed off with lemon juice or vinegar before eating. The salt used, of course, was not processed, and it contained the normal amount of magnesium and other minerals of seawater, so it did not affect blood-pressure as precipitously as modern, "free-running" industrial salt.

What caused the population of Ikaria to dwindle? Domestic and foreign emigration has been a constant drain. The unpredictable availability and expense of transportation, as well as the allure of economic opportunity and modern amenities in the mainland and abroad played an important role. Local recreation and social interaction on the island was mostly limited to the numerous communal, open-air feasts linked to various religious holidays, when the consumption of sheep and goat meat cooked in public areas and accompanied by the strong local wine was the usual fare, supplemented by game, mostly from flocks of migratory birds. As to fish, however, it was the traditional fare in funeral wakes. It still is in many parts of Greece. Meat was for festive occasions.

One wonders whether Ikaria residents and the mainland physicians they rarely visited ever imagined there would come a day when an atrocious, so-called "correct Mediterranean Diet" would be invented abroad and falsely attributed to islanders.

As to the documented, predominantly leftist political leanings of the island's residents, they are, to some extent, connected with internal social issues. They include the common resentment of seafood catchers and eaters against meat eaters, perceived as social injustice because of the highly envied socio-economic status of livestock owners and consumers versus the "proletariat" status of fishermen. Meat, particularly red meat, was a status symbol, an indication of financial success and prominence.

The importance of these perceptions is reflected in centuries-old folk songs and poems, where, for example, a father urges his son not to become a revolutionary and risk losing his chances at the enviable local status of a sheep and goat owner. There is no popular folk song extolling the social status of a skillful fisherman or a productive producer of tomatoes and beans. It is clear that nutrition based on foods of animal origin was the most desirable one, and those who could afford it were usually the best looking and most envied individuals.

It is also worth reminding researchers that Greece had rampant tuberculosis infection rates in the first half of the 20th century. The victims included some prominent members of the Communist Party, who were internally exiled by dictators and royalists to "desert island" detention camps, including Ikaria in the 1930s to late 1950s. Some of them are known to have denounced their ideology and their comrades in exchange for hospitalization in state-operated sanatoria for tubercular patients, which were built and operated only on mountain areas—not by the seaside where a more affordable diet of grains, vegetables and fish was available.

In the days before antibiotics the only cure for the dreaded disease was restful confinement, large quantities of locally produced fresh, full-fat milk, and lots of fresh meat and eggs…not low-fat, low-cholesterol "Mediterranean" foods.

So there is plenty of fat lamb on the island of Ikaria, festivals featuring lamb are frequent, and life on the island was so limited (might we say boring?) that the young people left in droves, leaving a concentration of older folks eating mostly natural foods, some of whom lived long. These facts make it difficult to conclude that a low-fat diet is a longevity diet, or even that Ikarians enjoy remarkable longevity at all.

SO FAR WE HAVE LOOKED at four "Blue Zones"—regions that have lots of long-lived people—Sardinia, Okinawa, Costa Rica, and Ikaria. What have we learned so far about the characteristics of these centenarians?*

What we have learned is that these healthy folks eat plenty of animal foods and animal fats, especially lard. They eat organ meats and their dairy foods are raw. And by and large, they avoid modern processed junk food.

Now we turn our attention to a very different Blue Zone, Loma Linda, home of the largest concentration of Seventh-Day

---

* Maybe the most important thing is to live in a place that ends with the letter A. Just kidding.

Adventists in the world. The religion is strongly against smoking, alcohol and eating "unclean" foods like pork. We can conclude that the Seventh-Day Adventists are definitely not eating lard.*

Their religion also discourages—but does not prohibit—consumption of meat, rich foods, caffeinated drinks and even stimulating condiments and spices.

In Buettner's chapter on Loma Linda in *The Blue Zones*, his exacting research comprises interviews with an energetic centenarian named Marge; Dr. Ellsworth Wareham, age ninety, who pioneered open-heart procedures and is still helping out with surgeries; and a family that is bringing their children up as vegetarians on lots of nuts and soy foods.

Dr. Wareham became a vegan in middle age because he says he found nice smooth arteries in vegetarians (yet they still needed heart surgery). He must not be familiar with the International Atherosclerosis Project, which found that vegetarians had just as much atherosclerosis as meat eaters.[21] He uses soy milk and egg substitutes and eats lots of nuts. He's a lucky man: he has a colleague who is "just as careful" with his diet but has had cancers of the prostate and the neck and two heart attacks.

The California Adventists have been the subject of two long studies, according to which "as a group the Adventists currently lead the nation in longest life expectancy." According to the study, Adventists contracted lung cancer at a rate of only 21 percent compared to a control group (which contained some smokers), and had a lower incidence of other cancers, as well as less heart disease and diabetes.[22]

Buettner concludes that vegetarians live longer because they eat lots of nuts (he visits a health food store that has bins of nuts from floor to ceiling), avoid meat (which causes heart diseases because it contains lots of saturated fat), and drink lots of water. We "know with certainty [that] consuming fruits and vegetables and whole grains seems to be protective for a wide variety of cancers."[23] Being a vegetarian or eating a lot of nuts will get you about two extra years of life, he claims.

However, as in the other chapters in *The Blue Zones*, we don't learn many details about the Adventist diets. Buettner does mention that only about 4 percent of Adventists are strictly vegan and these individuals are thirty to thirty-two pounds lighter than nonvegetarian Adventists of the same height—does that mean they are frail?

Many of the Adventist oldsters grew up on farms, and at least in the past, they consumed raw milk—in fact, it was the advocacy of Adventists that ensured the right to purchase raw milk in stores in California. Are they still consuming raw milk, eating cheese and butter, and eating eggs? We never find out.

---

* They do, however, live in a place that ends with the letter *A*.

And the Adventists are certainly not disease-free. According to one doctor Buettner interviewed, "Some Adventists get personally offended if they get colon cancer or some other disease. They have a reputation for avoiding these things now, of course, but it begs the question, what do you expect to die of? And when we looked, we found that, by and large, the proportions of deaths from different causes in Adventists are about the same as everybody else. It is just that they die later."[24] Does this have anything to do with the fact that they don't drink or smoke or consume caffeine? Or with the fact that some of them avoid meat?

The bottom line of the Adventist studies: on average, Adventist men live 7.3 years longer and Adventist women live 4.4 years longer than other Californians. Remember that only 4 percent of those Adventists are vegans, and that they are being compared with the entire California population, which includes many who smoke, drink alcohol, take drugs, drink coffee and eat junk food. Adventists in California as a whole are highly educated and prosperous white people, a group with better longevity than uneducated, poor, nonwhite people.

And contradictions abound. For example, while the first Adventist Health Study showed reduced all-cause mortality and increased longevity for Adventists, the 2016 European Prospective Investigation into Cancer and Nutrition–Oxford (EPIC-Oxford) cohort study did not show an all-cause mortality advantage for British vegetarians.[25]

Statistician Russell Smith analyzed the existing studies on vegetarianism and discovered that while there have been ample investigations that show, quite unsurprisingly, that vegetarian diets significantly decrease blood cholesterol levels, few studies have evaluated the effects of vegetarian diets on mortality. In a review of some three thousand articles in the scientific literature, Smith found only two that compared mortality data for vegetarians and nonvegetarians.[26]

One was a 1978 study of Seventh-Day Adventists. By ignoring a large portion of the data and through statistical manipulation, researchers computed "odds ratios" showing that mortality increased as meat or poultry consumption increased (but not for cheese, eggs, milk or fat attached to meat). But when Smith analyzed total mortality rates from the study as a function of the frequencies of consuming cheese, meat, milk, eggs and fat attached to meat, he found that the total death rate *decreased* as the frequencies of consuming cheese, eggs, meat and milk *increased*.[27]

The second study, published by Burr and Sweetnam in 1982, showed that the annual death rate from heart disease among vegetarians was only 0.01 percent lower than that of nonvegetarians, yet the authors described that difference as "substantial." The difference in all-cause death rate was in the opposite direction, namely higher for vegetarians, especially female vegetarians.[28]

The claim that vegetarians have lower rates of cancer compared to nonvegetarians has been squarely contradicted by a 1994 study comparing Adventist vegetarians with the general population.[29] Researchers found that although vegetarian Adventists have the same or slightly lower cancer rates for some sites—for example, slightly lower rates of breast cancer—the rates for numerous other cancers are much higher than the general U.S. population standard, especially cancers of the reproductive tract. Seventh-Day Adventist females had more Hodgkin's disease (131 percent), more brain cancer (118 percent), more malignant melanoma (171 percent), more uterine cancer (191 percent), more cervical cancer (180 percent), and more ovarian cancer (129 percent) on average.

In an interview with Buettner, at the offices for the Adventist Health Study in Loma Linda, study researchers claimed, "We found that the Adventists who ate meat had a 65 percent increased risk of [colon cancer] compared to vegetarian Adventists." But a study of cancer incidence from EPIC-Oxford found that the incidence of colon cancer was higher in vegetarians.[30]

As for overall health in vegans and vegetarians, a 2014 study found that these groups have more cancer, more allergies, more mental illness and more tooth decay. They need more health care and have a poorer quality of life.[31]

THE BIG QUESTION: is it low meat consumption that most contributes to good health or is it avoidance of alcohol, tobacco, caffeine and junk food? To answer this question, let me introduce yet another Blue Zone, this one in the north island of New Zealand. I call it the Maria (pronounced *MAR-y-a*) Blue Zone, after the auburn-haired Maria family, which came to New Zealand from the Azores. Nicholas Maria, who settled in New Zealand in the 1860s, died at age 93 after a life of many adventures; his wife lived on for several years after his death.

His son, Albert, died young at age 75—a tragic death from a blocked prostate, as they could not get him to the doctor in time (250 miles away from his farm in the far north of New Zealand). Albert's wife, Eva, lived to age 95.

Albert and Eva had six children. Son Roger died in his nineties; son Owen died at age 102 and was still farming in his late nineties; daughter Phyllis (mother of my husband) came very close to 102; daughter Enid died "young," in her eighties; daughter Jessie died in her nineties; daughter Winnie is still alive at age 98.

Eva Maria's brother died at age 104. Two aunts died in their late eighties.

My husband also married into longevity: both his mother-in-law and father-in-law (family name of Grimes) lived into their nineties, and their daughter Joyce lived to age 91. Their other daughter, Margaret, died at age 81. My husband's father (family name Morell) lived alone until age 98 and died at age 100. In fact, every one of these long-lived people lived on their own until close to the time of their death. My husband is 92 and still does tractor work on our farm.

This was a family of clean-living people: none of them smoked, most of them never drank and—surprisingly—none of them had the English habit of drinking a lot of tea, let alone coffee. But they sure did eat meat. They consumed a typical New Zealand diet of meat (lamb, beef, pork), organ meats, eggs, fish, shellfish and of course oodles of deep yellow grass-fed New Zealand butter on everything. Sugar consumption was moderate and no one drank soft drinks. The milk they consumed on the farm was raw.

This family prided itself on vegetable consumption—no meal was complete without four or five vegetables on the plate. But we should not confuse a diet containing a lot of vegetables with what's called a "plant-based" diet as Buettner does. Theirs was a meat-based diet garnished with vegetables, and the vegetables were dressed with butter and salt.

And oh yes, they all got cod liver oil as kids.

Many of these long-lived folks were farmers. Typically, they killed a lamb on Thursday or Friday. The organ meats were consumed that evening, and the roast or leg was served for Sunday dinner. Leftovers became curry and hash in the new week. The butcher sold blood sausage, and fast-food stores sold fish 'n' chips fried in tallow. They collected fresh mussels and oysters in New Zealand's pristine ocean waters, and fished for trout in New Zealand's clear streams. The prized parts of the trout were the roe (a powerful superfood) and the vitamin A–rich flesh behind the eyes—my husband tells me they always ate this part of the fish immediately on catching it. The skin-on filets were dipped in batter and fried in tallow. Once a physician told Aunt Sybil, Albert's sister, then in her eighties, not to do such a terrible thing, not to eat fats nor her home-fried fish. "But I like my fats," she said.

The Maria Blue Zone provides us with the right formula for longevity: real food including plenty of superfoods like organ meats, animal fats, raw dairy foods, grass-fed butter, and seafood, along with moderate habits. Renunciation of delicious, satisfying food is not necessary for good health while young, nor for good health well into old age.

THE QUESTION IS WHY? Why does Buettner insist that the secret to longevity is a plant-based diet low in fat and high in plant foods when both the published scientific evidence and his own experiences visiting the Blue Zones show the opposite?

The answer emerges in his acknowledgments, where he thanks his mentors—all of them ensconced in mainstream medicine—for "keeping me on the path of science and off the short cuts of conjecture and hyperbole." The Blue Zone project was largely funded by the National Institute on Aging, part of the National Institutes of Health, which has firmly embraced the USDA's Dietary Guidelines for Americans. According to these guidelines, a healthy diet 1) emphasizes vegetables, fruits, whole grains, and fat-free or low-fat milk and milk products; 2) includes lean meats, poultry, fish, beans, eggs and nuts; 3) is low in saturated fats, trans fats, cholesterol, salt and added sugars; and 4) balances the calories from foods and beverages with calories burned through physical activities to maintain a healthy weight.*

This prescription leaves out all the healthy, nutrient-dense foods that have sustained human beings throughout the world, including the elderly living in the Blue Zones: organ meats; shellfish, fish liver oils; animal fats like butter and lard; soaked and soured grains; fermented foods; gelatinous bone broth; raw whole dairy products; and generous amounts of salt.

The Blue Zone project also received funds from Davisco Foods International, producer of industrial dairy products including low-fat cheese, whey protein, whey protein isolates and whey protein fractions—hardly the type of benefactor that would sanction raw whole dairy products sold directly from the farm to the consumer.

The notion that fat-free foods constitute the key to longevity falls squarely in the category of "conjecture and hyperbole." The Blue Zone project constitutes damage control against the burgeoning interest in traditional foods, and the dawning realization that government-sanctioned dietary guidelines are nothing but a pack of lies designed to keep the hospital beds full.

---

* What is a healthy weight? The answer is, not too thin, especially as you age. "Excess" body fat, especially in women, prevents frailty and helps compensate for a decline in energy supply as we age. Also, during periods of illness, excess body fat seems to be beneficial. For example, patients suffering from heart disease have better chances of survival if they are obese rather than slim. For more information, visit www.smartbmicalculator.com.

CHAPTER 9

What to Eat?

Translating the Wisdom of Our Ancestors into a Healthy Modern Diet

THE STUDY OF traditional diets from around the world reveals the fallacy of modern diet plans—whether the low-protein, low-fat, high-carbohydrate diet promoted by government agencies or the high-protein, low-fat, low-carbohydrate diets advocated by major spokesmen for "paleo" or "ancestral" diets. These and other approaches—raw food, vegetarian, juicing, blood type, metabolic typing, gluten-free* and other fad diets that come and go—are dietary schemes that share little with the way human beings have eaten for thousands of years.

Given the bewildering variety of traditional diets, is it possible to come to any conclusions at all about how to eat? In fact, we can—it *is* possible to formulate basic principles to guide us through the maze of modern food choices. And eating according to the principles of traditional

diets does not mean we have to eat weird foods like insects, seal oil, fish heads and fermented bones. There are modern ways to obtain the nutrients we need using foods that appeal to us—and, more importantly, appeal to our children.

THE FIRST AND FUNDAMENTAL principle of traditional diets is that they contained no industrially processed or refined food. In Dr. Price's day, the list of processed food ingredients included white sugar, white flour, canned condensed milk, canned foods and—just coming on the market—industrial seed oils made from cottonseed and corn. The list is much longer today. In addition to white sugar, we have various refined sweeteners including corn syrup, maltodextrin, sugar alcohols and high-fructose corn syrup; refined white flour appears in breads, pasta, crackers, cookies and

---

* Some people need to avoid commercial products containing gluten-containing grains, but the gluten-free movement is also a fad embraced by industrial food processors.

pastries; and dangerously rancid industrial seed oils,* which form the basis of all processed foods—chips, crackers, bread, pastries, candy bars, cereals, fried foods, margarines, shortenings and spreads. The average Westerner gets a major portion of his calories from these empty ingredients.

We've also figured out how to process the life out of wholesome foods like milk—through pasteurization and homogenization—and grains—through the extrusion process to make breakfast cereals.

Add to these the thousands of additives that permeate everything from baby food to fruit juice to bread—many of them not labeled, and Americans consume about nine pounds of food additives per year, including artificial sweeteners, MSG and other artificial flavors, artificial colorings, dough conditioners, preservatives, starches, antifreeze† and fiber. These give taste, color and texture to insipid processed foods and lengther their shelf life. Also lurking in our foods are industrial and agricultural chemicals, pesticides and herbicides, including those inserted into seeds through genetic engineering.

To enumerate the harmful effects of industrial food ingredients is beyond the scope of this book, but the evidence clearly indicts all these products as bad for the human body, incapable of supporting good health. Healthy traditional people never ate these things, and as soon as these food-like substances were introduced into their diets—often by well-meaning missionaries—their health began to decline.

SECONDLY, ALL TRADITIONAL DIETS contained animal products. This was Dr. Price's greatest disappointment. He had hoped to find an isolated culture living entirely on plant foods, but had to admit that all traditional people ate animal foods and, in fact, went to considerable trouble and risk to obtain animal foods.‡ Some groups, such as the Eskimos and Inuit of the far north, ate a diet composed almost entirely of meat and fish, while other groups, including agriculturists in Africa and the slave classes in the South Pacific, consumed only small amounts of animal foods.

Most cultures from around the world

---

* Today's processed oils come mostly from soy and canola, which contain high levels of omega-3 fatty acids; these break down into highly toxic fragments during high-temperature processing or cooking.

† All commercial ice cream contains "food-grade" antifreeze in the form of propylene glycol, said to be nontoxic in small amounts.

‡ Some will object that the Jains in India do not eat animal foods, having adopted a policy of "do no harm" to the extent that they wear masks over their mouths so as not to inadvertently kill any flying insects. However, the Jains consume milk products—traditionally whole, raw milk products, which supply vitamins B_{12}, A, D, and K, along with calcium and other nutrients less available from plant foods. In addition, they ingest large amounts of microscopic insect parts and insect feces in rice, pulses and other foods when these foods are not fumigated as they are in the Western world. The Sikhs of northern India, living on meat products as well as milk and grains, tend to be taller and more robust compared to their vegetarian neighbors in the south of India.

consume a diversity of animal foods—meat, poultry, eggs, fish, shellfish and insects, and have a particular advantage when milk products are included in the diet;* at the same time, most cultures also consume high-carbohydrate foods in the form of grains or tubers—in fact, is several cultures we have explored, the high-carbohydrate food is considered the "food" or the "meal," while animal foods form the basis of the accompanying relish or sauce.

This is good news for modern peoples—we do not need to adopt an extreme diet to re-create the dietary habits of healthy traditional groups. A healthy diet contains both animal foods and high-carb plant foods, and avoids the fringes of too much animal food or too much plant food.†

One important point: the animal foods were always consumed with the fat—milk with its cream, eggs with the yolks, meat and birds with their fat and fatty organs, fish and shellfish when they were fattest. Fats and organ meats provide vitamin A and many cofactors needed for protein assimilation; too much lean meat leads to "protein poisoning"[‡1] or, as the American Indians put it, "rabbit starvation." Modern practices of consuming lean meat, skimmed milk, egg whites without the yolks, skinless chicken breasts or protein powders can lead to immune system dysfunction, fatigue, chronic pain, frequent infections, reduced visual acuity and many other symptoms of vitamin A deficiency—even cancer and heart disease.

Again, this is good news! Lean meat and skinless chicken breasts are inedible, egg whites without their yolks are disgusting, and skimmed milk is thin and insipid. Low-fat and fat-free foods, as well as protein powders, are processed with numerous chemicals and additives to make them palatable. Fortunately, we don't have to eat any of these yuck foods to be healthy. Quite the contrary: full-fat foods are not only satisfying but also support good health in many ways; they should be the basis of any diet.

Animal foods provide nutrients that plant foods do not contain—vitamin B_{12} and the fat-soluble vitamins A,§ D, and K_2.

---

* Archeologists have found evidence of dairy farming throughout the Mediterranean region in the form of milk fat residue on pottery shards dating back nine thousand years.

† Otzi, the five-thousand-year-old skeleton that emerged from a melting glacier, had a good meal shortly before he died. It consisted of ibex meat; einkorn wheat, possibly in the form of bread; some sort of fat, which might have been from bacon or cheese; and bracken, a common fern. Otzi ate a balanced diet!

‡ A 1988 paper published in the *Journal of Archaeological Science* warns against "the debilitating and potentially serious consequences of excess protein consumption when reconstructing palaeodiets and subsistence strategies." The authors note that coastal hunter-gatherers needed added fat or carbohydrates in their diet to avoid an excessive protein intake.

§ Carotenes in plant foods are the precursors of vitamin A, but they are not good sources of vitamin A for humans. Human beings convert carotenes to vitamin A with difficulty, and some people's bodies do not make this conversion at all.

Moreover, minerals such as zinc, calcium, copper, magnesium and iron, as well as vitamin B_6, are much more easily absorbed from animal foods. Zinc deficiency is usually the first deficiency to show up in those practicing vegetarianism—zinc is critical for reproduction and clear thinking, and helps form over one hundred enzymes, including enzymes involved in detoxification* and mineral metabolism. The best sources of zinc are red meat and shellfish.

Animal foods are also our best source of calcium; in fact, primitive peoples had only two good sources of calcium—milk products and bones. Those groups that did not have access to calcium-rich milk took pains to eat animal bones, either fermented or ground to a powder and added to their food. Milk products give human beings a distinct advantage if for no other reason than they provide abundant calcium in easily assimilated form. Plant foods do contain calcium but also compounds that block calcium absorption; and they are not as rich in calcium as milk and milk products; it takes at least forty carrots or over three cups of cooked spinach to match the 800 milligrams of calcium in five cups of milk.

NUTRIENT-DENSE: THESE TWO words sum up Dr. Price's findings about traditional diets. Price took samples of traditional foods back to his laboratory in Cleveland, Ohio, and analyzed them for vitamin and mineral content. He found very high levels of minerals in traditional diets—calcium, magnesium, phosphorus, copper, potassium, iron and iodine—and equally high levels of water-soluble vitamins—vitamin C and the range of B vitamins. Levels of minerals and water-soluble vitamins were at least four times higher in the diets of non-industrialized people.

Most surprising were the high levels of fat-soluble vitamins—A, D, and K_2—which occur uniquely in animal fats, organ meats, fatty fish, shellfish and fish liver oils. Butter, cream and egg yolks are delicious sources of these vitamins, especially if the animals are raised outside on pasture. So-called "primitive" diets contained at least ten times more of these fat-soluble vitamins than the modern American diet—and that was in the 1940s. The discrepancy is certainly larger today with the advent of industrial agriculture and the practice of removing every bit of fat from our meat, poultry and dairy products.

Vitamins A, D, and K_2[†] are sadly absent in today's diets of processed foods based in vegetable oils, and yet they are key to virtually every process in the body—from protecting us against infectious disease and cancer to ensuring good

---

* One zinc-containing enzyme is alcohol dehydrogenase, needed to process alcohol.

† Dr. Price referred to vitamin K_2 as Activator X or the Price Factor, because he did not know exactly what it was; subsequent research reveals this fat-soluble vitamin to be vitamin K_2, the animal form of vitamin K_1.

eyesight and hearing. Without these fat-soluble vitamins, we cannot make hormones, including sex hormones and the feel-good chemicals that ward off depression. Most important, vitamins A, D and K_2 ensure robust and harmonious bone and muscle development during the growing years; vitamin K_2 supported by vitamins A and D creates bone density and prevents the sealing of the growth plates in the long bones too early, so that we grow tall; plentiful vitamin K_2 in utero and during development ensures wide and strong development of the facial bones, so that the dental palate is large, the teeth are straight, the cheekbones wide and the face attractive. Vitamin K_2 puts calcium in the bones and teeth, where it belongs, and prevents it from depositing in the soft tissues, including the arteries, where it does not belong. Plentiful vitamin K_2 in the saliva, along with adequate dietary calcium and phosphorus, prevents tooth decay.

Vitamins A, D and K_2 work together—vitamins A and D tell the cells to make certain proteins; vitamin K_2 then activates proteins after signaling by vitamins A and D. Taking too much of one of these vitamins can lead to deficiencies of the other two; we need to obtain the fat-soluble vitamins from food, where they tend to occur together, and not from isolated vitamins or supplements.

These fat-soluble vitamins occur in weird foods like insects, intestines and seal oil, but also in delicious foods like pâté, liverwurst, scrapple, caviar, oily fish, shrimp, oysters, mussels, duck and goose fat, pork lard, butter, cream and egg yolks—the very foods the diet dictocrats tell us not to eat are the foods that supply these critical nutrients. Eating like our ancestors ate means including as many and as much of these foods in our diet as we can.*

Because we simply don't eat as many organ meats and weird foods as traditional people do, a good practice is to include a natural cod liver oil in the diet to supply vitamins A and D, along with vitamin K_2–rich foods like aged cheese, duck and goose fat, duck and goose liver, and butter and egg yolks from pasture-fed animals. Butter centrifuged to make a butter oil and emu oil (in capsules) are other rich sources of vitamin K_2.

SHOULD WE COOK? Animals don't cook their food, and neither should we, say the raw foodists. True, animals don't cook, but neither do they wear clothes and shoes, live in houses, talk, write, create works of art, and fill their lives with ritual and process. We are not animals but human beings, and all human societies cook some or even most of their food, even the inhabitants of the frozen north, and even inhabitants of the tropics who do not need to build fires for warmth.

Many plant foods are indigestible or

---

* In Russia and European countries, various types of sausage serve as vehicles for organ meats—sausage is a way of making offal taste good! But in the United States, federal law prevents the addition of "meat by-products" to sausage. Those by-products go into pet food instead.

even poisonous to humans unless they are cooked, especially grains, legumes, many tubers and dark leafy greens—consuming a lot of raw vegetable juice is not a formula for good health. Cooking liberates minerals and other nutrients so that we get more energy and nutrition from plant foods. Gentle cooking unfolds the tightly wound proteins in meat, making them more available to enzymatic breakdown.

At the same time, every culture we have looked at consumes some of its animal protein raw—raw meat, raw fish and shellfish, raw dairy products. Cooking destroys vitamin B_6, which is more plentiful and more available in animal foods. Heating of milk is particularly harmful; raw milk contains enzymes to ensure the complete assimilation of every single nutrient in the milk. The heat of pasteurization destroys all these enzymes, turning a food that is easy to digest and assimilate into a food that is very difficult to digest and likely allergenic.

Many cultures relished weird raw foods like muktuk and organ meats straight from the kill, but there are less challenging ways of getting our raw animal protein: steak tartare, carpaccio, oysters, sushi, raw milk and delicious raw cheese. At the same time, you do not need to subject yourself to raw kale or raw vegetable juices; rough vegetables only yield their goodness when well cooked and garnished with fat, especially butter.

ALL TRADITIONAL CULTURES consumed lacto-fermented foods. There are no exceptions to this rule. From the fermented fish of the Inuit and Eskimos to poi and similar foods in the South Pacific to sour beers in Africa to delicate pickles in the Asian diet, all traditional cultures took in plenty of healthy bacteria by eating these raw fermented foods. Only in recent years has science confirmed the role of beneficial bacteria in the gut, and raw lacto-fermented* foods help replenish that bacteria every day.

Lacto-fermented foods also provide enzymes that help with digestion, sparing our own bodies from energy-intensive enzyme production. As much as 70 percent of all our energy goes into digestion, and anything that can reduce that energy load translates to more energy for the human being. The Eskimos valued fermented foods for giving strength and stamina; the Africans drank lacto-fermented sorghum beer to give them more energy when working in the hot sun. The fact that fermented foods provide digestive enzymes explains the phenomenon of increased energy with raw, lacto-fermented foods and beverages.

Typically, lacto-fermented foods and beverages are consumed with rich cooked foods—a glass of sour kombucha is heavenly with a slice of quiche, and gherkins

---

* In lacto-fermentation, bacteria convert the sugars in foods and beverages to lactic acid; in alcoholic fermentation, yeasts convert the sugars in foods and beverages into alcohol. Both lactic acid and alcohol are preservatives—but lactic acid doesn't make you drunk! While it's not good to have lactic acid buildup in the muscles, lactic acid in the digestive tract supports healthy bacteria and good digestion.

go perfectly with pâté. Sour fermented foods help with digestion of fatty foods, and also provide enzymes to make up for any enzymes lost in cooking. In fact, think of lacto-fermented foods as super-raw foods which more than compensate for any enzymes lost in cooked food.

It's easy to include lacto-fermented foods in the diet. Many brands of raw lacto-fermented sauerkraut* and pickles are available today, as are probiotic drinks like kombucha and sparkling kefir beverages; these foods are also easy and fun to make. Raw cheese, traditionally made salami, yogurt and gravlax are other delicious lacto-fermented foods.

GRAINS ARE A HOT TOPIC these days. In fact, they seem to be the enemy du jour, shunned by paleo dieters and the gluten-free crowd. But as we have seen, all traditional cultures in the temperate regions of the world consumed grains—even the "Stone Age" Australian Aborigines. And archeological research has found evidence of grain consumption in Paleolithic campfires. Starch grains found on grinding stones dating back thirty thousand years have shown up in Paleolithic sites in Italy, Russia and the Czech Republic.[2]

Widespread intolerance of grains is a recent phenomenon, and it's probably no coincidence that these problems have followed several decades of insistence on large amounts of whole grains in the form of rough quick-rise whole wheat bread, granola, muesli, oat bran and extruded whole-grain breakfast cereals.[†]

Traditional cultures took great care with seed foods—grains, legumes, nuts and other seeds—by soaking, souring, culturing and fermenting, often for days. These seed foods are also cooked, at the beginning of the process or during, but usually at the end. All these processes release the goodness in grains, minimize irritants and antinutrients, and make them more digestible. Even gluten is broken down by the proper preparation processes. Researchers in Italy have found that even diagnosed celiacs can consume genuine sourdough bread without adverse effects.[3]

The sour grain preparations of Africa are an acquired taste for Westerners, but there are several ways of consuming properly prepared whole grains that are acceptable to our tastes—even to children. Oatmeal soaked overnight in slightly acidulated warm water and then cooked, served with butter or cream and maple syrup, is

---

* There are more beneficial bacteria in a spoonful of raw sauerkraut than there are in a whole bottle of probiotic pills.

† The high-temperature, high-pressure process of extrusion, used to make breakfast cereals shaped like O's, flakes and strands, does to the delicate proteins in grains what pasteurization does to the delicate proteins in milk—warps and distorts them so that they become highly allergenic and even toxic. Evidence indicates that extruded breakfast cereals are especially toxic to the nervous system—yet millions of schoolchildren in the United States begin their day with these grain products. Extruded grains also disrupt gut flora.

delicious; once you taste real sourdough bread, all other bread will seem insipid in comparison. Brown rice can be soaked several hours before cooking. If consumed only occasionally in the context of a nutrient-dense diet, white rice and bread made from white flour (preferably sourdough) are easier to digest and actually better choices than rough whole grains.

HOW MUCH FAT SHOULD WE EAT?
We've seen a lot of variation in traditional diets. For the Inuit and Eskimo, fat can comprise up to 80 percent of dietary calories; for some groups in Africa, fat content is much lower, probably in the range of 30 percent. Whatever the level in the diet, these fats are mostly animal fats or highly saturated coconut or palm oil.

Some people do very well on high-fat diets—which stabilize blood sugar and maximize the intake of fat-soluble nutrients. Other people have trouble digesting lipids and feel better on a diet that is lower in fat. Most people do best when fat contributes between 40 to 60 percent of total calories. For a diet of 2,400 calories per day, that translates into about twelve tablespoons of fat, including the fat on meat, in egg yolk, and in whole dairy products, in addition to cooking fat and added fats like butter.

Our bodies definitely need the saturated and monounsaturated fat that we get from animal fats and traditional oils obtained from olives, coconuts or palm fruit—we need these fats for everything from our cell membranes, to mitochondria function, to energy storage, to hormone production. If we do not get enough of these fats from our diet, the body can make them out of carbohydrate foods. Since there is a limit to the amount of protein we can ingest—about 20 percent of calories—the remaining 80 percent of calories must be divided between fats and carbohydrates. If we lower the amount of fat we eat, the deficit must be made up with carbohydrates.

Getting our fat from carbohydrates can work in the context of a diet where the animal foods supply adequate fat-soluble vitamins. In many regions of Africa, animal food and fat consumption is low, but the animal foods they do eat are rich in nutrients—foods like insects, shrimp pastes and organ meats. These foods are not acceptable to Western palates, but fortunately, we have access to many sources of animal fat in the West—from the fat on our meat to whole dairy products to butter, cream and egg yolks.

As we have seen, the ideal diet contains a wide variety of animal and plant foods; the ideal diet also contains a wide variety of saturated and monounsaturated fat sources—meat fats including lard, tallow and bacon fat; poultry fats from chicken, duck and goose; egg yolks; butter, cream, whole milk and cheese; and olive oil, coconut oil and palm oil.

Traditional cultures consumed many sources of saturated and monounsaturated fats; what they did not consume were seed oils containing high levels of polyunsaturated fatty acids. Unfortunately, most modern people are getting most of their fats from these unstable oils—which are completely new to the human diet. While we need small amounts of polyunsaturated fatty acids in our diet, too much can lead to imbalances on the cellular level; and a surfeit of polyunsaturated fatty acids from vegetable oils has been implicated in most of today's chronic disease, from heart disease and cancer to infertility and premature aging.

Polyunsaturated oils are major ingredients in all processed foods, in cooking oils, and in margarines, shortenings and spreads. They have no place in the human diet. We can get the small amounts of polyunsaturated fatty acids (called essential fatty acids or EFAs) we need from animal fats and healthy traditional oils extracted from olives, coconuts and palm fruit.

YOU'VE HEARD ABOUT OMEGA-3 and omega-6 fatty acids. We need both in small amounts in balance, ideally about two to three times more omega-6 than omega-3. We get omega-6 from nuts, grains and seeds as well as from animal fats like butter, and omega-3 mainly from seafood, organ meats and egg yolks.

Unfortunately, most modern diets contain large quantities of omega-6 from industrial seed oils—these oils can be almost 100 percent omega-6—and not enough omega-3. However, too much omega-3 is not a good idea either—we've seen problems such as stroke and bleeding in the Inuit and Eskimo diet with too much omega-3, and that can happen in modern diets when people take too much fish oil or flaxseed oil.

A balance of small amounts of omega-6 and omega-3 is key, and easy to achieve by simply eliminating all industrial seed oils from the diet and including seafood and small amounts of cod liver oil.

ALL TRADITIONAL PEOPLES consumed salt—evaporated from salt springs or seawater, or mined from underground deposits. Salt was the original item of trade, not only in Europe but also in Africa, Australia and the Americas.* When salt was not available, traditional peoples consumed seawater, animal blood and even animal urine; or they burned sodium-rich plants and added the ashes to their food.

We need salt to digest our food— chloride to make hydrochloric acid for digesting meat and sodium to activate enzymes for digesting carbohydrates. We also need sodium for brain function, adrenal function, regulation of blood pressure, and production of a variety of hormones. Sodium is also key to cellular function,

---

* Throughout history, governments have fought wars to obtain access to salt and controlled people by restricting salt. One great advantage of living in the modern age is the worldwide availability of inexpensive salt.

needed to maintain electrolyte and fluid balance.*

We need about one and one-half teaspoons of salt per day to satisfy the body's requirements for sodium and chloride—more when working in the hot sun or when under stress. Again, that's good news for modern people—we don't need to forego salt to be healthy; quite the contrary—salt is vital for good health.

What's different about modern salt is that it is refined to remove all the magnesium and trace minerals naturally present in salt; best to use an unrefined salt that has not been stripped of minerals through modern processing. Salt should be gray, pink or beige, not stark white. Fortunately, many varieties of unprocessed salt are available today.

SKIN AND BONES—TRADITIONAL cultures ate these parts of the animal, along with muscle and organ meats. Our bodies contain two main types of protein—muscle protein and collagen. In fact, we have more collagen in our bodies than muscle. Collagen is what holds us together, creates the framework for our bones, forms the basis of strong tendons and joints, surrounds our organs, lines the intestinal tract, interlaces our fatty tissue and undergirds our skin.

By "bones" we mean the collagenous portions, the gristle, joints and connective tissue. Traditional cultures consumed these portions, usually by cooking the bones, heads and feet of animals to make a nourishing broth. Think of bone broth as melted collagen, an elixir that provides the building blocks for your own collagen.

We can get collagen by boiling down rhinoceros skin to make a glue, or by eating muktuk, but a more acceptable way to nourish our collagen is to make gelatin-rich broth from chicken, fish, beef or pork bones (including the collagen-rich feet) and using that for delicious sauces, gravies, soups and stews. It's also important to eat skin—crispy chicken skin or satisfying *chicharónnes* (pork rinds). That's right, old fashioned foods like *gribenes* (crispy duck or chicken cracklings) and jellied pig's feet are health foods!

TRADITIONAL CULTURES PREPARED for the next generation; this is the final principle of nourishing traditional diets. They recognized the fact that health was not just about feeling good in the present, but also about ensuring that future generations would be healthy and strong.

Dr. Weston A. Price is unique among early investigators in his practice of asking the people he studied about special or sacred foods they consumed to ensure healthy offspring. Dr. Price's investigation showed that so-called primitive people understood and practiced preconception nutritional programs for *both* parents.

---

* Twenty-seven percent of the body's salt is in the bones. Osteoporosis results when the body does not get enough salt, among other factors.

Many tribes required a period of premarital nutrition, and children were spaced to permit the mother to regain her full health and strength, thus assuring subsequent offspring of physical excellence.* Lactating women, as well as the maturing boys and girls, also ate special foods in preparation for future parenthood. Dr. Price found these foods to be very rich in fat-soluble vitamins A, D, and K_2—foods like liver, organ meats, animal fats, gelatinous soups, fish eggs, fish liver oils and whole raw milk, cheese and butter from grass-fed animals.

These practices put modern man to shame; we are very careless in the way we bring children into the world, and when something goes wrong, we blame it on one of the three G's—germs, genes or God. Traditional cultures knew better; they knew that the responsibility for bringing healthy children into the world rested squarely on their shoulders.

EVERYTHING THAT TRADITIONAL peoples did with their food resulted in the maximization of nutrients—everything from their agricultural practices to their food choices to their preparation techniques. We can do the same with our modern diets—it just requires care in purchasing our food and attention to detail.

Traditional Diets Maximized Nutrients	Modern Diets Minimize Nutrients
Foods from fertile soil	Foods from depleted soil
Organ meats preferred over muscle meats	Muscle meats preferred, few organ meats
Natural animal fats	Processed vegetable oils
Animals on pasture	Animals in confinement
Dairy products raw and/or fermented	Dairy products pasteurized or ultrapasteurized
Grains and legumes soaked and/or fermented	Grains refined, extruded, improperly prepared
Soy foods, long fermented, consumed in small amounts	Soy foods industrially processed, large amounts
Bone broths	MSG, artificial flavorings
Unrefined sweeteners	Refined sweeteners
Lacto-fermented vegetables	Processed, pasteurized condiment
Lacto-fermented beverages	Modern soft drinks, coffee, tea
Unrefined salt	Refined salt, low salt
Natural vitamins occurring in foods	Synthetic vitamins, taken alone or added to food
Traditional cooking	Microwave cooking, irradiation
Traditional seeds, open pollination	Hybrid seeds, GMO seeds

* Price reported that in cultures throughout Africa and the South Seas, the native people considered it shameful to have a child more than once every three years. The practice of spacing children—either with natural birth control methods, through a system of multiple wives, or even through abstinence in marriage—accords very well with modern science. A 2006 study published in the *Journal of the American Medical Association* found that the ideal interval between babies was at least eighteen months but not more than five years.

And healthy eating requires no renunciation. A traditional diet is satisfying and delicious; it is an inclusive diet, not one that excludes major food groups. A healthy traditional diet includes wonderful foods like pâté, caviar and butter; whole milk and cheese; grains and legumes; sauces and gravies; generously applied salt; refreshing lacto-fermented foods; healthy soft drinks; and even naturally sweetened desserts.

The rewards are great: freedom from aches and pains; increased energy and mental acuity; protection against chronic disease; optimism and the lifting of depression; a graceful and energetic old age; and, most important, healthy children to carry on wise food traditions for future generations.

CHAPTER 10

Recipes

THE CHALLENGE FOR cooks and parents is translating the culinary habits of traditional peoples—for some of whom the greatest delight is consuming bloody quivering raw liver or crunching into raw kidney freshly plucked from a slaughtered goat—into foods that Westerners (especially Western children) can enjoy. The following recipes are designed to pique your curiosity and challenge your cooking habits—and demonstrate the fact that truly traditional foods can be both nutritious and delicious.

Grains

Sorghum Porridge

Sorghum is a common grain throughout Africa. It needs to be carefully soaked prior to cooking to neutralize antinutrients.

Serves 4

1 cup whole-grain sorghum
2 tablespoons whey, yogurt, vinegar or fresh lemon juice
1 teaspoon ground cardamom
½ teaspoon ground cumin
½ teaspoon sea salt
Sorghum syrup, for serving
Butter or ghee, for serving

Use a grain mill to grind the sorghum into a coarse flour. Mix with about 2 cups water and the whey—the mixture should be soupy; add more water if necessary. Cover and allow to ferment at room temperature for 24 hours.

In a medium saucepan, bring 2 cups water to a boil. Stir in the fermented sorghum, cardamom, cumin and salt. Bring to a simmer and cook gently, uncovered, for 30 minutes, stirring frequently, until the porridge is soft and creamy.

Scoop into bowls as you would oatmeal and serve with sorghum syrup and butter or ghee.

Llymru

This ancient Welsh recipe works best if you use the traditionally milled oatmeal from Scotland, such as the Oatmeal of Alford brand (available in the U.K.) or Bob's Red Mill Scottish oatmeal. Porridges of long-soaked oats are a fixture in northern climates. The Welsh version, *llymru*, eventually gave us the word "flummery," or pudding, made with the gelatinous soaking water (see page 240). In England it was sometimes called "wash brew" because the thick gray liquid resembled dishwater.

Llymru was from early times considered healthy and strengthening, and was valued as a healing food for invalids right up until the twentieth century.

Serves 4 to 6

2 cups Scottish oatmeal

1 cup buttermilk or kefir

Raw whole milk or cream, for serving

In a medium bowl, stir together the oats, buttermilk and 1 cup water; the mixture should have a liquid consistency. Set aside at room temperature for 2 nights, then pour through a fine-mesh strainer set over a bowl. Let the strained liquid stand for several hours, then pour off the surface water. Transfer the llymru to a medium saucepan and simmer, stirring frequently, for 40 minutes. Serve with raw whole milk or cream.

Sowens and Swats

Traditional cultures were not so foolish as to eat coarse oat bran; instead they made sowens by soaking the oat bran for a long time to remove the starch. The rough bran is then discarded or fed to chickens. The starch, or *sowens,* is cooked to make a thin porridge, somewhat like cream of wheat, and the liquid or swats is similar to African beers, very sour and smelly but actually refreshing to drink—a real energy booster.

Makes 2 cups sowens and 2 cups swats

2 cups oat bran

½ teaspoon salt

Butter or milk, for serving

Put the oat bran in a medium bowl, add 4 cups water, cover and set aside to soak at room temperature for 3 days. Strain the mixture through a fine-mesh strainer set over a bowl, pressing the bran to remove all the liquid, and discarding the solids. Set the liquid aside to stand for another day so the starchy matter (the sowens) settles to the bottom of the bowl. Pour off the liquid (the swats) that rises to the top and set the sowens aside. You should have about 2 cups swats and ⅓ cup sowens.

In a medium saucepan, bring 2 cups water to a boil with the salt. Add the starchy sowens and simmer, stirring frequently, for about 20 minutes. The result is a thin, smooth porridge.

Serve with butter or milk or use to make flummery (page 240).

Acorn Porridge

Acorn porridge—usually referred to as "acorn"—is a smooth, thick paste redolent of peanut butter. Typically the acorn is cooked in a large pot over an open fire and stirred continuously with a long stick.

The preparation of acorn flour in traditional cultures was a long and tedious process of shelling, grinding, and leaching. Today we can purchase flour already prepared in this manner. Use only acorn flour that has been carefully leached to remove tanins, such as Acorno brand.

Serves 4

1 cup filtered water
½ cup acorn flour
Pinch of sea salt
Pure maple syrup, for serving

In a small saucepan, bring the water to a boil. Stir in the acorn flour and salt. Reduce the heat to maintain a simmer and cook, stirring continuously, for about 15 minutes. Thin with a little water if necessary. Remove from the heat, cover, and set aside for 10 minutes.

Serve with maple syrup.

Acorn Griddle Cakes

Makes about 12

⅔ cup acorn flour
⅓ cup unbleached all-purpose flour
1 teaspoon baking powder
½ teaspoon salt
1 tablespoon honey, warmed
1 egg, beaten
3 tablespoons butter, melted, plus more as needed
Pure maple syrup, for serving

In a medium bowl, combine the acorn flour, all-purpose flour, baking powder and salt. In a separate large bowl, beat together the honey and egg. Add the dry ingredients to the egg mixture, alternating with ¾ cup water, until the mixture forms a smooth batter. Beat in the melted butter.

Heat a griddle or cast-iron skillet over medium heat and grease the surface with a little butter. Place several spoonfuls of batter onto the hot griddle and cook for about 5 minutes, then flip the griddle cake and cook for 5 minutes more. Continue until all the batter is cooked.

Serve with melted butter and maple syrup.

Cricket Flour Pancakes

Many traditional cultures consumed insects, which are a great source of protein, fat, vitamins and minerals, but for most people, these morsels are an acquired taste. Here's an easy way to include insects in your diet and make your pancakes more nutrient-dense at the same time. Crickets have a distinct aftertaste, so the salt and spices in this recipe are a must. Cricket flour can be purchased on the Internet. Be sure to buy a product that is pure cricket flour, not one that has added fillers (such as "cricket protein"). Also note: people who are allergic to shellfish should not consume insects.

If you own a grain grinder, you can grind your spelt or emmer berries immediately before soaking. Otherwise purchase the flour from a health food store and keep in the freezer until use.

Makes about 24

2 cups freshly ground spelt or emmer flour
2 cups plain whole-milk yogurt or kefir
¾ cup cricket flour
1 teaspoon baking soda
½ teaspoon sea salt
½ teaspoon ground cinnamon
¼ teaspoon ground cloves
1 tablespoon maple sugar
3 eggs, beaten
1 teaspoon pure vanilla extract
2 tablespoons butter, melted, plus more for serving
Filtered water, as needed
Pure maple syrup, for serving

In a medium bowl, stir together the spelt flour and the yogurt until completely blended. Cover and set aside on the kitchen counter overnight.

The next morning, beat the three eggs, and then blend in the cricket flour, baking soda, salt, cinnamon, cloves maple sugar, eggs, vanilla, melted butter and enough filtered water to obtain a pancake-batter consistency.

Heat a griddle or cast-iron skillet over medium heat and grease the surface with a little butter. Add the pancakes several spoonfuls at a time to the skillet or griddle. Cook for about 5 minutes, then flip and cook for 5 minutes more. Serve with melted butter and maple syrup.

Alternatively, place the cooked pancakes on a baking sheet and dehydrate in a warm oven until completely warm and crisp. These make a nutritious, easily digested snack for schoolchildren and athletes.

Yogurt Dough

This makes a good all-purpose crust for Steak and Kidney Pie (page 219) or for Yogurt Dough Fried in Ghee (page 214). For a lighter effect, use a larger proportion of unbleached all-purpose flour. If you own a grain grinder, you can grind your spelt or emmer berries immediately before soaking. Otherwise purchase the flour from a health food store and keep in the freezer until used.

Makes enough for 1 double-crust or 2 single-crust pies

1 cup plain whole-milk yogurt

1 cup (2 sticks) unsalted butter or ghee, at room temperature

3 cups freshly ground spelt or emmer flour

½ cup unbleached all-purpose flour

2 teaspoons sea salt

In the bowl of a stand mixer fitted with the paddle attachment (or in a large bowl using a spoon or a hand mixer), beat together the yogurt and butter. Add the spelt flour, all-purpose flour and salt and mix to make a very thick dough. Form the dough into a ball, place in a bowl, cover with a clean kitchen towel and leave in a warm place for 12 to 24 hours. If not using immediately, wrap the dough ball in parchment or waxed paper and store in the refrigerator for up to 7 days.

Soups and Stews

In any culture that has iron pots—starting with ancient Babylon—long-simmered soups and stews are a fixture of the cuisine. Anything could go into the pot: meat, organ meats, fat, blood, milk, grains, legumes or vegetables. Even groups that did not have metals were able to cook stews in vessels made of clay or ingenious clay-covered cooking baskets.

Slow Cooker Succotash

"Succotash" comes from the Narragansett word *sohquttahhash*, meaning "broken corn kernels." Modern succotash made from sweet corn and lima beans is a far cry from the traditional stew, which consisted of dog meat, bear fat, corn and beans. Here is a version that uses pork and pork fat with plenty of seasonings—it's almost like a Native American chili.

Serves 8 to 10

1 cup dried heritage beans, soaked overnight in warm water, drained and rinsed
2 pounds pork shoulder or pork butt, cut into small pieces
1 pig's foot or ham hock
1 pound pork fat (not rendered), cut into very small pieces
1 28-ounce can diced tomatoes with juices
1 teaspoon sea salt
1 teaspoon dried sage
1 teaspoon dried oregano
½ teaspoon red pepper flakes
2 garlic cloves, smashed
Filtered water
½ cup coarse masa flour

Place all the ingredients except the masa flour in a slow cooker and add enough water to cover everything. Cover and cook on low for about 8 hours. During the last 30 minutes, stir in the masa flour.

Before serving, remove the pig's foot or hock, let cool, then cut up the meat, skin and cartilage and return them to the pot. Mix well; taste, adding more salt and red pepper flakes as needed.

Sustancia

Sustaining *sustancia*, considered very important for pregnant women and the elderly, is a rich stew of pork shanks cooked with a variety of organ meats, including liver, kidney, ears, cheek, brain and heart. Most of these are difficult, if not impossible, to obtain. This version uses pork shanks, liver and heart and is easy to make using a slow cooker.

Serves 10 to 12

2 pork shanks or pig's feet
About ½ pound pork or beef liver, cut into small pieces
About ½ pound pork or beef heart, cut into small pieces
2 tablespoons lard
1 28-ounce can chopped tomatoes with juices
1 teaspoon dried oregano
1 teaspoon green peppercorns
¼ teaspoon red pepper flakes
½ to 1 teaspoon sea salt
2 garlic cloves, smashed
Filtered water
1 medium onion, chopped, for garnish
2 poblano peppers or jalapeños, seeded and chopped, for garnish
1 bunch cilantro, chopped, for garnish
Cooked rice, for serving (optional)

Place the pork shanks or feet, liver, heart, lard, tomatoes, oregano, peppercorns, red pepper flakes, salt and garlic in a slow cooker. Add filtered water to cover. Cover and cook on low for 8 hours or up to overnight.

Remove the shanks and set aside to cool, then remove all the meat, cartilage and skin and chop them very small. Return them to the slow cooker and reheat on low. Taste and add more salt and red pepper flakes as needed.

Serve garnished with the onion, poblanos and cilantro, with cooked rice, if desired.

Filipino Menudo

Serves 6 to 8

Sea salt

2¼ pounds pork shoulder or butt, cut into large pieces

1 teaspoon sea salt

½ pound pork liver

3 tablespoons lard

1 onion, diced

2 garlic cloves, minced

Freshly ground black pepper

1 28-ounce can tomatoes, with juices

1 14-ounce can garbanzo beans, drained, or 2 cups cooked garbanzo beans

¼ cup raisins

2 potatoes, peeled and diced

Bring a large pot of lightly salted water to a boil. Add the pork meat and return the water to a boil. Boil the pork meat for 5 minutes, then remove it and set aside to cool. Remove 1 cup of the cooking liquid from the pot and set aside; return the remaining liquid to a boil.

Add the pork liver to the pot and boil until tender, 7 to 10 minutes. Drain the liver and set aside to cool.

Once the pork meat and liver have cooled to the touch, cut them into bite-size pieces, keeping them separate; pat dry and set aside.

In a large heavy saucepan or flame-proof casserole, melt the lard over medium heat. Add the onion and garlic and cook, stirring, until tender, about 5 minutes. Add the pork and cook, stirring, for 5 minutes. Season with salt and pepper. Add the tomatoes and reserved pork cooking liquid; cover and cook for 10 minutes. Stir in the liver, garbanzo beans, raisins, and potatoes, adding a little water if necessary; cover and simmer until the potatoes are fork-tender, about 10 minutes.

Korean Short Ribs

Serves 4

4 pounds beef short ribs (preferably cut Korean-style)

3 to 4 tablespoons lard

¼ cup soju (Korean rice liquor) or vodka

2 cups homemade beef broth

2 tablespoons maple sugar

½ cup naturally fermented soy sauce

2 tablespoons gochujang (Korean red chile paste)

1 small Asian pear, peeled, cored and diced

6 garlic cloves, peeled and mashed or minced

1 tablespoon grated fresh ginger

2 star anise pods

1 tablespoon arrowroot powder mixed with 1 tablespoon water

4 cups cooked rice (white or brown)

6 green onions, halved lengthwise, for garnish

Kimchi (page 237), for serving

In a heavy cast-iron Dutch oven, melt the lard over medium heat. Pat the short ribs dry with paper towels. Working with two ribs at a time, brown them in the lard for 2 to 3 minutes per side. Transfer to a platter and repeat with the remaining ribs.

Add soju (or vodka) to the pot, bring to a boil and scrape any browned bits from the bottom of the pan. Add beef broth and bring to a boil. Stir in the maple sugar, soy sauce and gochujang to the pot, scraping up any browned bits from the bottom, and stir until smooth. Add the pear, garlic, ginger and star anise. Return the ribs to the pot, cover and simmer, turning the ribs occasionally, for about 3 hours, or until the meat is falling off the bone.

Use a slotted spoon to transfer the ribs to a serving dish and keep them warm while you prepare the sauce.

Bring the liquid in the pot to a boil and cook until it has reduced to about 2 cups and coats a wooden spoon. Stir in the arrowroot mixture so the sauce becomes a thick glaze.

Divide the cooked rice among four heated serving plates or bowls, place the ribs on the rice, and spoon the sauce over the ribs. Garnish with green onions and serve with kimchi alongside.

Ghanaian Groundnut Stew

Adapted from The Anthropologists' Cookbook

African soups and stews often contain ground peanuts, along with meat and often dried insects or whole small fish. The fish give a decidedly fishy taste that might not go down well with Westerners, so they are completely optional; if you're omitting them, just add sea salt to taste.

You can use unrefined red palm oil or refined white palm oil. The red palm oil, too, has a distinctive taste, so you might want to try this dish first with refined white palm oil. Common side dishes for this stew include chopped onion, fried onion, chopped banana, chopped green pepper and fried shredded coconut.

Serves 4 to 6

4 cups diced raw chicken or beef
1 medium onion, chopped
1 28-ounce can diced tomatoes with juice
3 garlic cloves, smashed
½ teaspoon cayenne pepper
1 cup peanut butter (smooth or crunchy)
½ cup palm oil (see headnote)
4 to 6 cups homemade chicken or beef broth
½ cup dried salted anchovies (optional)
Sea salt
Cooked rice, for serving

Preheat the oven to 350°F.

Pat the chicken or beef dry with paper towels. Melt the palm oil in a large skillet. Working in batches, fry the meat in the palm oil until browned on all sides. Remove with a slotted spoon and set aside on a large plate. Add the onion to the pan and cook, stirring, until golden, then remove with a slotted spoon and set aside with the meat. Add the tomatoes and garlic and cook over high heat, stirring continuously, until slightly reduced.

Meanwhile, heat the broth in an ovenproof casserole. Whisk the peanut butter into the broth until melted and smooth. Add the meat, onion and tomato-garlic mixture and mix well. Season with the cayenne and dried fish (if using). Cover and transfer to the oven.

Bake until the meat is tender, about 1 hour. Taste and season with sea salt before serving.

Serve the stew with rice and the side dishes of your choosing.

Chicken Adobo with Chicken Livers and Gizzard

Adobo is a well-known Filipino stew, typically made with chicken or pork marinated in vinegar, garlic, bay leaves, black peppercorns and soy sauce. This version includes the livers and gizzard of the chicken.

Serves 6 to 8

1 whole chicken, 3-4 pounds, cut into pieces

Liver from the chicken, membrane removed, cut into 6 to 8 pieces and patted dry

Gizzard from the chicken, membrane removed, cut into 6 to 8 pieces and patted dry

About ¼ cup lard, plus more as needed

1 tablespoon annatto seeds

1 medium onion, halved and sliced

4 cups coconut vinegar

3 garlic cloves, crushed

2 bay leaves

1 teaspoon whole black peppercorns

¼ cup naturally fermented soy sauce

Cooked rice, for serving

In a large cast-iron skillet, melt the lard over medium high heat. Add the annatto seeds and cook for about 4 minutes—the lard will take on a red coloring from the seeds. Remove the seeds with a slotted spoon.

Add the chicken pieces to the pan and cook until golden on both sides. Remove with a slotted spoon and set aside. Add the liver and gizzard and cook until browned, adding more lard to the pan if necessary. Remove with a slotted spoon and set aside. Add the onion and cook in the lard remaining in the pan until golden.

Return the chicken pieces, liver and gizzard to the pan. Add the vinegar, garlic, peppercorns, bay leaves and soy sauce and bring to a boil. Reduce the heat to maintain a steady simmer and cook, uncovered, stirring occasionally, until the chicken is cooked through and the liquid has reduced to a thick sauce, about 45 minutes.

Serve with rice.

Thai Mung Bean Noodle Soup

Mung bean noodles are a great Asian alternative to grain-based noodles.

Serves 4

2 ounces mung bean noodles

4 ounces ground pork

2 tablespoons lard

2 garlic cloves, very finely minced

About 4 cups homemade chicken broth

4 or 5 pieces small dried mushrooms, soaked for 10 minutes in cold water, drained, and coarsely chopped (optional)

1 tablespoon naturally fermented fish sauce, such as Red Boat

½ teaspoon coconut sugar or maple sugar

2 teaspoons naturally fermented soy sauce

½ teaspoon freshly ground white pepper

3 spring onions, chopped

¼ cup fresh cilantro leaves, chopped

Put the noodles in a bowl, add cold water to cover, and set aside to soak for 10 minutes, until softened. Drain the noodles and cut them into 2-inch pieces.

Meanwhile, form the pork into about 12 small balls and set aside on a plate.

In a medium saucepan, melt the lard over medium heat. Add the garlic and fry, stirring to prevent burning, for 30 seconds.

Add the broth and bring to a boil over high heat. Add the balls of pork and cook for 1 minute. Add the noodles and mushrooms (if using) and stir thoroughly. Stir in the fish sauce, soy sauce, sugar and white pepper.

Remove from the heat and ladle into bowls. Garnish with the spring onions and cilantro.

Nutrient-Dense Snacks

Raw Liver Pills

Hate liver? Can't imagine eating raw liver? Then try these.

Makes 48 to 60

butter or lard for greasing
About ½ pound sliced liver

Grease a baking sheet with butter or lard. Cut the liver into ¼-inch cubes. Spread the liver in a single layer over the prepared baking sheet and place in the freezer. Once frozen, store in small plastic bags. Swallow the cubes like vitamins, with water.

Liver Biscuits

Here's a way to get liver into your children without them even knowing!

Makes about 24

2 cups freshly ground spelt or emmer flour (see note on page 204)
2 cups plain whole-milk yogurt or kefir
½ cup desiccated liver (available from Radiant Life)
½ teaspoon baking soda
2 teaspoons sea salt
2 teaspoons ground cardamom
1 teaspoon ground cumin
3 tablespoons maple sugar or pure maple syrup
3 eggs, beaten
2 tablespoons butter, ghee, or lard, melted, plus more as needed
Filtered water
Honey, for serving (optional)

In a medium bowl, mix the spelt flour and the yogurt or kefir, stirring until completely blended. Cover and set aside at room temperature overnight.

The next morning, beat the eggs. Blend in the remaining ingredients and enough filtered water to obtain a pancake-batter consistency.

Heat a griddle or cast-iron skillet over medium heat and grease the surface with a bit of butter. Spoon the batter onto the hot griddle and cook for about 5 minutes, then flip and cook for 5 minutes more. Transfer the pancakes to a baking sheet and dehydrate in a warm oven.

Serve with butter and honey, if desired.

Yogurt Dough Fried in Ghee

African mothers consider these tasty snacks very important for their children to eat at least two times per week—so much better for them than Goldfish crackers!

Makes about 3 cups

1 recipe Yogurt Dough (page 205)
About ½ cup or more plain or spiced ghee

Pinch the dough into pieces of about 1 teaspoon each.

In a large skillet, melt the ghee over medium heat. Fry the dough in batches (do not crowd the pan), then use a slotted spoon to transfer them to a paper towel–lined plate to drain and cool. Repeat with the remaining dough, adding more ghee if necessary.

Store in an airtight container in the refrigerator for up to 2 weeks.

Note: As a variation, you can knead a little desiccated liver, cricket flour (see page 203), or grated raw cheese into the warm dough before pinching into pieces.

Pemmican

Genuine pemmican is very difficult to make—it requires cutting the lean meat from an entire animal into thin strips and drying it in front of a fire, rendering all the fat of the animal, tanning the skin and sewing it into a bag, pounding all the meat into a fine powder, drying berries in the sun, placing the meat and berries in the bag, pouring in the rendered fat, and sewing the end of the bag securely with thread made of sinew! Not something that modern hunters and food enthusiasts are likely to do.

Here is a recipe that takes the drudgery out of pemmican production. The addition of sea salt is not strictly kosher, but it will make your pemmican more palatable.

Makes about 3 pounds

lard for greasing
2 pounds lean ground beef
2 cups tallow (beef or sheep fat)
2 cups dried fruit, such as raisins, currants or cranberries
Sea salt

Preheat the oven to about 180°F. Grease two baking sheets with tallow.

Spread the ground beef over the prepared baking sheets and dry in the oven until hard and crispy, about 8 hours.

Working in batches, transfer the dried meat to a high-speed blender and grind it into a powder. (A food processor will not work for this—you need to use a blender with a strong motor and a sharp blade.)

Melt the tallow in a small saucepan, then let cool. In a large bowl, mix the meat powder, melted tallow, and dried fruit. Season with salt. Spoon the pemmican into ramekins, cover, and store in the refrigerator for up to 2 weeks. (Pemmican may also be stored in the freezer.)

Serve the pemmican spread on sourdough toast or crackers, or cooked in a pan to make a kind of hash.

Cricket Tacos

Makes about 8

1 pound ground beef

½ cup medium sherry

2 garlic cloves, minced

½ cup cricket flour (see page 203)

2 teaspoons chili powder

Sea salt

8 corn tortillas

About ½ cup lard

2 cups grated mild cheese, such as Jack cheese

Fermented Tomato Salsa (page 238), for serving

In a cast-iron skillet, brown the beef over medium high heat, breaking it up with a wooden spoon as it cooks, until crumbly. Add the sherry and bring to a boil. Add the garlic, cricket flour and chili powder and season with salt. Boil a few minutes until the sauce has reduced and thickened. Use a rubber spatula to transfer the meat mixture from the skillet to a bowl.

In the same pan, melt about ¼ cup of the lard over medium-high heat. Place a few tortillas in the pan to coat one side with the lard. Turn and fill each with about 2 tablespoons of the meat mixture. Fold the tortillas in half to enclose the filling. Fry on both sides until golden—it helps to press the tacos flat with a bacon press. Transfer the tacos to a paper towel–lined plate to drain. Repeat with the remaining tortillas and filling, using more lard as necessary.

Serve with salsa (page 238).

Organ Meats

The key to preparing organ meats is making them acceptable to Western palates—that is, making offal taste good. Fortunately, there are many traditional ways of doing so.

Scrapple

Scrapple, also known by the Pennsylvania Dutch name *pannhaas* or "pan rabbit," is a dish with roots dating back before Roman times. It was traditionally made on butchering day with pork scraps and trimmings to avoid waste. The meat and the broth it is cooked in are combined with cornmeal, flour and spices and spooned into rectangular pans to form congealed loaves. Scrapple is a true ethnic dish of the mid-Atlantic states of Delaware, Maryland, New Jersey, Pennsylvania and Virginia, and is usually served at breakfast. Unfortunately, most recipes for scrapple today do not call for organ meats, and contain questionable ingredients such as condensed milk and vegetable oil. This recipe is more genuine!

Makes about 2 loaves

2 to 3 pounds pork butt, preferably skin on, cut into chunks, or 1 pig's head

2 pig's feet

1 pig's heart, cut into several pieces (optional)

2 medium onions, coarsely chopped

6 garlic cloves, chopped

4 to 6 ounces pork liver, sliced

Sea salt and freshly ground black pepper

6 tablespoons lard

2 cups cornmeal, or more as needed

½ cup buckwheat flour

2 teaspoons dried sage

1 teaspoon paprika

¼ teaspoon cayenne pepper

If using a pig's head, scrape off any bristles, split the head in half, and remove the brain and eyes. Wash well in cold water. Place the pig's head or pork butt, pig's feet, heart (if using), onion and garlic into a large pot and add water to cover. Bring to boil, skimming off any scum that rises to the top. Reduce the heat to maintain a simmer and cook for 3 hours, or until the flesh is very tender and (in the case of the head and feet) falling off the bone. Let the meat cool slightly in the pot, about 10 minutes. Remove the meat with a slotted spoon and transfer it to a large bowl, reserving the broth in the pot. Set the meat aside until cool enough to handle, then remove all the meat, skin and tendons from the pig's feet and head or butt and finely dice.

Meanwhile, pat the liver dry and rub with salt and pepper.

In a large cast-iron skillet, melt 2 tablespoons lard over medium-high heat. Add the liver and cook for about 2 minutes per side. Remove from the pan and let cool. Finely dice the liver; set aside.

In a medium saucepan, bring the broth to a boil. Slowly add the cornmeal. Cook, stirring frequently, for about 30 minutes, adding more cornmeal or water to get a thick but still soupy consistency. Stir in the flour and sage, paprika and cayenne and season with salt. Add the diced meat and liver to the pot and mix well.

Pack the mixture into loaf pans and smooth the surface. Cover with plastic wrap and let cool. Refrigerate the scrapple until set, at least 3 hours. Melt the remaining 4 tablespoons lard and pour over the scrapple and return it to the refrigerator. The scrapple will keep in the refrigerator for several days or can be frozen for longer storage.

To serve, cut into slices and fry in lard until well browned. Serve with eggs for breakfast. Some people like to eat their scrapple like pancakes, smothered in maple syrup!

Steak and Kidney Pie

This traditional dish from the British Isles is surprisingly good served hot at dinner or eaten cold the next day!

Serves 6 to 8

1 beef kidney or 2 lamb kidneys

Juice of 2 lemons

About 2 pounds skirt steak, cut into strips about ½ inch by 2 inches

About 1 cup unbleached all-purpose flour, plus more as needed

Sea salt and freshly ground black pepper

About ½ cup tallow (beef or sheep fat) or lard

8 ounces mushrooms, sliced

1 medium onion, quartered and sliced

½ cup brandy or red wine

2 cups homemade beef or veal broth

1 teaspoon naturally fermented fish sauce, such as Red Boat

1 recipe Yogurt Dough (page 205)

2 tablespoons butter, melted

Trim any membranes from the kidneys, slice them lengthwise, and then cut them into ¼-inch-thick slices. Transfer to a bowl, toss with the lemon juice, cover and marinate in the refrigerator for several hours. Remove and pat dry with paper towels.

In a large cast-iron skillet, melt about ¼ cup of the tallow or lard. Put the flour in a shallow bowl and season with salt and pepper. Dredge the kidney pieces in the seasoned flour. Fry the kidney pieces in the tallow or lard, turning to cook both sides, until well browned. Remove with a slotted spoon and set aside. Dredge the skirt steak pieces in the seasoned flour and, working in batches, fry them in the tallow or lard, adding more as needed. Remove with a slotted spoon and set aside. Add the mushrooms and onion to the pan and cook, stirring, until well browned. Remove with a slotted spoon and set aside.

In the same pan, melt 1 to 2 tablespoons more tallow. Add 3 to 4 tablespoons of the seasoned flour and cook well in the fat. Add the brandy or red wine, stirring it into the flour with a wire whisk. Add the broth, mix in well with the whisk, and allow to boil down until you have a thick gravy. Stir in the fish sauce, then season with black pepper and more salt, if needed. Stir the kidney, meat, and mushrooms and onion until well mixed. Allow to cool.

Divide the yogurt dough into two pieces, one slightly larger than the other. Dust a pastry cloth with unbleached flour and roll out the larger piece of dough as thinly as possible. Line an 8-inch pie pan with the dough. Use scissors to trim the dough, leaving about ½ inch overhanging the edge of the pie pan. Fill the pie with the meat mixture. Roll the remaining dough into a round that is slightly larger than the pie pan. Pinch the edges of the lower and upper crusts together. Pierce the upper crust a few times with a knife and brush it with the melted butter.

Bake at 350°F for about 40 minutes, or until the crust is well browned and the meat mixture is bubbling.

Brawn

Headcheese, or brawn, is not cheese but the tender meat of a pig's head, and often the feet or hocks, set in jellied broth. A version of this dish is found in every European country, Russia and many parts of Asia, as well as in Canada and certain regions of the United States. A variety made with added vinegar is known as souse.

Serves 12 or more

1 pig's head, or 2 to 3 pounds fatty pork, cut into chunks

2 pig's feet

2 pork hocks

½ cup vinegar

3 bay leaves

1 tablespoon whole black peppercorns

Sea salt

Mustard, for serving

If using a pig's head, scrape off any bristles, split the head in half, and remove the eyes and brain.

Put all the ingredients except for the salt in a large pot. Add just enough water to cover. Bring to a boil, skimming any foam that comes to the top, then reduce the heat to maintain a simmer, cover, and simmer for 6 to 8 hours, or until the meat is falling off the bones. Use a slotted spoon to transfer the meat to a large bowl; leave the cooking liquid in the pot. Use your fingers to remove the meat, skin and cartilage from the head, feet and hocks. Chop or dice the meat, skin and cartilage and season with salt. Distribute the meat between two large rectangular glass pans.

Meanwhile, boil the cooking liquid until it has reduced by about 2 inches.

Allow to cool. Strain the cooking liquid through a fine-mesh sieve and pour it over the meat to completely cover. (Reserve any remaining cooking liquid for other uses.) Cover and refrigerate overnight until set.

To serve, cut the brawn into squares and accompany with mustard. Leftovers may be frozen.

Bone Marrow on Toast

Serves 4

8 marrow bones, about 1½ inches thick
¼ cup sea salt, plus more as needed
8 small slices sourdough bread, toasted
1 medium red onion, quartered and very thinly sliced
coarse sea salt

In a large saucepan, combine 2 quarts water and the sea salt and heat over medium heat until the salt has dissolved. Allow to cool.

Place marrow bones in the salt water and refrigerate for at least 24 hours. (This will change the marrow from an off-putting brown to an attractive white color.)

Preheat the oven to 400°F.

Remove the marrow bones, pat dry, and arrange them in a single layer on a rimmed baking sheet. Roast for about 20 minutes.

To serve, place 2 bones on each plate, along with 2 small slices of sourdough toast, a pile of sliced onion, and a small pile of coarse sea salt. Spread the marrow on the bread, sprinkle with salt and top with sliced onion.

Crispy Chicken Livers

Serves 4

2 pounds chicken liver, cut in half and cleaned of any membrane

1 cup unbleached all-purpose flour

2 teaspoons sea salt

½ teaspoon freshly ground black pepper

½ to 1 cup lard

1 medium onion, quartered and thinly sliced

4 garlic cloves, minced

½ cup dry or medium sherry

¼ cup naturally fermented soy sauce

1 cup homemade chicken broth

Cooked rice, mashed potatoes, or Cassava Fufu (page 233), for serving

Rinse the livers and pat dry. In a shallow bowl, combine the flour, salt, and pepper. Dredge the livers in the flour, shaking off any excess.

In a medium cast-iron skillet, melt the lard over medium-high heat—it should be at least 1 inch deep in the pan. Working in batches, fry the livers, turning as needed, until crisp. Remove from the pan with a slotted spoon and drain on paper towels. Add the onion and garlic to the fat remaining in the pan and cook, stirring continuously, until golden. Remove with a slotted spoon.

Pour off any excess fat and deglaze the pan with sherry. Add the soy sauce and broth and cook until the liquid has reduced to a thick sauce. Return the onion, garlic and chicken livers to the pan and stir to coat everything with the sauce.

Serve over rice, mashed potatoes, or fufu.

Cooking with Blood

Many cultures use blood as an ingredient in cooking—not just the Maasai, who extract blood from their living cattle, but European cultures as well, from Hungary to the British Isles. American Indians filled the stomachs of the animals they killed with finely cut-up organ meats, shredded fat and blood. And blood from chickens and pigs is used throughout the South Seas and the Caribbean.

We know that blood is a rich source of vitamin D, and we can guess that it is a powerhouse of vitamin B_{12}, iron and many other vitamins and minerals.

Where to obtain this unique ingredient? Certainly not from a grocery store! You will need to know a farmer who can save you the blood from butchering chickens or pigs. You can also order frozen pig's blood from Philippine grocers through the Internet. It comes in 10-ounce containers, so these recipes are adjusted for this quantity.

Blood Pancakes

Blood pancakes feature in many European cuisines, from Finland to Switzerland.

Serves 12

2 cups plain whole-milk yogurt

3 cups freshly ground whole-grain flour, such as barley, rye, or spelt, or a mixture

10 ounces pig's blood (see headnote)

2 eggs, beaten

2 tablespoons molasses, warmed

½ teaspoon sea salt

1 teaspoon finely ground white pepper

1 teaspoon ground marjoram

4 tablespoons (½ stick) butter, melted

Naturally sweetened jam, for serving

In a medium bowl, mix the yogurt and the flour—the mixture will be very thick. Stir well to make sure that all the flour is moistened. Cover and set aside at room temperature overnight.

The next morning, gradually beat in the blood and remaining ingredients to form a very thick batter.

Heat a large cast-iron skillet over medium heat and grease the surface with a little butter. Spoon several spoonfuls of thick batter into the pan and cook for 2 to 3 minutes per side. Remove from the pan and repeat with the remaining cakes.

Serve with naturally sweetened jam.

British Black Pudding

Makes 3 pounds

1½ cups steel-cut (pinhead) oats

1½ cups water, slightly warmed

2 tablespoons vinegar

2½ teaspoons salt

20 ounces fresh pig's blood (see headnote, page 223)

2 cups finely diced or grated pork fat

1 large yellow onion, finely chopped

1 cup whole milk

1½ teaspoons freshly ground black pepper

2 teaspoons ground allspice

Put the oatmeal in a medium bowl and add the warm water and vinegar. Cover and set aside to soak overnight at room temperature.

The next day, preheat the oven to 325°F. Grease two glass loaf pans (that hold 5 to 6 cups) with lard. Even better, use a Le Creuset 2-quart terrine pan.

Drain the soaked oats, discarding the water.

Stir 1 teaspoon of the salt into the blood. Pour the blood through a fine-mesh sieve set over a large bowl to remove any lumps. Stir in the fat, onion, milk, pepper, allspice and remaining 1½ teaspoons salt. Add soaked oats and mix to combine. Fill the prepared loaf pans or terrine pans, cover with foil or lid, and bake for 1 hour, until firm. Let cool completely. Refrigerate for up to 1 week. The blood pudding may also be frozen.

To serve, cut a slice about ½ inch thick off the loaf (and, if desired, shape the slice into 2 round patties, as you would for an English breakfast, below). Fry in melted lard until the edges are slightly crisped and browned.

English Breakfast

This hearty breakfast has nourished generations of English yeomen and lasses.

Serves 2

4 British Black Pudding patties (page 224)
2 tablespoons lard
4 sausage links
2 slices Canadian bacon
2 slices sourdough bread, crusts removed
2 small tomatoes, halved crosswise
4 eggs
1 teaspoon finely minced fresh parsley

Melt the lard in a large cast-iron skillet and fry the blood sausage over medium heat. Transfer to two heated plates and keep warm in a low oven or warming drawer. In sequence, fry the sausages, Canadian bacon, bread, and tomatoes (cut-side down), adding more lard if necessary, and dividing them between the plates. Finally, fry the eggs to your taste.

Place the eggs on top of the bread. Sprinkle the plates with parsley and serve.

Spicy Blood Meat Loaf

Serves 8

2 cups sourdough bread crumbs, plus more if needed

1 cup heavy cream

4 tablespoons (½ stick) butter

1 medium onion, finely chopped

1 carrot, finely chopped

1 celery stick, finely chopped

¼ teaspoon red pepper flakes

1 teaspoon dried thyme

1 teaspoon cracked black pepper

1 teaspoon sea salt

2 pounds ground beef

10 ounces pig's blood (see headnote, page 223)

2 eggs

1 tablespoon naturally fermented fish sauce, such as Red Boat

1 7-ounce jar tomato paste

Preheat the oven to 350°F.

Put the bread crumbs in a large bowl and pour over the cream. Mix well and set aside to soak.

In a medium skillet, melt the butter over medium heat. Add the onion, carrot and celery and cook, stirring, until soft. Add the red pepper flakes, thyme, black pepper and salt and stir well.

Add the sautéed vegetables to the bowl with the soaked bread crumbs. Add the ground beef, blood, eggs and fish sauce. Mix well with your hands. Form the mixture into a loaf and place it in a rectangular glass baking dish. Spread the tomato paste over the loaf. Pour about ½ cup water into the pan. Bake for about 1½ hours. To serve, cut into slices.

Boudin Noir (French-Style Black Pudding)

Recipe courtesy Angie Minno

Serves 6

Butter, for greasing

½ cup diced pork fat

1 apple, cored and minced

1 onion, minced

2 cups sourdough bread crumbs

3 eggs, beaten

½ cup heavy cream

10 ounces pig's blood (see page 223)

1 tablespoon brandy

2 teaspoons *quatre-épices* (see Note)

1 teaspoon sea salt

Freshly ground black pepper

1 pound ground beef or pork

Preheat the oven to 350°F. Grease a 6-cup glass loaf pan. Bring a kettle of water to a boil, then keep the water at a simmer.

In a medium skillet, render the pork fat over medium heat. Add the apple and onion and cook until soft. Set aside.

In a large bowl, mix the bread crumbs, eggs, cream, blood, brandy, *quatre-épices,* salt and pepper to taste. Add the sautéed apple and onion and the rendered fat from the pan and mix well.

Put the ground meat in a separate large bowl and gradually mix in the bread crumb mixture (it mixes in more evenly this way). Transfer the mixture to the prepared loaf pan, patting it into an even layer, cover the top with foil (make sure it doesn't come in contact with the mixture), and set the loaf pan in a roasting pan. Set the pan on the oven rack and carefully pour in water from the kettle to come about halfway up the sides of the loaf pan. Bake for 35 to 45 minutes, or until completely set.

Note: You can make your own quatre-épices *by mixing ground white pepper, allspice, ginger and cloves.*

Cajun-Style Black Pudding

Recipe courtesy Angie Minno

Serves 6

½ cup diced pork fat

3 celery sticks, minced

1 onion, minced

2 cups sourdough bread crumbs

3 eggs, beaten

½ cup heavy cream

10 ounces pig's blood (see headnote, page 223)

1 teaspoon salt

½ teaspoon freshly ground black pepper

½ teaspoon freshly ground white pepper

1 tablespoon paprika

1 tablespoon oregano

2 teaspoons ground celery seeds

2 or 3 garlic cloves, minced

1 pound ground beef, veal or pork

Preheat the oven to 350°F. Grease a 6-cup glass loaf pan. Bring a kettle of water to a boil, then keep the water at a simmer.

In a large skillet, render the pork fat over medium heat heat. Add the celery and onion and cook until soft. Set aside.

In a large bowl, mix the bread crumbs, eggs, cream, blood, salt, black pepper, white pepper, paprika, oregano, celery seeds, and garlic. Add the sautéed vegetables and all the fat from the pan and mix well.

Put the ground meat in a separate large bowl and gradually mix in the bread crumb mixture (it mixes in more evenly this way). Transfer the mixture to the greased loaf pan, patting it into an even layer. Cover the top with foil (make sure it doesn't come in contact with the mixture), and set the loaf pan in a roasting pan. Set the pan on the oven rack and carefully pour in water from the kettle to come about halfway up the sides of the baking dish. Bake for 35 to 45 minutes, or until completely set.

Blood Soup

Blood soup is traditionally made with duck or goose blood after butchering day. Here's a variation that uses pig's blood instead.

Serves 8 to 10

½ cup dried prunes, chopped

½ cup raisins

20 ounces pig's blood (see headnote, page 223)

2 cups crème fraîche or sour cream

2 quarts stock made from chicken, duck or goose bones, strained and cooled

¼ teaspoon marjoram

¼ teaspoon ground allspice

Sea salt

Reserved meat picked off the bones used to make the stock, finely chopped

Preheat the oven to 250°F. Warm the reserved meat in the oven.

Bring a small saucepan of water to a boil. Place the chopped prunes and raisins in a bowl and pour the boiling water over the fruit to cover. Set aside.

Pour the cooled stock into a medium saucepan. Whisk the blood and crème fraîche into the stock. Add the marjoram, allspice and salt to taste. Heat over low heat, very slowly, stirring very frequently. You need to warm the soup to serving temperature, but if it gets too hot, the blood will curdle.

Drain the dried fruit. Arrange a pile of the warmed meat and the dried fruit in soup bowls. Pour the soup over and serve immediately.

Seafood

Potted Shrimp

Many cultures preserved meat and seafood in fat. Potted shrimp from the British Isles is one example.

Makes about 2 cups

1 pound small shrimp, peeled and deveined
½ cup (1 stick) plus 2 tablespoons salted butter, melted
3 tablespoons medium or dry sherry
1 teaspoon finely grated lemon zest
2 tablespoons finely chopped fresh chives

In a medium skillet, melt 2 tablespoons butter over medium heat. Add the shrimp and cook until they turn pink and are cooked through. Add the sherry and lemon zest to the pan and cook until the liquid thickens and coats the shrimp. Allow to cool and stir in the chives. Divide the shrimp between two 1-cup ramekins, pressing down so they are level and about ½ inch below the rim. Pour the melted butter over the shrimp to cover, dividing it evenly between the ramekins. Refrigerate. Keeps at least two weeks.

Serve with sourdough toast.

Mussels with Coconut Milk

Serves 4

1 14-ounce can full-fat coconut milk

2 tablespoons naturally fermented fish sauce, such as Red Boat

Juice of 2 limes

1 teaspoon red pepper flakes

2 garlic cloves, minced

1 tablespoon minced fresh ginger

About 4 pounds fresh mussels

Place all ingredients except the mussels in a large pot. Bring to a simmer over medium heat and cook for several minutes. Add the mussels to the pot, cover and cook about 5 to 7 minutes until the mussels open—be careful not to overcook them or the mussels will become tough.

Divide the mussels among four bowls, discarding any that did not open, and pour the cooking liquid over them. Serve immediately.

Oyster Stew

Serves 6

2 pints raw shucked oysters in their liquor

1 cup unbleached all-purpose flour

Sea salt and freshly ground black pepper

4 tablespoons (½ stick) or more butter

2 cups homemade fish broth

1 cup crème fraîche or heavy cream

1 teaspoon naturally fermented fish sauce, such as Red Boat

About 2 tablespoons finely minced fresh chives

Drain the oysters, reserving their liquor, pat dry and cut into three or four pieces each. Put the flour in a shallow bowl and season with salt and pepper.

Dredge the oysters in the seasoned flour.

In a medium skillet, melt the butter over medium heat. Working in batches, add the dredged oyster pieces and fry for just 2 to 3 minutes adding more butter if necessary. Be careful not to overcook the oysters or they will be tough. Remove from the pan with a slotted spoon and repeat with the remaining oysters.

Meanwhile, in a saucepan, combine the reserved oyster liquor, fish broth, crème fraîche and fish sauce and bring to a simmer over medium heat. Add the oysters and serve immediately, garnished with the chives.

Salmon Roe Canapés

Fish eggs are highly valued as a fertility food in cultures throughout the globe. Here's a particularly delicious way to enjoy this nutrient-dense food.

Serves 4

8 small thin slices sourdough bread, crusts removed
½ cup (1 stick) butter, melted
½ cup crème fraîche or sour cream
⅓ cup wild salmon caviar (roe)
1 tablespoon chopped fresh dill

Preheat the oven to 250°F.

Brush the bread with the melted butter, set the slices on a baking sheet and bake until crisp.

Place 2 teaspoons of the crème fraîche on each piece of bread and top with 2 teaspoons of the salmon caviar. Sprinkle fresh dill on top and serve.

Vegetables

Cassava Fufu

Cassava is a staple food throughout Asia, Africa and Central and South America; in fact, it is a dietary staple for more than half a billion people worldwide. Cassava contains cyanide compounds that must be neutralized by proper preparation before it can be eaten. Traditionally this was accomplished by soaking the cassava roots in water, grinding them into a paste, spreading the paste and drying in the sun for about five hours. Commercial cassava is oven dried to produce a flour with cyanide levels less than ten parts per million. Cassava also contains the mineral-blocking antinutrient phytic acid, which is considerably reduced by cooking. Cassava flour is a good source of resistant starch, which passes through the small intestine undigested and is broken down by bacterial fermentation in the colon to produce butyric acid, an important fatty acid for the immune system.

There are numerous ways of preparing cassava; *fufu*, common to Ghana, is one of the simplest. A search of the Internet will provide many modern recipes using cassava flour in gluten-free recipes for bread, muffins and similar foods.

Serves 6

2 cups cassava flour

Place the cassava flour in a bowl and stir in 1 cup water, mixing as well as possible to avoid lumps. Bring 2 cups water to a boil in a small saucepan. Slowly add the cassava flour paste, stirring continuously with a wooden spoon or paddle. The mixture should be thick and perfectly smooth. Form it into balls and serve with Ghanaian Groundnut Stew (page 210).

Fried Okra

Okra is a common vegetable in Africa, Asia and the American South. The mucilaginous interior of the pods contains soluble fiber considered helpful for feeding children and mitigating malnutrition. The pods are cooked, pickled, eaten raw or included in salads. In the southern United States, okra is typically fried—a delicious way to eat this challenging vegetable. Fried okra is often served with shrimp.

Serves 4

About 1½ pounds fresh okra

1 cup buttermilk or plain whole-milk yogurt

About 1 cup unbleached all-purpose flour

1 teaspoon paprika

1 teaspoon sea salt

1 teaspoon freshly ground black pepper

¼ teaspoon cayenne pepper

About 2 cups lard or rendered bacon fat, for frying

Trim the ends off the okra and cut the pods crosswise into rounds. Put them in a bowl, add the buttermilk, and soak for a few minutes. Place in a colander to drain.

In a shallow bowl, combine the flour, paprika, salt, black pepper, and cayenne. Dredge the okra pieces in the seasoned flour.

In a heavy-bottomed deep skillet, melt the lard or bacon grease and heat it over medium high heat to 350°F. Working in small batches, add the dredged okra slices and fry for 2 to 3 minutes, or until well browned. Use a slotted spoon to transfer the okra to paper towels to drain. Serve hot.

Yam Fritters

Serves 4

About ½ cup lard or refined palm oil

2 cups grated peeled yam

½ cup arrowroot powder

½ teaspoon sea salt

½ teaspoon freshly ground black pepper

¼ teaspoon cayenne pepper

In a large cast-iron skillet, melt the lard or heat the palm oil over medium-high heat.

In a medium bowl, mix the grated yam, arrowroot, salt, black pepper, and cayenne. Carefully place three or four spoonfuls of the yam mixture in the hot fat and fry until golden brown on both sides. Remove with a slotted spoon and drain on paper towels. Repeat with the remaining yam mixture. Serve hot.

Swiss Chard

Like so many green vegetables, chard needs careful preparation to minimize the antinutrients it contains. This medieval recipe shows that our ancestors understood this principle.

Serves 6

About 4 pounds chard, stems removed and leaves cut into fine strips

½ pound salt pork, cut into thin strips about the size of matchsticks

4 cups homemade chicken broth

2 tablespoons minced fresh parsley

2 tablespoons minced fennel

Sea salt

Soak the chard in cold water for about 1 hour, then drain in a colander, rinse, and leave in the colander to drain until somewhat dry.

Meanwhile, in a large saucepan, combine the salt pork and broth and bring to a boil. Add the chard and cook, uncovered, for about 15 minutes. Stir in the parsley and fennel.

Season with sea salt and serve immediately.

Fermented Condiments

Authentic Kimchi

Makes 2 to 3 quarts

1 head napa cabbage

½ cup coarse sea salt

Filtered water, cold

2 or 3 daikon radishes, peeled and cut into thin matchsticks

4 scallions, ends removed and cut into 1-inch pieces

⅓ cup gochagaru (Korean red chile powder)

¼ cup naturally fermented fish sauce, such as Red Boat

¼ cup minced fresh ginger

6 to 8 garlic cloves, minced

Cut the cabbage in half lengthwise and remove core, then slice it crosswise into 2-inch-thick pieces. Place the cabbage in a large bowl, sprinkle with the coarse salt, and toss until the salt is well distributed. Add enough cold water to just cover the cabbage. Cover the bowl with plastic wrap and let sit at room temperature for 12 to 24 hours.

Drain the cabbage in a colander and rinse under cold water. Gently squeeze out the excess liquid and set aside.

Place the daikons, scallions, chile powder, fish sauce, ginger and garlic in a large bowl and stir to combine. Add the cabbage and toss until the cabbage is thoroughly coated with the mixture. Pack the mixture tightly into two quart-sized widemouthed mason jars. Seal the jars and let sit in a cool, dark place for 24 hours. Open the jars to let the gases escape, then reseal and refrigerate for at least 48 hours before eating. The kimchi will keep in the refrigerator for many months.

Fermented Tomato Salsa

Makes 1 quart

2 to 3 tablespoons extra-virgin olive oil, plus more for greasing

10 Roma (plum) tomatoes, halved lengthwise and seeded

4 large garlic cloves, minced

2 jalapeños, seeded and diced

1 small bunch cilantro, chopped

2 tablespoons fresh lemon or lime juice

1 teaspoon cumin seeds, roasted in the oven and then ground to a powder

½ teaspoon dried oregano

Pinch of cayenne pepper

1 tablespoon unrefined sea salt

¼ cup homemade whey (see Note)

Preheat the broiler. Grease two baking sheets with olive oil.

Place the tomatoes skin-side down on the baking sheets and sprinkle with the olive oil and minced garlic. Place under the broiler until the tomatoes begin to brown. Let the tomatoes cool and then chop them into ¼-inch dice. Transfer to a large bowl, add the jalapeños, cilantro, lemon juice, cumin, oregano, cayenne, salt and whey and mix well. Pack the mixture into a quart-sized widemouthed mason jar. Seal the jar and leave at room temperature for 2 days, then transfer to the refrigerator. The salsa will keep for up to 2 months.

Note: To make homemade whey, line a strainer with a clean thin dish towel and set it over a bowl. Place 1 quart plain whole-milk yogurt in the strainer, cover, and leave on the counter overnight. The whey will drip into the bowl. Store the whey in a glass jar in the refrigerator. Use the remaining "yogurt cheese" for Coeur à la Crème *(page 239).*

Desserts

Coeur à la Crème

Serves 4

Yogurt cheese, from making fresh whey (see page 238)

1 cup crème fraîche

½ cup honey, warmed

¼ cup brandy

1 teaspoon pure vanilla extract

½ teaspoon grated lemon zest

1 cup heavy cream, whipped

2 pints strawberries, washed, tops removed and quartered lengthwise

¼ cup maple sugar

¼ cup balsamic vinegar

Line a 7¼-inch *Coeur à la Crème* mold (available on the Internet) with cheesecloth, leaving enough overhanging the edges to fold over the top. In a large bowl, combine the yogurt cheese, crème fraîche, honey, brandy, vanilla and lemon zest, mix well and gently fold in the whipped cream. Carefully transfer the mixture to the mold and fold the overhanging cheesecloth over the top. Cover with plastic wrap, place on a rack set in a rimmed baking sheet (to catch the juices that drip out of the holes in the mold), and refrigerate for at least 4 hours.

Meanwhile, in a bowl, toss the strawberries in the maple sugar and leave at room temperature for about 1 hour. Toss with the vinegar, cover, and refrigerate.

To serve, invert the *Coeur à la Crème* onto a serving plate and surround it with the strawberries.

Flummery

Serves 4

¼ cup honey, warmed

2 tablespoons Scotch whisky or brandy

Zest of 2 organic oranges

2 cups swats (page 201), at room temperature

¼ cup maple sugar

¼ cup fresh orange juice (from about 2 oranges)

2 teaspoons gelatin

1 cup heavy cream, whipped

In a small bowl, mix the honey, whisky and orange zest; set aside.

In a small pan over medium heat, sprinkle the gelatin over the orange juice; stir constantly until the gelatin is dissolved. Allow to cool slightly.

In a medium bowl, mix the swats with the maple sugar and orange juice mixture. Divide the mixture among 4 ½-cup ramekins or molds and refrigerate until set.

Dip the molds in hot water to loosen the flummery, then invert them onto individual serving plates. Pour the honey mixture over the top and garnish with whipped cream.

Chestnut Cookies

Makes 18 to 20

1 cup arrowroot powder, plus more for dusting

1½ cups chestnut flour

½ cup maple sugar

1 teaspoon vanilla powder

½ teaspoon sea salt

½ cup (1 stick) unsalted butter, sliced, at room temperature

Preheat the oven to 350°F. Grease a baking sheet with a little butter and dust it with arrowroot powder.

In a food processor, combine the chestnut flour, arrowroot powder, maple sugar, salt and vanilla powder. Pulse until well combined. Add the butter slices and process until well blended.

Shape the dough into 1-inch balls and place them on the prepared baking sheet. Flatten each cookie with a fork. Bake for about 25 minutes until lightly browned. Let cool on the pan on a wire rack before removing from the pan.

Acknowledgments

No book can come from one person alone, and *Nourishing Diets* in particular owes much to others.

First, the two Mary's: the late Mary Enig, PhD, my original partner and colleague, whose collaboration gave *Nourishing Traditions* legitimacy and accuracy; and Mary Evans, my literary agent, whose support and faith in my work has resulted in this and two other books, *Nourishing Broth* and *Nourishing Fats*.

For all three books, it has been an absolute pleasure to work with Karen Murgolo and Brittany McInerney at Grand Central. I appreciate their expert input, but even more their hands-off approach, always respecting my message and point of view. Ivy McFadden did a superb job of editing a long and complicated manuscript, checking all the names of eighteenth- and nineteenth-century diarists and making sure that everything was accurate and correct. Thank you to Yasmin Mathew, our production editor.

For the chapter on the Aborigines of Australia, I am much indebted to Arabella Forge who lent me books on early Australia that I would not otherwise have found, and which led me on a path to discovery of Aboriginal land management techniques. Philip Higsdon provided the fascinating detail about aboriginal consumption of kangaroo milk.

A number of years ago, Don Cote provided valuable information and leads that resulted in my first article on the Native Americans; more recently, Ellen O'Brien waded through the six volumes of *History, Conditions and Prospects of the Indian Tribes of the United States*, published in 1852, for nuggets concerning food and hunting.

Anore Jones spent many years living north of the Arctic Circle in Alaska and wrote two wonderful books, *The Fish We Eat* and *The Plants We Eat*. She graciously gave me much valuable feedback on the chapter concerning the native peoples of Alaska, Canada and Greenland. Thanks also to Paal Røiri who provided input on carbohydrate consumption among the Inuit. Chris Masterjohn's work on *pibloktoq* provided important insights into the Eskimo diet.

Sylvia Onusic, PhD, helped me find many references, particularly in connection with South Seas diets.

As for the Asian diet, help came from all sides. Mr. and Mrs. Eugene Yen provided input in my original article on China, as did Steven Gist for the section on Japan, Tina Parks and Hea Young Kuhn for the section on Korea and Tom and Nee Sinclair for the section on Thailand. Agnes Bunagan provided important insights into the Philippine diet.

In the chapter on Europe, the late Katherine Czapp provided inspiration for the section on Russia as did Cristiano Nisoli for the section on the Mediterranean diet.

Finally, I am most grateful for the patience and support of my husband, Geoffrey Morell, the source of information on the Maria Blue Zone. He spent many evenings providing a nourishing diet *for me* during the last few weeks dedicated to finishing *Nourishing Diets*.

Sally Fallon Morell
January 28, 2018

Notes

Introduction

1   www.westonaprice.org/about-us/dr-weston-a-price-movietone.
2   www.westonaprice.org/the-paleo-diet-by-loren-cordain, accessed September 27, 2017.
3   www.westonaprice.org/the-paleo-solution-by-robb-wolf, accessed September 27, 2017.
4   W. W. Newcomb Jr., *The Indians of Texas*, University of Texas Press, 1961.
5   Weston A. Price, *Nutrition and Physical Degeneration* (San Diego: The Price-Pottenger Nutrition Foundation, 1945), 161–162.

Chapter 1: Australian Aborigines

1   www.nt.gov.au/health/healthdev/health_promotion/bushbook/volume2/chap3/before.html, accessed February 14, 2017.
2   T. L. Mitchell, *Three Expeditions into the Interior of Eastern Australia* (London: T and W Boone, 1839), 90.
3   Bill Gammage, *The Biggest Estate on Earth: How Aborigines Made Australia* (Sydney, Australia: Allen & Unwin, 2011).
4   Ibid., 151.
5   Ibid., 151.
6   John McKinlay, *McKinlay's Journal of Exploration in the Interior of Australia (Burke Relief Expedition)* (Melbourne, F.F. Bailliere 1862), 50.
7   Mitchell, 90.
8   Charles Sturt, *Narrative of an Expedition into Central Australia* (T and W Boone, 1849), 69.
9   H. L. Roth, "On the Origin of Agriculture," *Journal of the Anthropological Institute of Great Britain and Ireland* (1886): 132.
10 Gammage, 292–293.
11 Ibid., 294.
12 A. C. Ashwin, *From Australia to Port Darwin with sheep and horses in 1871* (Royal Geographic Society of Australia [SA], 1932), 5.
13 Bruce Pascoe, *Dark Emu, Black Seeds: Agriculture or Accident?* (Broome, Australia: Magabala Books Aboriginal Corporation, 2014), 29.
14 Ibid., 29.
15 Ibid., 30.
16 Ibid., 44.
17 G. A. Robinson, *The Journals of George Augustus Robinson*, vol. 4 (1841), 207.
18 R. Gerritsen, *Australia and the Origins of Agriculture* (Oxford: Archaeopress, 2008), 84.
19 Pascoe, 36.
20 R. G. Kimber, "Resource Use and Management in Central Australia," *Australian Aboriginal Studies*, no. 2 (1984): 19.
21 Pascoe, 39.

22 Ibid., 44.

23 Ibid., 52.

24 Ibid., 52.

25 Ibid., 47.

26 Jolanda Nayutah and Gail Finlay, *Minjungbal: The Aborigines and Islanders of the Tweed Valley,* (Lismore, Australia: North Coast Institute for Aboriginal Community Education, 1988).

27 B. Gott, "Aboriginal Fire Management in S.E. Australia: Aims and Frequency," *Journal of Biogeography,* no. 32 (2005): 1204.

28 Mitchell, vol. 2, 211–212.

29 D. Frankel, "An Account of Aboriginal Use of the Yam Daisy," *The Artefact,* vol. 7 (June 1982): 43–45.

30 Ibid.

31 Pascoe, 44.

32 Ibid., 33.

33 Gerritsen, 2008, 50.

34 Mitchell, 1939, vol. 2, 61.

35 J. Kirby, *Old Times in the Bush of Australia: Trials and Experiences of Early Bush Life in Victoria: During the Forties* (Victoria, Australia: G. Robertson and Company, 1897), 28.

36 Nayutah and Finlay.

37 Pat and Sim Symons, *Bush Heritage* (Queensland: Pat and Sim Symons, 1994).

38 Ibid.

39 Glen Leiper, *Mutooroo Plant Use by Australian Aboriginal People* (Eagleby, Australia: Eagleby South State School, 1984).

40 Symons.

41 Leiper.

42 www.burkeandwills.net.au/Journals/Wills_Journals/Wills_Journal_June_1861.htm, accessed February 20, 2017.

43 P. K. Latz, *Bushfires and Bushtucker: Aboriginal Plant Use in Central Australia* (Alice Springs, Australia: IAD Press, 1995).

44 Symons.

45 Ibid.

46 Leiper.

47 Symons.

48 Leiper.

49 Symons.

50 Leiper.

51 Nayutah and Finlay.

52 Symons.

53 Leiper.

54 Symons.

55 Ibid.

56 Leiper.

57 Symons.

58 Leiper.

59 Pascoe, 45.

60 Ibid., 106.

61 Leiper.

62 Janette Brand Miller, *Tables of Composition of Australian Aboriginal Foods* (Canberra, Australia: Aboriginal Studies Press, 1993).

63 Ibid.

64 Leiper.

65 Symons.

66 I. M. Crawford, *Traditional Aboriginal Plant Resources in the Kalumburu Area: Aspects in Ethno-economics* (Perth: Western Australian Museum, 1982).

67 Leiper.

68 W. J. Peasley, *The Last of the Nomads* (Western Australia: Fremantle Press, 1983), 145.

69 Symons.

70 W. Jackson, *The Australian Captive* (Cincinnati: Henry W. Derby, 1853).

71 *The Sydney Gazette and New South Wales Advertiser*, December 23, 1804.

72 Symons.

73 Ibid.

74 Mitchell 1839, vol. 2, 153.

75 Pascoe, 42.

76 Ibid., 42.

77 M. Archer, "Confronting Crises in Conservation"; D. Luney and C. Kickman (eds.), *A Zoological Revolution: Using Native Fauna to Assist in Its Own Survival* (Royal Zoological Society of New South Wales and the Australian Museum, 2002), 20.

78 Leiper.

79 Personal communication, Philip Higson.

80 Gammage, 282.

81 Symons.

82 Leiper.

83 J. M. Naughton et al, "Animal Foods in Traditional Australian Aboriginal Diets: Polyunsaturated and Low in Fat," *Lipids*, no. 21 (November 1986): 684–690.

84 Personal communication, Leon Abrams, MA.

85 Latz.

86 Symons.

87 Latz.

88 M. Young, *The Aboriginal People of the Monaro*, 2nd ed. (New South Wales: Department of Environment and Conservation, 2005), 246.

89 P. M. Rouja et al, "Fat, Fishing Patterns, and Health Among the Bardi People of North Western Australia," *Lipids*, no. 38 (2003): 399–405.

90 Gammage, 282.

91 B. Wright, "The Fish Traps of Brewarrina," Aboriginal Health Conference, NSW, September 1983, 89; Pascoe, 54.

92 Sturt, 68.

93 Price, 168.

94 Kirby 1897, 35–36.

95 Pascoe, 57.

96 Ibid., 56.

97 Ibid., 57.

98 Ibid., 96–97.

99 Ibid., 76.

100 W. V. MacFarlane, "Aboriginal Desert Hunter/Gatherers in Transition," *The Nutrition of Aborigines in Relation to the Ecosystem of Central Australia*, CSIRO, Melbourne, 1978.

101 Latz.

102 Ibid.

103 Pascoe, 68.

104 I. Walters, "Some Observations on the Material Culture of Aboriginal Fishing in the Moreton Bay Area: Implications for Archaelolgy," *Queensland Archaeological Research*, University of Queensland, Brisbane, vol. 2 (1985): 51.

105 Pascoe, 142–143.

106 T. Watkin, *1788: Comprising A Narrative of the Expedition to Botany Bay and A Complete Account of the Settlement at Port Jackson* (Melbourne, Australia: Text Publishing, 2009), 65.

107 Pascoe, 82

108 Gammage, 2.

109 Latz.

110 Gammage, 9.

111 E. Hassell, "Notes on the Ethnology of the Wheelman Tribe of Southwestern Australia," *Anthropos* no. 31 (1936): 698–700.

112 W. J. Peasley, *The Last of the Nomads* (North Freemantle, Australia: Freemantle Press, 1983), 127.

113 Latz.

114 Symons.

115 L. Head, "Landscapes Socialized by Fire," *Arch in Oceania* no. 29 (1994): 172–181.

116 Pascoe, 116–117.

117 T. G. H. Strehlow, *Aranda Traditions* (Melbourne, 1947), 30–31.

118 Gammage, 131.

119 Pascoe, 80.

120 Grey, 2009, 6–7.

121 Sturt, 1833, vol. 1, 22, in Pascoe, 79.

122 Pascoe, 92.

123 Ibid., 97.

124 Ibid., 96–97.

125 Sturt, 1849, 111.

126 Price, 193.

127 Arnold de Vries, *Primitive Man and His Food* (Chandler Book Co., 1952), 69.

128 Ibid., 72.

129 Price.

130 W. Buckley, *The Life and Adventures of William Buckley. 1852* (Melbourne: The Text Publishing Company, 2002), 70.

131 MacFarlane.

132 Price.

133 Richard Guilliatt, "Out of Nowhere." *The Weekend Australian Magazine*, October 25–26, 2014, 12–16.

134 *Anangu Way* (Alice Springs, Australia: Nganampa Health Council, Inc., 1991).

Chapter 2: Native Americans

1   S. Boyd Eaton, MD, with Marjorie Shostak and Melvin Konner, MD, PhD, *The Paleolithic Prescription: A Program of Diet & Exercise and a Design for Living* (Harper & Row); Loren Cordain, PhD, and S. Boyd Eaton, MD, "Evolutionary Aspects of Diet: Old Genes, New Fuels. Nutritional Changes Since Agriculture," *World Review of Nutrition and Dietetics* (1997): 81.

2   Jean Carper, *USA Weekend.*

3   Elizabeth Somer, MA, RD, "Stone Age Diet," *SHAPE*, October 1998.

4   http://thepaleodiet.com/what-to-eat-on-the-paleo-diet-paul-vandyken, accessed March 24, 2017.

5   http://robbwolf.com/what-is-the-paleo-diet, accessed March 17, 2017.

6   Price, 73–102.

7   Price.

8   Álvar Núñez Cabeza de Vaca, *The Narrative of Cabeza de Vaca*, Rolena Adorno and Patrick Charles Pautz, eds. (University of Nebraska Press, 2003), 68.

9   Ibid., 107.

10 Fray Gaspar Jose de Solis, *Diary of a Visit of Inspection of the Texas Missions Made by Fray Gaspar Jose de Solis in the Year 1767–1768*, trans. Margaret K. Kress, *Southwestern Historical Quarterly*, vol. 35, 44.

11 Samuel Hearne, *A Journey from Prince of Wales's Fort in Hudson's Bay to the Northern Ocean in the Years 1769, 1770, 1771, 1772; New Edition with Introduction, Notes and Illustrations* (Hard Press, 2016), 407.

12 Arnold De Vries, *Primitive Man and His Food*, Chandler Book Company, Chicago, Illinois, 1952, 19.

13 Ibid., 20.

14 Ibid., 20.

15 Ibid., 20.

16 Ibid., 21.

17 www.online-literature.com/darwin/voyage_beagle/10, accessed March 24, 2017.

18 Price, 243.

19 De Vries, 19.

20 Ibid., 19.

21 Cabeza de Vaca, 121–122.

22 Ibid., 136.

23 Ibid., 137.

24 Ibid., 151.

25 Ibid., 148–149.

26 Newcomb, 139.

27 Ibid., 164.

28 Eaton, 80.

29 USDA data, prepared by John L. Weihrauch with technical assistance of Julianne Borton and Theresa Sampagna.

30 Vilhjalmur Stefansson, *The Fat of the Land* (MacMillan Company, 1956), 138.

31 Frances Densmore, "Chippewa Customs," *Bureau of American Ethnology*, bulletin 86, 43.

32 Steffanson, 30–31.

33 Hearne, 152.

34 Ibid., 119.

35 Ibid., 129.

36 Ibid., 129.

37 Ibid., 130.

38 J. H. Howard, "Yanktonai Ethnohistory and the John K. Bear Winter Count," *Plains Anthropologist Memoire* no. 11, vol. 21–73, part 2 (1816).

39 Hearne, 199.

40 Ibid., 354.

41 Ibid., 207.

42 Ibid., 380.

43 Ibid., 325.

44 Ibid., 209.

45 Ibid., 425.

46 Ibid., 466.

47 Ibid., 111.

48 Ibid., 116.

49 Ibid., 378.

50 Ibid., 404.

51 Ibid., 381.

52 Ibid., 380.

53 Ibid., 273.

54 Ibid., 256.

55 Ibid., 214. Arnold De Vries, *Primitive Man and His Food*, Chandler Book Company, Chicago, Illinois, 1952, 19.

56 Ibid., 385.

57 Beverly Hungry Wolf, *The Ways of My Grandmother*, reprint edition (New York: William Morrow Paperbacks, 1998), 183–189.

58 John Fire Lame Deer and Richard Erdoes, *Lame Deer Seeker of Visions* (New York: Simon & Schuster, 1972), 122.

59 Stefansson, 27.

60 Hungry Wolf.

61 Ibid.

62 William Byrd, *The Dividing Line Histories of William Byrde II of Westover*, ed. Kevin Joel Berland, (Chapel Hill: University of North Carolina Press, 2013), 176–177.

63 Inez Hilger, "Chippewa Child Life," *Bureau of American Ethnology*, bulletin 146, 96.

64 Byrd, 176–177.

65 Price, 264.

66 Ibid., 75.

67 Mary Ulmer and Samuel E. Beck, *Cherokee Cooklore* (Museum of the Cherokee Indian, 1951).

68 William Campbell Douglass, MD, *The Milk Book* (Second Opinion Publishing, 1994), 215.

69 www.worldcat.org/title/gastronomia-prehispanica-en-mexico-pre-hispanic -gastronomy-in-mexico-la-gastronomie-prehispanique-au-mexique-prakolumbinische -gastronomie-in-mexiko/oclc/254028251, accessed March 17, 2017.

70 C. W. Hesseltine and H. L. Wang, *Indigenous Fermented Food of Non-Western Origin* (Berlin/ Stuttgart: J Cramer, 1986), ch. 18.

71 Newcomb, 116.

72 *History, Condition & Prospects of the Indian Tribes of the United States, Collected & Prepared under the Direction of the Bureau of Indian Affairs*, vol. 4 (1852): 157.

73 Newcomb, 294.

74 *History, Condition & Prospects of the Indian Tribes of the United States, Collected & Prepared under the Direction of the Bureau of Indian Affairs*, vol. 2 (1852): 64, 176.

75 Hearne, 380.

76 Ibid., 386

77 Personal communication with Florence Shipek, expert on the Californian coastal Indians.

78 *History, Condition & Prospects of the Indian Tribes of the United States, Collected & Prepared under the Direction of the Bureau of Indian Affairs*, vol. 6 (1852), 83.

79 Ulmer and Beck.

80 Hearne, 379.

81 Densmore, 39.

82 "Wildman" Steve Brill with Evelyn Dean, *Identifying and Harvesting Edible and Medicinal Plants* (New York: Hearst Books 1994), 220.

83 Personal communication with Florence Shipek.

84 Ulmer and Beck.

85 Garcilaso de la Vega, *The Florida of the Inca* (University of Texas Press, 1951), 421.

86 I. W. Brown, "Salt and the Eastern North American Indian: An Archeological Study. Lower Mississippi Survey," bulletin No. 6, Peabody Museum, Harvard University, 1980.

87 P. M. Kraemer, "New Mexico's Ancient Salt Trade," www.elpalacio.org/articles/winter12/salttrade-v82-no1.pdf, accessed June 21, 2017.

88 David Perlman, "Stone Basins May Be Miwok Salt 'Factory,'" www.sfgate.com/news/article/Stone-basins-may-be-Miwok-salt-factory-3277185.php, accessed June 21, 2017.

89 Pascoe, 61.

90 Charles C. Mann, *1491: New Revelations of the Americas Before Columbus*, 2nd ed. (Vintage Books, 2011), 367–369.

91 Hearne, 333.

92 Ibid., 479.

93 M. Kat Anderson, *Tending the Wild: Native American Knowledge and the Management of California's Natural Resources*, reprint ed. (University of California Press, 2013).

Chapter 3: The Far North

1 Price, 59–72.

2 De Vries, 29.

3 Ibid., 31.

4 Ibid., 31.

5 Price, 65.

6 H. Brody, *Living Arctic: Hunters of the Canadian North* (Seattle: University of Washington Press, 1987), 55.

7 A. Hoygaard, *Studies on the Nutrition and Physio-Pathology of Eskimos* (Oslo, 1940), 21.

8 Ibid., 20.

9 Ibid., 23.

10 Ibid., 24.

11 Ibid., 26.

12 V. Stefansson, "Adventures in Diet," *Harper's Monthly Magazine*, November 1935.

13 Anore Jones, *Qualuich Niginaqtuat, Fish That We Eat*, Report for the U.S. Fish and Wildlife Service, Office of Subsistence Management, Fisheries Resource Monitoring Program (2006), 67.

14 www.foodista.com/blog/2012/02/15/stinky-foods-10-weird-facts-about-kiviak, accessed April 4, 2017.

15 http://ngm.nationalgeographic.com/2006/01/arctic-hunters/ehrlich-text, accessed April 4, 2017.

16 Høygaard, 20.

17 P. Gadsby and L. Steel, "The Inuit Paradox," *Discover Magazine*, October 2004.

18 S. M. Budge et al, "Blubber fatty acid composition of bowhead whales, Balaena mysticetus; Implications for diet assessment and ecosystem monitoring," *Journal of Experimental Marie Biology and Ecology*, no. 359 (2008): 40–46; U. Strandberg et al, "Vertical fatty acid profiles in blubber of a freshwater ringed seal—Comparison to a marine relative," *Journal of Experimental Marine Biology and Ecology*, October 2011;407(2): 256–265.

19 E. Mikkelsen and P. Sveistrup, "The East Greenlanders' possibilities of existence, their production and consumption," *Meddelelser om Gronland*, 1944, 134(2):245.

20 W. Bogoras, "The Chukchee: Material culture. Memoires of the American Museum of Natural History" in *The Jesup North Pacific Expedition*, vol. III, part 1 (1904), 200.

21 J. Murdoch, "On Some Popular Errors in Regard to the Eskimos," *The American Naturalist*, vol. 21, no. 1 (January 1887), 9–16.

22 Brody, 56–57.

23 Paal Røiri, Eskimo-kostholdets betydning for dødeligheten av hjerteog karsykdommer Hvilken betydning har det store inntaket av protein og mettet fett, langkjedete omega-3 fettsyrer samt det ubetydelige inntaket av karbohydrater? En dokumentasjon av at gjeldende norske kostholds-retningslinjer ikke er i pakt med foreliggende forskningsresultater, og bør revideres. *Fremlagt for Institutt for Ernæringsforskning*, Medisinsk fakultet, Universitetet i Oslo, den 30. Oktober 2002.

24 Ibid.

25 K. J. Ho et al, "Alaskan Arctic Eskimo: responses to a customary high fat diet," *American Journal of Clinical Nutrition* 25 (August 1972), 737–745.

26 Ibid., 738.

27 Anore Jones, *Nauriat Niginaqtuat, Plants that We Eat*, Indian Health Service Contract Number 243-79-0220, 1983, 127–129.

28 Høygaard, 124–126; P. Heinbecker, "Studies on the Metabolism of Eskimos," *Journal of Biological Chemistry*, vol. LXXX, no. 2, 461–475.

29 Jones, 57c.

30 Høygaard, 23.

31 Jones.

32 Stefansson, "Adventures in Diet."

33 A. Bertelsen, "Animalske antiscorbulica I gronland," *Hospitalstidende* 1911 (54): 537–545.

34 J. R. Geraci and T. G. Smith, "Vitamin C in the Diet of Inuit Hunters from Holman, Northwest Territories," *Arctic*, June 1979; 32(2): 137.

35 Høygaard, 44.

36 Gerarci and Smith.

37   Stefansson, "Optimal Eating," November 1935, http://idoportal.blogspot.com/2008/06/optimal
       -eating-vilhjalmur-stefansson.html, accessed January 27, 2018.

38   https://prezi.com/etcsjdsjwxsl/seal-blood-inuit-blood-and-diet-a-biocultural-model-of-ph,
       accessed April 9, 2017.

39   www.webmd.com/a-to-z-guides/sodium-na-in-blood#1, accessed April 9, 2017.

40   Høygaard, 20.

41   Ibid., 24.

42   Gatsby and Steel.

43   J. G. Fodor et al, "'Fishing' for the Origins of the 'Eskimos and Heart Disease' Story: Facts or
       Wishful Thinking?" *Canadian Journal of Cardiology*, vol. 30, issue 8 (August 2014): 864–868;
       A. Høygaard, "Studies on the nutrition and physio-pathology of Eskimos," *Norsk. Viden-skaps-
       Akad. Skr. Mat. Naturv*, 1941.

44   Høygaard, 70.

45   E. R. Pinckney and C. Pinckney, The potential toxicity of excessive polyunsaturates. *American
       Heart Journal* June 1973;85(6): 723–736.

46   Høygaard, 76.

47   Ibid.

48   http://nutritiondata.self.com/facts/ethnic-foods/9974/2, accessed April 4, 2017.

49   E. F. Foulks, "The Transformation of Arctic Hysteria," in *The Culture-Bound Syndromes: Folk
       Illnesses of Psychiatric and Anthropological Interest*, R. C. Simons and C. C. Hughes, eds. (D.
       Reidel Publishing Company, 1985), 310.

50   D. Landy, "Pibloktoq (Hysteria) and Inuit Nutrition: Possible Implication of Hypervitaminosis
       A," *Soc Sci Med*, 1985;21(2): 173–185.

51   Høygaard, 29.

52   Foulks.

53   J. Banhuus-Jessen, "Arctic Nervous Diseases," *Veterinary Journal* 1935;91: 339–350, 379–390.

54   A. F. C. Wallace and R. E. Ackerman, "An Interdisciplinary Approach to Mental Disorder among
       the Polar Eskimos of Northwest Greenland," *Anthropologica*, New Series, vol. 2, no. 2 (1960):
       249–260.

55   A. F. C. Wallace, "An Interdisciplinary Approach to Mental Disorder Among the Polar Eskimo of
       Northwest Greenland," *Anthropologica* 1960;11(2): 1–12.

56   Høygaard, 78.

57   Ibid.

58   J. Robert-Lamblin, "Meat: the Staple Diet for Arctic Peoples," *Centre National de la Recherche
       Scientifique*, France, 1993.

59   P. Helmes, "Changes in disease and food patterns in Angmagssalik," *Circumpolar Health 81:
       Nordic Council for Arctic Medical Research* 1998;33: 243–251.

Chapter 4: The South Seas

 1   Price, *Nutrition and Physical Degeneration*, 103–128.

 2   D. L. Oliver, *Ancient Tahitian Society, vol. I* (University Press of Hawaii, 1974), 287.

 3   Price, 109.

 4   Personal communication with Kay Baxter.

 5   Ibid.

6   J. C. Beaglehole, ed., *The Journals of Captain James Cook on His Voyages of Discovery. Vol. 2*, Hakluyt Society Extra Series no. 35 (Cambridge, UK: Cambridge University Press, 1961), 442–423, in Oliver, 274–275.

7   N. J. Pollock. "Food Classification in Three Pacific Societies: Fiji, Hawaii, and Tahiti," *Ethnology*, 1986 April, 25(2): 107–117.

8   Oliver, 435–437.

9   D. Lepofsky, "Gardens of Eden? An Ethnohistoric Reconstruction of Ma'ohi (Tahitian) Cultivation," *Ethnohistory*, December 1999;46(1): 1–29.

10 Ibid.

11 Ibid.

12 Ibid.

13 https://en.wikisource.org/wiki/The_Endeavour_Journal_of_Sir_Joseph_Banks/Manners_and _customs_of_South_Sea_Islands._1769, accessed April 30, 2017.

14 Lepofsky, 1999.

15 Antonio Pigafetta; James Alexander Robertson, trans., *Magellan's Voyage Around the World, Volume 1* (Arthur H. Clark Company, 1906), 64–100.

16 www.cookislands.org.uk/pukapuka.html#.WQJoY73rw3E, accessed April 27, 2017.

17 Oliver, 229.

18 I. A. Prior et al, "Cholesterol, coconuts, and diet on Polynesian atolls: a natural experiment: the Pukapuka and Tokelau island studies," *Am J Clin Nutr*, 1981 Aug;34(8): 1552–1561.

19 M. M. Tedder and J. L. O. Tedder, *Yams: A Description of Their Cultivation on Guadalcanal in the Solomon Islands* (Noumea, New Caldonia: South Pacific Commission, June 1974).

20 Oliver, 236.

21 Ibid., 234.

22 Ibid., 220–221.

23 https://en.wikisource.org/wiki/The_Endeavour_Journal_of_Sir_Joseph_Banks/Manners_and _customs_of_South_Sea_Islands._1769, accessed April 30, 2017.

24 Price, 127.

25 www.telegraph.co.uk/news/worldnews/1578329/Spam-at-heart-of-South-Pacific-obesity-crisis .html, accessed April 30, 2017.

26 www.westonaprice.org/get-involved/letters-winter-2000, accessed April 30, 2017.

Chapter 5: Africa

1   Price, *Nutrition and Physical Degeneration*, 130.

2   Ibid., 134.

3   Ibid., 130–131.

4   Ibid., 133.

5   Ibid., 150.

6   Ibid., 133.

7   Ibid., 147.

8   H. Leon Abrams Jr., "The Preference for Animal Protein and Fat: A Cross Cultural Survey," in *Food and Evolution*, Marvin Harris and Eric B. Ross, eds. (Philadelphia: Temple University Press, 1987).

9   Price, 137.

10 Ibid., 150.

11 Steffanson, *The Fat of the Land*, 130–131.

12 G. Prentice, *British Medical Journal*, December 15, 1923, 1181.

13 H. A. Dirar, *The Indigenous Fermented Foods of the Sudan: A Study in African Food and Nutrition* (Wallingford, UK: CAB International, 1993), 399.

14 Ibid., 1.

15 Ibid., 9.

16 Ibid., 42.

17 Ibid., 36.

18 Ibid., 30.

19 Ibid., 52.

20 Ibid., 53.

21 Ibid., 53.

22 Ibid., 55–72.

23 Ibid., 160.

24 Ibid., 243–247.

25 Ibid., 312.

26 Ibid., 311.

27 C. W. Hesseltine and H. L. Wang, *Indigenous Fermented Food of Non-Western Origin* (Berlin/ Stuttgart, Germany: J. Cramer, 1986), chapter 18.

28 Personal communication with Leslie Kosar, 2002.

29 Dirar, 412–427.

30 Ibid., 388–396.

31 Ibid., 387.

32 Ibid., 396–401.

33 Ibid., 401–402.

34 Ibid., 402.

35 Ibid., 403–404.

36 Ibid., 405.

37 Ibid., 406–407.

38 Ibid., 407–408.

39 Ibid., 409.

40 Ibid., 409.

41 Ibid., 345–383.

42 Ibid., 29.

43 E. Williams and P. Williams, "Uganda West Nile District," in *Western Diseases: Their Emergence and Prevention*, H. C. Trowell and D. P. Burkitt, eds. (London: Edward Arnold Publishers, Ltd, 1981), 188–193.

44 M. Gelfand, "Zimbabwe," in *Western Diseases: Their Emergence and Prevention*, H. C. Trowell and D. P. Burkitt, eds. (London: Edward Arnold Publishers, Ltd, 1981), 194–203.

45 G. V. Mann, "Studies of a surfactant and cholesteremia in the Maasai," *Am J Clin Nutr*, 1974 May;27(5): 464–469.

Chapter 6: Asia

1 I. Veigh, MA, PhD, trans., *Huang Ti Nei Ching Su Wen: The Yellow Emperor's Classic of Internal Medicine* (Baltimore: The Williams & Wilkins Company, 1949), 55–56.

2   F. J. Simoons, *Food in China: A Cultural and Historical Inquiry* (Boca Raton, Florida: CRC Press, 1991), 64.

3   www.atchuup.com/bizarre-things-found-in-chinese-wal-mart, accessed May 12, 2017.

4   www.dailyrotten.com/archive/2003/_2003-01-04.html, accessed July 1, 2017.

5   http://arachnophiliac.info/burrow/news/scorpion_king.htm, accessed July 1, 2017.

6   Simoons, 339.

7   Z. Y. Chen et al, "Breast Milk Fatty Acid Composition: A Comparative Study Between Hong Kong and Chongqing Chinese," *Lipids*, 1997;32(10): 1061–1067.

8   http://ricepedia.org/culture/history-of-rice-cultivation, accessed November 24, 2017.

9   http://ricepedia.org/china, accessed November 24, 2017.

10 Emiko Ohnuki-Tierney. *Rice as Self* (Princeton: Princeton University Press, 1994).

11 C. W. Hesseltine and H. L. Wang, eds. *Indigenous Fermented Foods of Non-Western Origin*, published for the New York Botanical Garden in Collaboration with the Mycological Society of America (Berlin/Stuttgart, Germany: J Cramer, 1986), 322.

12 Simoons, 375.

13 P. E. Tyler, "Lacking Iodine in Their Diets, Millions in China Are Retarded," *New York Times*, June 4, 1996, A1–A10.

14 K. C. Chang, ed., *Food in Chinese Culture* (New Haven, CT: Yale University Press, 1977).

15 Simoons, 87.

16 S. I. Sugiyama, "Fermented Soy Bean Products," IFI NR. 2, (1990): 19–24.

17 Food and Agriculture Organization of the United Nations, "Fermented Cereals: A Global Perspective" (FAO Agricultural Services Bulletin), 1999, chapter 3.

18 Simoons, 381.

19 K. H. Steinkraus, ed., *Handbook of Indigenous Fermented Foods* (New York: Marcel Dekker, 1977), 305.

20 "China the hardest hit by global surge in cancer, says WHO report"; www.scmp.com/news /china/article/1422475/china-hardest-hit-global-surge-cancer-says-who-report, accessed June 30, 2017.

21 "Stroke Rate Higher in Chinese People," www.everydayhealth.com/heart-health/stroke-rates -higher-in-chinese-people-9783.aspx, accessed June 30, 2017.

22 Tyler.

23 "The China Project: The Most Comprehensive Study Ever Undertaken on Diet and Health," *Spectrum*, March–April 1997: 27.

24 T. C. Campbell and C. Junshi, *The Cornell Project in China*.

25 C. Ruan et al, "Milk composition in women from five different regions of China: the great diversity of milk fatty acids," *J Nutr.* 1995 Dec;125(12): 2993–2998.

26 Campbell and Junshi, 56.

27 Ibid., 56.

28 www.prnewswire.com/news-releases/china-beef-cattle-farming-industry-and-beef-market -report-2015-2019-300134710.html, accessed May 12, 2017.

29 J. Ridgewell, *A Taste of Japan* (Thompson Learning, 1993).

30 Countess Morphy, ed., *Recipes of All Nations* (New York: Wm H. Wise & Company, 1935).

31 Personal communication with Jane Greenberg.

32 Ridgewell.

33 Ibid.

34 Ibid.

35 Ibid.

36 Ibid.

37 H. Okuyama et al, "Dietary fatty acids—the N-6/N-3 balance and chronic elderly diseases. Excess linoleic acid and relative N-3 deficiency syndrome seen in Japan," *Progressive Lipid Research*, 1997;35(4): 409–457.

38 Morphy.

39 www.biwa.ne.jp/~y-isono/trad/tradeg.html.

40 Ridgewell.

41 Ibid.

42 H. Toshima et al, *Lessons for Science from the Seven Countries Study* (Springer, 1994).

43 www.wcrf.org/int/cancer-facts-figures/data-cancer-frequency-country, accessed June 30, 2017.

44 T. Takezaki et al, "Dietary factors and lung cancer risk in Japanese: with special reference to fish consumption and adenocarcinomas," *British Journal of Cancer* 2001; 84(9): 1199–1206.

45 Ridgewell.

46 George V. Mann, ed., *Coronary Heart Disease, The Dietary Sense and Nonsense* (London: Veritas Society, 1993).

47 T. Suzuki et al, "Epidemiology of osteoporosis: incidence, prevalence, and prognosis," *Nihon Rinsho*, 1998 Jun;56(6): 1563–1568.

48 T. J. Moore, *Lifespan: What Really Affects Human Longevity* (New York: Simon & Schuster, 1990).

49 M. G. Marmot and S. L. Syme, "Acculturation and coronary heart disease in Japanese-Americans," *Am J Epidemiol*, 1976 Sep;104(3): 225–247.

50 www.fftc.agnet.org/library.php?func=view&id=20110729162248, accessed May 12, 2017.

51 www.pressian.com/news/article.html?no=10793, *Pressian*. In Korean. Retrieved May 13, 2017.

52 Michael J. Pettid, *Korean Cuisine: An Illustrated History* (London: Reaktion Books, 2008), 166.

53 A. E. Hirst et al, "A comparison of Atherosclerosis of the Aorta and Coronary Arteries in Bangkok and Los Angeles," *Am J Clin Path*, 1962;38(2): 162–170.

54 A. Harras, ed., *Cancer Rates and Risks*, 4th ed. (U. S. Department of Health and Human Services, National Institutes of Health, 1996).

55 www.wcrf.org/int/cancer-facts-figures/data-cancer-frequency-country, accessed July 1, 2017.

56 P. Srisawat, *The Foods of Thailand* (Berkeley, California: SLG Books, 1998).

57 H. M. Hauck et al, *Food Habits and Nutrient Intakes in a Siamese Rice Village, Studies in Bang Chan* (Ithaca, New York: Cornell University Press, 1958).

58 G. S. Manning et al, "Fasciolopsis buski in Thailand," *Amer J Trop Med Hyg* 1970;19:4: 613–619.

59 T. Papasarathorn et al, "Effects of garlic, onion, red pepper and green pepper pickled in vinegar upon the development of pig Ascaris eggs," *Public Health Alumni Bull* (Thailand), 1963;3:2: 1010.

60 R. Dissamarn et al, "Viability of larvae of *Trichinella Spiralis* in some common Thai dishes," *J Med Assoc Thailand* 1966;49:12: 985.

61 E. Sadun et al, "The effect of maklua (*diospyros mollis*) in the treatment of human hookworm," *J Parasit* 1954;40:1: 49–53.

62 R. Oliart et al, "Effects of Dietary Polyunsaturated Fatty Acids on Sucrose-Induced Cardiovascular Syndrome in Rats," American Oil Chemists Society Annual Meeting, Chicago, IL, May 1998.

Chapter 7: Europe

1 J. Bottero, *Mesopotamian Civilizations*, vol. 6. (Winona Lake, Ind.: Eisenbrauns, 1995).

2 N. Nasrallah, *Delights from the Garden of Eden: A Cookbook and a History of the Iraqi Cuisine* (Sheffield, UK: Equinox Publishing, 2003), 22.

3 D. R. Brothwell, *Food in Antiquity* (Baltimore: Johns Hopkins University Press, 1997).

4 www.youtube.com/watch?v=ofiwRzoYrdw, accessed May 27, 2017.

5 Avicenna, *The Canon of Medicine*, book 2, quoted in S. Niknamian, "Iran's Traditional Foods," *Wise Traditions in Food, Farming and the Healing Arts*, Winter 2016.

6 H. Moradi et al, "Avicenna viewpoint about health preservation through healthy nutrition principles," *Iran J Public Health*, 2013;42(2): 220–221.

7 R. Lacey and D. Danzinger, *The Year 1000: What Life Was Like at the Turn of the First Millennium, An Englishman's World* (Boston: Little, Brown and Company, 1999), 9–10.

8 P. Camporesi, *Bread of Dreams: Food and Fantasy in Early Modern Europe*, D. Gentilcore, trans. (Chicago: University of Chicago Press, 1996), 123.

9 Price, 23–57.

10 C. A. Wilson, *Traditional food east and west of the Pennines* (Norwich, UK: Page Bros, Ltd, 1991), 61.

11 F. M. McNeill, *The Scots Kitchen: Its Lore and Recipes*, 1929.

12 G. Markham, *The English Housewife* (Kingston, Ontario: McGill-Queen's University Press, 1986).

13 D. Pool, *What Jane Austen Ate and Charles Dickens Knew* (New York: Simon & Schuster, 1993), 207.

14 P. Montagné, *Larousse Gastronomique* (New York: Clarkson Potter, 2001), 592.

15 E. Campion, *Two Bokes of the History of Ireland* (1570), quoted in R Sexton, *A Little History of Irish Food* (Gill and MacMillan, 2001), 29.

16 McNeill.

17 M. R. Best, introduction to *The English Housewife*, xlvi.

18 Wilson, 49.

19 M. Berriedale-Johnson, *Olde Englishe Recipes* (Essex, UK: Judy Piatkus (Publishers) Limited of Loughton, 1981), 13.

20 Ibid., 10.

21 Ibid., 122.

22 J. D. Pennant, *More Llandegai Recipes* (Sackville Printing Works), 5.

23 "Gastrologue," *The Scotsman Magazine* (1920).

24 McNeill.

25 S. Mennell, *All Manners of Food* (Illini Books, 1996), 303.

26 Wilson, 59–60.

27 J. Burnett, "Plenty and Want: A Social History of English Diet from 1815 to the Present Day," lecture delivered to the British Dietetic Association on Saturday, October 15, 1966.

28 V. Holsinger et al, "Whey Beverages: A Review," *Journal of Dairy Sciences*, vol. 57 (August 1974): 849–859.

29 McNeill.

30 Mennell, 46.

31 Best, xxv.

32 C. B. Heiatt et al, *Pleyn Delit: Medieval Cookery for Modern Cooks* (Toronto, Ontario: University of Toronto Press, 1997), xx.

33 Markham.

34 Best, xliii.

35 Ibid., xxxvi.

36 Sally Mitchell, *Daily Life in Victorian England* (Westport, Connecticut: Greenwood Press, 1996), 122.

37 Basil Dmytryshyn, *Medieval Russia: A Source Book, 850–1700*, 3rd ed. (Harcourt Brace, 1991).

38 Joyce Toomre, ed., *Classic Russian Cooking, Elena Molokhovets' A Gift to Young Housewives*, (Indiana University Press, 1992).

39 The author is indebted to Katherine Czapp for a large part of the information in this section, taken from "Eating by the Seasons in Russia," *Wise Traditions in Food, Farming and the Healing Arts*, the quarterly magazine of the Weston A. Price Foundation, Spring 2008, www.westonaprice .org/health-topics/traditional-diets/eating-by-the-seasons-in-russia, accessed May 29, 2017.

40 W. C. Willett et al, "Mediterranean diet pyramid: a cultural model for healthy eating," *American Journal of Clinical Nutrition*, June 1995 61(6S): 1402S–1406S.

41 A. Keys, "Mediterranean diet and public health: personal reflections," *American Journal of Clinical Nutrition* 1995 61(suppl): 1321S–1323S.

42 Ibid.

43 A. Keys, "Coronary heart disease in seven countries," *Circulation*, 1970;41 (Suppl 1).

44 R. H. Smith, *Diet, Blood Cholesterol and Coronary Heart Disease: A Critical Review of the Literature*, vol. 2 (November 1981), 4–49.

45 F. Pérez-Llamas et al, "Estimates of food intake and dietary habits in a random sample of adolescents in southeast Spain," *Journal of Human Nutrition and Diet*, December 1996 9:(6): 463–471.

46 A. Alberti-Fidanza, "Dietary studies on two rural Italian population groups of the Seven Countries Study. 1. Food and nutrient intake at the thirty-first year follow-up in 1991," *European Journal of Clinical Nutrition* February 1994 48(2): 85–91.

47 P. Artusi, *Science in the Kitchen and the Art of Eating Well*, English translation ed. (Lorenzo Da Ponte Italian Library, 2003).

48 Morphy, *Recipes of All Nations*, 779–781.

49 T. Barer-Stein, PhD, *You Eat What You Are: People, Culture and Food Traditions* (Willowdale, Ontario: Firefly Books, 1999).

50 E. S. Machlin, *The Classic Cuisine of Italian Jews* (New York, Dodd, Mead and Company, 1981), 83–87.

51 http://www.food-links.com/typical-naples-campagna-foods-in-italy/, accessed January 17, 2018.

52 Personal communication with Roberta Wearmouth, 2004.

53 Keys, "Mediterranean diet and public health: personal reflections."

Chapter 8: True Blue Zones

1 D. Buettner, *The Blue Zones: Lessons for Living Longer from the People Who've Lived the Longest* (National Geographic Society, 2008), 15.

2 G. M. Pes et al, "Male longevity in Sardinia," *European Journal of Clinical Nutrition* 69 (April 2015): 411–418.

3 https://www.revolvy.com/main/index.php?s=Sarda%20pig, accessed January 18, 2018.

4 https://gain.fas.usda.gov/Recent%20GAIN%20Publications/Regional%20Report%20-%20Okinawa _Osaka%20ATO_Japan_3-24-2014.pdf, accessed July 4, 2017.

5   http://pubs.royle.com/article/Nutritional+Assessment+In+Vegetarians+And+Vegans%3A+Questi ons+Clinicians+Should+Ask/1246906/0/article.html, accessed July 4, 2017.

6   http://pdfsr.com/pdf/nutrition-for-the-japanese-elderly, accessed April, 2017.

7   http://nourishedkitchen.com/hara-hachi-bu, accessed July 5, 2017.

8   Deborah Franklyn, "Take a Lesson from the People of Okinawa," *Health*, September 1996, 57–63.

9   http://okicent.org, accessed July 4, 2017.

10 www.today.com/id/33293475/ns/today-today_health/t/american-future-lifespans-greatly-exaggerated/#.WPKViL3rw3E, accessed April, 2017.

11 www.westonaprice.org/health-topics/soy-alert/how-much-soy-do-okinawans-eat-2, accessed July 5, 2017.

12 L. Rosero-Bixby et al, "The Nicoya region of Costa Rica: a high longevity island for elderly males," *Vienna Yearb Popul Res.* 2013;11: 109–136.

13 G. Baker, "Costa Rica: Land of the Centenarians," *Wise Traditions in Food, Farming and the Healing Arts*, Spring 2017.

14 http://island-ikaria.com/about-ikaria/Ikaria-BlueZone, accessed April, 2017.

15 Dan Buettner, The Island Where People Forget to Die, *New York Times Magazine*, October 24, 2014, http://www.nytimes.com/2012/10/28/magazine/the-island-where-people-forget-to-die. html?pagewanted=all&_r=0, accessed January 18, 2018.

16 https://greekcitytimes.com/ikaria-land-of-free-range-goats-not-sheep, accessed April, 2017.

17 http://search.aol.com/aol/video?q=Ikaria%2C+sheep%2C+youtube&s_it=video-ans&sfVid =true&videoId=AAE3BCDAAF9B868FCDC8AAE3BCDAAF9B868FCDC8&v_t=client97 _inbox, accessed April 2017.

18 www.researchgate.net/publication/281521429_Determinants_of_All-Cause_Mortality_and _Incidence_of_Cardiovascular_Disease_2009_to_2013_in_Older_Adults_The_Ikaria_Study _of_the_Blue_Zones, accessed July 4, 2017.

19 https://en.wikipedia.org/wiki/MedDietScore, accessed July 4, 2017.

20 www.westonaprice.org/get-involved/letters-winter-2009.

21 General findings of the International Atherosclerosis Project, *Lab Invest*, 1968 May;18(5): 498–502.

22 https://en.wikipedia.org/wiki/Adventist_Health_Studies, accessed July 4, 2017.

23 Buettner, 130.

24 Ibid., 163.

25 P. N. Appleby et al, "Mortality in vegetarians and comparable nonvegetarians in the United Kingdom," *Am J Clin Nutr*, 2016 Jan;103(1): 218–230.

26 www.westonaprice.org/health-topics/abcs-of-nutrition/vegetarianism-what-the-science-tells-us, accessed July 5, 2017.

27 R. L. Phillips et al, "Coronary heart disease mortality among Seventh-Day Adventists with differing dietary habits: a preliminary report," *Am J Clin Nutr*, 1978 Oct;31(10 Suppl): S191–S198.

28 M. L. Burr and M. Sweetnam, "Vegetarianism, dietary fiber and mortality," *American Journal of Clinical Nutrition*, 1982, 36: 873.

29 Mills, 1136S–1142S.

30 T. J. Key et al, "Cancer incidence in vegetarians: results from the European Prospective Investigation into Cancer and Nutrition (EPIC-Oxford)," *Am J Clin Nutr*, vol. 89, no. 5 (May 2009): 1620S–1626S.

31 N. T. Burkert and others. Nutrition and Health—The Association between Eating Behavior and Various Health Parameters: A Matched Sample Study. Published: February 7, 2014 DOI: 10.1371/journal.pone.0088278; AMCN 27 Dec 2011, 712–738.

Chapter 9: What to Eat

1 D. Noli and G. Avery, "Protein Poisoning and Coastal Subsistence," *Journal of Archeological Science* 1988, 15: 395–401.

2 "Paleolithic Humans Had Bread Along with Their Meat," http://www.nytimes.com/2010/10/19/science/19bread.html, accessed July 10, 2017.

3 R. Di Cagno et al, "Gluten-free sourdough wheat baked goods appear safe for young celiac patients: a pilot study," *J Pediatr Gastroenterol Nutr*, 2010 Dec;51(6): 777–783.

Index

About the Author

SALLY FALLON MORELL is the author of the bestselling cookbook *Nourishing Traditions* (with Mary G. Enig, PhD), *Nourishing Broth* (with Kaayla T. Daniel, PhD, CCN), and *Nourishing Fats*. As president of the Weston A. Price Foundation, she is the number one spokesperson for the return of traditional nutrient-dense foods to American tables. Visit her blog at nourishingtraditions.com